KIDS,

HERBS,

HEALTH

LINDA B. WHITE, M.D., AND SUNNY MAVOR, A.H.G.

Other Health Books by Interweave Press

Women's Herbs, Women's Health
By Christopher Hobbs, L. Ac. and Kathi Keville

Handmade Medicines: Simple Recipes for Herbal Health
By Christopher Hobbs, L.Ac.

101 Medicinal Herbs: An Illustrated Guide
By Steven Foster

What the Labels Won't Tell You: A Consumer Guide to Herbal Supplements
By Logan Chamberlain, Ph.D.

Stress and Natural Healing
By Christopher Hobbs, L.Ac.

To order these books or receive a complete catalog of Interweave Press publications,
call 1-800-272-2193

The information in this book should not be used as a substitute for advice from a qualified health-care practitioner. Dosage information is provided as a general guide. Some medicinal herbs and other natural remedies may cause allergic reactions in susceptible individuals, and others may not be right to use for particular health conditions.

Cover design: Susan Wasinger
Illustrations: Susan Strawn Bailey, Gayle Ford
Book design: Dean Howes

Interweave Press
201 East Fourth Street
Loveland, CO 80537-5655
USA

White, Linda B. (Linda Blachly),
    Kids, herbs, and health : a parents' guide to natural remedies/
By Linda B. White and Sunny Mavor.
    p.   cm.
    Includes bibliographical references and index.
    ISBN 1-883010-53-5 (pbk.)
    1. Pediatrics—Popular works. 2. Children—Diseases—Alternative
treatment. 3. Naturopathy. 4. Herbs—Therapeutic use. I. Mavor,
Sunny, 1956— . II. Title.
RJ61. W 4661999
618.92–dc   98-53519
                                          CIP

Printed in the United States of America   618.92   9/3/99
First Printing: 10M:0199:QUE   WHi

ACKNOWLEDGMENTS

We both wish to thank our mentors: Ellen Dale, Jeanne Rose, Rosemary Gladstar, Ed Smith, Feather Jones, Brigitte Mars, Mindy Green, Rob McCaleb, Susun Weed, Amanda McQuade Crawford, Christopher Hobbs, Robyn Klein, Kathi Keville, Cascade Anderson Geller, Michael Moore, Michael Murray, Joseph Pizzorno, Dana Ullman, Ed Alstat, Francis Brinker, Michael Schmidt, and Bart Schmitt.

Many thanks go also to Debby Faes, P.A., for her invaluable assistance in separating fact from fiction. Thanks to the librarians at Exempla Lutheran Medical Center in Wheatridge, Colorado, for helping in our research. Much gratitude to Interweave Press for believing in this book from the start and to Susan Clotfelter and Doree Pitkin for their thoughtful editing.

Linda sends heartfelt thanks to Sunny Mavor for envisioning this book, for inviting me travel this road with her, for putting up with my idiosyncracies during the many months it took to write this beast, and for sharing her wisdom and her friendship.

Sunny extends a world of thanks and respect to Linda White, who is a delight to work with. In her wise approach, Linda is opening new doors for herbalists and physicians to work together.

DEDICATION

To my husband, Barney White, and our children, Alex and Darcy—three people who have loved and encouraged me and put up with all manner of home remedies.

—Linda B. White

To my loving family: My amazing husband, Doug, who has always let me be who I really am; my children, Skyler and Alyssa, who have blessed me beyond belief with their wisdom and love; and to my dad, who taught me as a child to be astounded at the beauty of wildflowers.

—Sunny Mavor

TABLE OF CONTENTS

Chapter 1

WHY NATURAL REMEDIES?

Most parents are alike in one respect: We want the best for our kids. We want the ideal diet, the safest neighborhood, the best school, and optimum health care. Usually we can identify the first three, though obtaining them can be a different story. But what about health care?

Parents are faced with a bewildering array of choices when it comes to their children's health. Magazine articles, radio and television shows, health professionals, friends, and grandmothers all offer advice. When illness strikes, it's hard to know which way to turn. The pediatrician? The acupuncturist? The herbalist? Grandma? Which remedy will help your child recover? Antibiotics? Echinacea? Chicken soup? Treating children is no longer as simple as remembering whether to starve a fever or feed a cold.

In this book, we try to clear some of the brush from your path. Speaking first as parents, second as physician and herbalist, we'll tell you how natural remedies have worked safely and effectively on our own children. Because we also know the dangers of a rigid do-it-yourself approach, we'll give you guidelines for seeking medical assistance, when to use natural therapies, and how to choose the right remedy for your child's particular needs. We've gleaned this information from herbal traditions, our experiences and those of others we trust, and all the scientific research we could find.

We believe that, armed with some knowledge, parents can choose natural medicines at least as easily as they can select from among the hundreds of over-the-counter cold medicines. More important still, these natural medicines are often better for your child. Not only can they ease symptoms, they can get at the root of the imbalance or deficiency that's causing illness. Most pharmaceuticals won't help your child recover from viral illnesses, nor will they enhance immune function. Herbal medicines can, and unlike many synthetic drugs, they do so with few, if any, side effects.

Regardless of what made you buy this book, we hope that you'll use it, take notes in it, keep it in the kitchen, bathroom, or sickroom. We'll take it as a high compliment if your copy winds up looking as well-loved and bedraggled as your child's favorite stuffed toy. Most of all, we hope that it provides you with practical information on not just curing your child's illnesses, but keeping your child strong and healthy.

Where Herbal Medicine Comes From

Even though natural remedies are now making headlines and network news shows, they're not newcomers. Humans have long used plants to ease their ailments. Traditional Chinese Medicine, which uses herbs, foods, and acupuncture to address illness, dates back nearly four thousand years. Ayurvedic texts from the same time prescribe herbs. European herbal traditions took cues from Middle Eastern and ancient Greek and Roman practice. Today, North American botanical remedies blend European traditions and the plant lore of Native Americans. Modern medical science is now proving that many traditional cures are not only effective, but safer than some pharmaceuticals.

Many herbal remedies have been proven successful over centuries of trial and error. Our ancestors stopped using the plants that failed to cure or caused harm, and handed down the remedies that worked. Because children tend to catch a lot of infectious diseases, they have participated in much informal herbal experimentation. It's likely that these children were just as vocal as yours about whether or not their medicine tasted good!

If herbal remedies are effective, why did people stop using them? Many cultures didn't. In a few countries, however, the United States among them, the rise of medical and pharmaceutical science, fueled by such truly miraculous discoveries as penicillin and vaccines, fostered a bias toward the new and technical. If it was old, cheap, and accessible to anyone, it simply couldn't be as good as what was expensive, rare, or had been subjected to rigorous testing by highly trained scientists. And sometimes, if scientists couldn't discover exactly *how* a plant remedy worked, they assumed that it lacked therapeutic value. Today, we know that medical science has logged many triumphs that improve children's lives. But we also know that science has not fully conquered disease, and that mysteries as perplexing as AIDS and as simple as the common cold persist.

The return to plant medicines is fueled by several trends: scientific confirmation of their effectiveness, an awareness of Western medicine's limits, a newly assertive attitude toward health care, and a yearning for a more natural lifestyle. Parents want their children to be seen as people, not disease-bearers. We want true health, not just the absence of illness. But with today's choices, it's hard to know how to proceed.

How to Use This Book

No single healing path is always right for everyone. Herbs can be beneficial, but they can interact with synthetic drugs, pre-existing conditions, or other herbs. For this reason, parents must use caution when adding herbs to a child's drug regimen. They must *not* abruptly replace a prescription medication with herbs unless they have consulted a physician. If your child has a chronic illness, is under a year old, or is already taking any prescription medicine, be sure to consult with your doctor about your decision to try herbal remedies. Your physician may have advised herbs for other patients, or may be able to recommend a qualified herbalist or other alternative practitioner.

Four Rules to Live By

Rule One: Talk with your children's doctor.

Remember that doctors intend to help. Generally speaking, pediatricians are not in the business for the money. They care for your sick child because doing so provides both personal satisfaction and professional challenge. No one wants to botch this job.

Whenever your child falls ill with more than a sniffle or low-grade fever, we urge you to consult a doctor. Ideally, he or she knows something about natural remedies or at least supports your desire to use them to nip mild illnesses in the bud. Even if your doctor views herbal medicines with outright disdain, you should still take your sick child to him or her, at least until you find a doctor more in sync with your viewpoint. *Please do not substitute this book for appropriate medical care.*

In each chapter, we include a section on signs and symptoms that warrant medical consultation. In some chapters, we include signs and symptoms that require immediate medical attention.

Rule Two: Learn about the safety of herbs before giving them to your child.

Probably one of your first questions is, "Are herbs safe for my children?" You want to support your child's life in a responsible and loving manner. We think that herbal remedies are an excellent way to do this.

But are all herbs safe for all children? No. Some plants, for example, foxglove, poison hemlock, and many others, are poisonous to humans. And some herbal medicines on the market today are appropriate for adults, but not for children. Even gentle herbs, taken at high doses for long periods, can cause problems for some users. But then, anything taken in excess can harm us, even water.

People who have problems with liver or kidney function are unable to eliminate drugs and herbs efficiently; parents of children with these disorders need extra medical guidance. And children

A HEALING HERITAGE, LOST AND FOUND

Many years ago, at the start of a series of herb classes, Sunny asked her students to explain what had ignited their interest in herbal medicine. Most said they wanted to become more involved in their own health care. Several sought to learn how to make their own medicines. Then one young woman named Catherine spoke.

Catherine had recently buried her beloved grandmother, her last remaining grandparent. After the funeral, the family gathered at the grandparents' farmhouse to swap stories. They told of the family's fortitude during the Great Depression. They shared the grandmother's favorite recipes and household hints.

Catherine wanted to know more about the recipes. In the farmhouse's kitchen, she searched through the many drawers and cabinets. What she found, however, were not books or file boxes of recipe cards, but drawer after drawer of small jars filled with dried herbs. When she asked her mother about these jars, her mother answered that Catherine's grandmother had shunned doctors, and instead had treated herself with plant medicines.

Why, Catherine wondered, hadn't she known this? Why hadn't her grandmother passed down her knowledge? In that time, her mother said, many considered the use of herbal remedies a sign of poverty and ingorance. Fearing scorn, Catherine's grandmother had kept her herbal wisdom a secret.

Many of our ancestors possessed some knowledge of healing herbs. By sharing our knowledge with you, we may help revive a tradition that you can pass on to your children and your children's children.

with allergies to certain plants may also react to closely related species used as medicinal herbs. Parents of kids on prescription medications need to be extra cautious.

So here's our qualified answer to the safety question: Gentle herbs, given within recommended guidelines, are safe for most people, including children. What this all means is that you must educate yourself about the herbs you're considering giving to your children.

The medicinal value of the herbs we recommend has been documented by years of traditional use, recent scientific research, or both. Although many herbs have been tested under experimental situations, only a fraction have undergone clinical trials, the term for studies involving humans. And the vast majority of those trials have been conducted on adults, not children. However, all the herbs we use in this book have a long history of safe use.

Rule Three: Look for quality in herbal remedies.

Before you buzz down to the health-food store to stock up on herbal remedies, we'd like you to know a few more things about the products you're likely to find there.

Be wary of products created for adults. These sometimes contain one or two herbs that have no history of safe use for children. In addition, liquid adult remedies often contain grain alcohol, which we recommend you not give your small child.

The taste test is all important. As an herbalist specializing in herbs for children, Sunny has learned the importance of blending herbs that are palatable. Kids simply will not tolerate the bitter taste of many medicinal plants. Put another way, yucky taste leads to poor compliance, but a child who likes her medicine will take it happily. This is especially important because, in order to be effec-

HERB SAFETY IN PREGNANCY AND NURSING

As a general rule, you should be extremely cautious about taking drugs or strong-acting herbs while pregnant or nursing, unless a qualified health practitioner recommends you do so.

Although many herbs stimulate uterine muscle in lab tests, the effects on actual pregnant women and their fetuses remain unknown. Furthermore, a woman's actual risk depends upon how much and for how long she takes an herb, her stage of pregnancy (the first trimester is the most critical period), and her tendency to miscarry. Plants containing the alkaloid berberine, such as goldenseal and Oregon graperoot, increase the risk of newborn jaundice. Harsh laxatives, including the herbs cascara sagrada, senna, rhubarb, and aloe vera as

well as over-the-counter drugs, should not be taken internally during pregnancy. The best guideline for taking herbs during pregnancy and nursing is, *ask a qualified practitioner first.*

In a nursing mother, chemical ingredients cross into her breast milk. This doesn't mean that you can't take gentle herbs and then nurse. Nursing women have eaten culinary and medicinal herbs probably since the world began. The consensus among herbalists is that nursing women can safely take the gentler herbs, including chamomile, catnip, ginger, fennel, and many of the others mentioned in Chapter 3. In fact, nursing is one of the most convenient ways to give sick infants small amounts of these herbs.

tive, most herbal formulas should be taken at least three times a day.

Consume carefully. It's crucial to completely read the label on herbal products. Consider not buying those that contain endangered, wild-harvested herbs if a cultivated source is available. Certified organic products are less environmentally harmful to produce; often they are of equal or higher quality. Look for an expiration date. As you become more experienced buying herbal remedies, you'll know whose product lines to trust.

You can make it yourself. Many healing herbs are easy to grow or gather from the wild; doing so assures freshness, although not necessarily potency. Herb gardening and "weed" gathering are activities you can pursue with your children; growing or collecting their own medicine may help them enjoy taking it when they are sick.

Rule Four: You know your child best. Trust your intuition if you feel the need to seek help.

Many run-of-the-mill childhood illnesses are benign, viral in origin, and self-limiting, meaning they go away without treatment. Even so, most parents want to do something, anything, to alleviate their sick child's discomfort. Fortunately, many home remedies can both hasten the healing process and reduce symptoms.

While we wish to affirm your ability to care for your sick child, we do not mean to suggest that you can always handle childhood illnesses at home. Whenever your child appears very ill, you need medical assistance. As a parent, you know when your child isn't right. One glance and you see that his eyes look glassy, his skin pale, his lips too red or too dry. You gather him in your arms and feel that his skin is hot and moist. He cries and you smell the illness on his breath. He won't eat. He alternately screams and sleeps. He sleeps far too little or far too much. His favorite toys don't interest him.

You know something's wrong. But how serious is it? Parents can easily lose objectivity, either over-reacting or denying that a problem exists. As a friend of Linda's—a British physician—says, "When one of my children falls ill, my brain's in a basket." To help you keep that rational edge, a list of signs of serious illness follows. If your child fits these, call your doctor. If you have doubts, call your doctor.

Each child is unique; so are the circumstances of each illness. While we've written this book with the best that our combined skills have to offer and the most current information to which we have access, it's no substitute for being there with your child, whom you know best. So if this book, or someone else, says your child's illness isn't serious, but your own gut instinct says it is—*or you have any doubts at all about your child's condition or treatment*—err on the side of caution and call your doctor, even if you feel silly doing so. Nothing is worth risking your child's well-being.

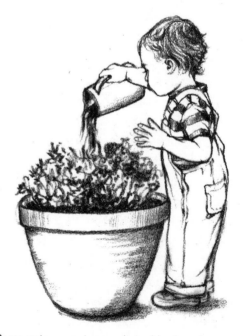

If you enjoy growing medicinal herbs, share your hobby with your children.

WHEN TO CALL A DOCTOR: EMERGENCY SIGNS AND SYMPTOMS

Contact your doctor *immediately* if your sick child:

Is under two months old

Is under three months old and has a fever

Has a fever that exceeds 104°F (40°C) at any age

Acts extremely irritable; nothing you do comforts her

Seems lethargic, i.e., weak, limp, apathetic, difficult to awaken

Becomes confused, delirious, or loses consciousness

Has a convulsion (loses consciousness, stiffens, rhythmically moves his extremities or otherwise postures abnormally, and loses bladder and/or bowel control)

Complains of stiff neck and headache and/or cannot touch his chin to his chest (early signs of meningitis)

Complains of severe pain in any part of his body

Has difficulty breathing—breathes fast, sucks in the skin at the hollow above her breastbone or between her ribs on each inhalation, sits with her chin thrust forward to breathe, has blue-tinged lips, or has possibly inhaled a foreign object

Has problems with balance or coordination

Becomes dehydrated, hasn't urinated for eight hours, cries without tears, has dry lips and mouth, has sunken eyes, and, if a baby, a sunken fontanel (soft spot).

Develops a rash that look like tiny bruises (a sign of serious blood infection)

Begins drooling. We're not talking about a drooling baby; we're talking about a drooling three-to-seven-year-old child with high fever, muffled voice, and difficulty swallowing. These are signs of epiglottitis, a potentially life-threatening infection of the flap of tissue that covers the windpipe during swallowing. Call 911.

May have ingested a poison. Call 911 or Poison Control.

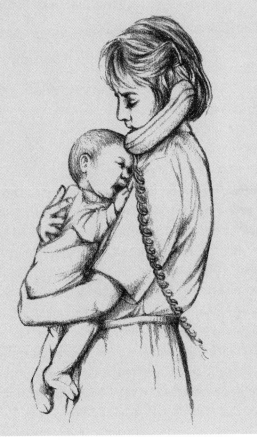

Chapter 2

Understanding Herbal Medicine

How do plant medicines work to heal your child? Plants, like everything else, are made of a wide variety of chemicals. Locked within the leaves, flowers, stems, and/or roots of medicinal plants are chemicals that act on the human body. Within the rhizome of the ginger plant, for example—the same plant that gives pumpkin pie its spice—are chemicals that increase the secretion of bile, tone the bowel, thin the blood, and reduce the stickiness of blood platelets. For parents, ginger's most important quality is its ability to quell nausea. However, this simple plant has also been researched for its antibacterial, antifungal, and pain-relieving abilities. It's easy to find in the grocery store, inexpensive, and tasty.

Ginger concentrates its medicinal compounds below the ground, where they're abundant enough that all you need to do is chop the fresh root and add it to cooking, or simmer it for several minutes to make a tea. In other plants, the beneficial chemicals are in the above-ground, or aerial, parts. The medicine in dried herbs evaporates quickly. While this rate is different for each plant and plant part, generally, the finer the plant material is chopped, and the more it is exposed to oxygen, heat, and light, the faster these beneficial chemicals take flight. If a dried herb has lost its characteristic scent—good or bad—that's nature's way of telling you its expiration date has passed. This is why we're reluctant to recommend powdered herbs. In addition, unless a powdered herb is tasty enough to be sprinkled on food, you will only be able to give it to your child if she can swallow capsules. We've found that kids have to be about six to seven years old to do this reliably.

Luckily, there are other ways of extracting and preserving the compounds, or constituents, that give herbs their healing power. Most fresh or dried herbs can be soaked in a water-and-glycerine or water-and-alchohol mixture for a few weeks to release their healing constituents. Then the mixture can be strained and the resulting liquid given to your child.

Ways to Take Herbs

Extracts into alchohol, called **tinctures**, and into glycerine, called **glycerites**, are only two of the many forms of herbs that you can give your child. The variety of herbal products and preparations can seem bewildering at first. It breaks down into three basic types:

(1) whole herbs in fresh or dried form, capsules, or tablets;
(2) various kinds of extracts, for which the herb has been soaked in or percolated through a liquid;
(3) an essential oil, which is a distilled, concentrated liquid form of the herb's volatile oils.

A guide to understanding the different forms and preparations, and the basics of making them, follows.

For All Uses

Fresh herbs. If you have an herb garden, you can use many herbs fresh. If you don't, a few beneficial herbs probably grow nearby whether you want them to or not—they're weeds. For example, you can use mint sprigs from your garden to garnish cold drinks or meals, and make them into a tea to soothe an upset tummy. You can crush fresh plantain, a ubiquitous lawn weed, and apply it to insect bites, stings, and wounds to hasten healing. As in cooking, if a medicinal recipe calls for dried herbs, and you wish to use fresh instead, substitute two times the amount. Why? Fresh herbs contain water. When botanical medicines are dried, they take up less volume.

Know your wild plants so you can identify them with certainty. Do your best to choose plants that are free of herbicides and pesticides.

Drying herbs is easy to do. Just hang them upside down in a clean, shady area until they are completely dried. You can also purchase dried leaves, flowers, and roots sold in bulk at many health-food stores.

Because this is how most people use herbs, the recipes in this book are formulated for dried herbs unless otherwise specified. Some herbs come prepackaged in plastic bags, jars, or tins. When you buy such herbs, it's better to purchase small quantities in whole form (whole roots, leaves, or flowers) rather than powdered. Leave them whole, stored in glass jars in a cool, dark area, until you need them. Just before using, crumble the leaves and flowers and grind the roots in a clean coffee grinder.

Infusions are teas made from dried or fresh leaves, stems, and flowers. For a children's hot tea, steep approximately one teaspoon of herbs in one cup of just-boiled water for three to five minutes.

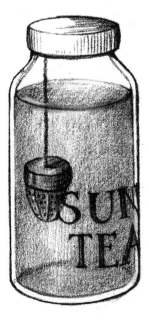

Medicinal tea, one of the simplest ways to take herbs, is as easy to make as regular tea.

Strain well; kids tend to be particularly touchy about floating matter in their tea. A coffee filter or a French coffee press works well.

You can also make cold infusions by steeping loose herbs in cool, pure water for four to eight hours in the refrigerator or outdoors. While Sunny prefers to put herbs in a stainless-steel tea ball or basket-type strainer, Linda puts them in a clean nylon stocking. Once the tea's ready, just pull out the tea ball or stocking.

Decoctions are teas made by simmering tougher plant parts—fresh or dried seed, root, or bark—in which the beneficial chemicals are more securely locked away. Use approximately two teaspoons of herb per two cups of water; we've found it inconvenient to make smaller quantities because it's too easy to boil the pot dry. Gently bring both herb and water to a boil. Cover and reduce heat to a low simmer for five to ten minutes. We recommend using a timer. As with an infusion, strain well before using.

For Internal Use

Capsules. Many herbal remedies are available for purchase in this form, but it's possible to make your own capsules at home. In fact, because powdered herbs quickly loose potency, Sunny prefers to do so. Discard store-bought capsules after one to two years.

To make your own capsules, you'll need empty 00-sized capsules, which are widely available at natural-foods stores, some pharmacies, and by mail order, and an electric coffee grinder. Grind the dried herbs in small batches and short bursts; then scoop the fine powder into the capsules. Sunny keeps an extra grinder on hand just for herbs; Linda cleans her coffee grinder with a drop or two of drinking alcohol to remove the coffee oils.

Tablets are made from powdered herbs plus inert fillers; chewable tablets often contain sugar

---

CAPSULE CAUTIONS

Be aware that children under seven often cannot swallow capsules correctly. If they try, they can end up with a throatful of bitter herb powder. Children under three also run the risk of choking on capsules or inhaling their contents. If a particular herb is available only in capsule form, open the capsule and mix the herb with applesauce, nut butter, honey, or any other pudding-like food your child enjoys.

---

or other sweeteners to make them taste good. If you give your children chewable tablets, especially if they contain vitamin C, insist that they brush their teeth afterwards to neutralize the acid and remove sugar.

Liquid extracts are usually made by soaking herbs for a period of time in a liquid. Because they are concentrated, extracts are more potent than bulk herbs. They're also easier to give to small children because you can blend them into favorite beverages. And with enough time and the right tools, you can make them yourself.

Tinctures are made with grain alcohol and distilled water. While tinctures are often appropriate medicines for adults, children are more sensitive to alcohol's effects, and most object to the taste. We don't know the long-term effects of giving alcohol, even in small doses, to children, so we prefer to give children glycerine extracts.

Some herbs, however, require extraction with a mix of alcohol and water to release their medicinal qualities. An example is California poppy, a calming herb that is helpful for children.

Glycerites. Glycerine derived from vegetable oils makes an excellent base and preservative for most children's herbal remedies. Kids tend to like

REMOVING ALCOHOL FROM TINCTURES

You can remove some, but not all, of the alcohol in tinctures by pouring the dose into a cup of just-boiled (not boiling) water. Let the alcohol evaporate for ten minutes. Losing some of the alcohol-based medicines along with the alcohol may be a worthwhile tradeoff. Cool the water and serve to your child.

its naturally sweet taste. Twenty years ago, when Sunny began studying herbal medicine, many herbalists mistakenly believed that glycerine poorly extracted plant constituents, and that herbal glycerites were weak and ineffective. In her own lab, she has found that glycerine actually serves as a good extractant for most of the herbs commonly used as children's remedies.

Vinegar extracts pale in potency compared to alcohol extracts and don't last as long. We don't use them often for making medicines, but we think they're fine for making tonics, mild herbal preparations that are taken regularly. Their advantages include vinegar's safety, a taste that's better than

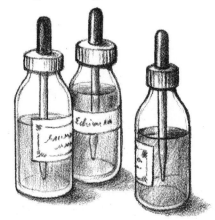

Glycerites are one of the most palatable ways to give kids herbs.

alcohol, suitability for foods such as salad dressing, and the ability to extract vitamins and minerals from fresh and dried herbs.

Vinegars can be made more quickly than tinctures and glycerites. We pour vinegar over nutrient-rich plants such as nettle, dandelion leaves, and the chopped roots of yellow dock and burdock. After a couple of days, we strain off the herbs and take the vinegar by the tablespoon, or mix it with oil for a salad dressing. Vinegar extracts remain potent in the refrigerator for only about one month.

Syrups. These thick, sugary solutions are fun to make at home, and because microorganisms can't grow in very concentrated solutions, they keep well. We don't recommend giving them to your child often, or at high doses, due to their high sugar content. We use syrups mainly for upper

MOTHER'S MILK

If you're a nursing mother, you've already got one of the easiest ways to give your child herbs. You can drink alcohol-free herbal extracts or teas and breast-feed some of the herb's goodness to your infant. First, however, make certain it's an herb that's safe to give your infant in this way.

The herbs consumed by a nursing mother are estimated to reach her bloodstream quickly and enter the milk supply in approximately fifteen to thirty minutes. Depending on variables such as the herb used, the mother's metabolism, and other factors, the strongest medicinal effect in the milk supply generally occurs in two to six hours. Herb residues may remain in the milk supply for up to forty-eight hours, and perhaps longer.

respiratory illnesses. Simmer soothing anti-cough herbs such as cherry bark, marshmallow root, and elecampane into a strong tea and add enough honey to make a thick, throat-coating emulsion.

For External Use

All kinds of small molecules, including the constituents of many herbs, can enter the bloodstream through the skin. If you're skeptical and have relatively tough skin, try putting a garlic poultice on the sole of one foot. Wait a couple hours, and then ask someone to smell your breath—you'll learn

that garlic is partly excreted through the lungs. When our children are sick (especially when nausea and vomiting thwart the use of oral medicines), we often use herbs externally in the following kinds of preparations.

Herb baths. For this huge batch of herbal tea, steep a handful of herbs in two quarts of hot water for at least ten minutes. Strain well, and pour the tea directly into the warm bath water.

You can also put a handful or two of herbs into a clean sock, knot the top, and throw the sock into the bath. Your child can use the sock as a sponge or bath toy. (If you have a small, nimble-fingered

WHAT ARE STANDARDIZED EXTRACTS?

When an herbal product says "standardized extract," it means that it is designed to have a consistent level of active ingredients from batch to batch. The manufacturer's goal is to create an herbal medication that has the same amount of activity in every bottle, despite the fact that the quantity of medicinal compounds in plants varies widely.

For example, Sunny's wild St.-John's-wort collection area in Montana has entirely different growing conditions than collection areas in the Pacific Northwest. Although both plant populations make good medicines, their levels of hypericin—one of the many active ingredients in the plant—is probably different.

Standardized extracts are somewhat controversial, because in many cases, more than one chemical, and often several chemicals working together, are what helps to restore health. Many herbalists believe that whole herbs are a better bet.

Standardized extracts are the products used

most often in clinical trials, where researchers need a way of ensuring that every patient gets the same dose. It's also easier for conventional doctors to recommend botanical medicines if they have clear guidelines about how much patients need to take to achieve therapeutic effects. Standardization provides such a tool.

Unfortunately, creation of these standardized products often requires chemical alterations with substances such as benzene, a powerful toxin, hexane, or other solvents produced from petroleum. You may not wish to support the use and production of these kinds of chemicals.

Some manufacturers "spike" their products by blending whole-herb material with additional concentrated or synthesized ingredients, usually the ones shown by research to have a particular medicinal effect. But you'll pay more for this process. And while your children deserve quality, we're not sure they need to take standardized or "spiked" extracts to get it.

child, you may want to think twice about using a sock—or muslin bag—lest you end up with a drain clogged with herbs.)

Foot baths. While your child's first foot bath may be short, he'll soon beg for this gentle healing method and remember it for years to come. We use foot baths for illnesses such as headaches, colds and flus, and to treat infections on the feet.

Steam inhalation. This old-fashioned technique sends warmth and moisture to dry, inflamed respiratory passages. Volatile herb constituents will rise with the steam, and many, such as thymol from thyme, have antiseptic properties. Because of the risk of burns, however, use herbal steams with caution; always put the pot of hot water on a table away from the stove. Commercial steamers can provide a more regulated temperature and flow of steam.

Essential oils. These are pure, concentrated extracts of volatile, aromatic herbs. Produced by heat or steam distillation, they require pounds of plant material for each ounce of oil, and their prices reflect this. (Don't, however, be tempted to purchase inexpensive, artificial fragrance oils, such as those offered at craft stores and supermarkets. Synthetic fragrances do not have the herbs' healing compounds.)

HEALING STEAM TREAT

What parent isn't busy? When our children have respiratory infections, we make one large pot of herbs serve three purposes. We steep a big batch of herbs for steam inhalation, and after the kids have inhaled the steam a few times—for several minutes each time—we strain most of the liquid into a warm bath or foot bath. We also save a few ounces for a healing cup of tea. For instructions on herbal steams, see Chapter 9, Colds.

While many manufacturers sell these oils without frightening cautions on the label, they are possibly the most hazardous of herbal products and require cautious, safe use and storage. Kathi Keville and Mindy Green, authors of *Aromatherapy: A Complete Guide to the Healing Art*, offer these safety guidelines for using essential oils with children: Never give your child essential oils internally, and do not apply undiluted essential oils to the skin. The delicious fragrance of oils may entice children to take a sip, so store them out of

ESSENTIAL OILS: AN HERBALIST IN THE SOUP

Most children tolerate essential oils—a few drops of them—in baths. But Sunny once made a big mistake that illustrates just how careful you have to be with essential oils. During her early years of herb experimentation, she came down with a fever. Either from lack of alertness or lack of knowledge, she poured the entire contents of a half-ounce bottle—more than one hundred drops—of peppermint oil into a hot bath and stumbled in. It smelled great and really opened up her sinuses. But within minutes, her skin starting itching terribly, and she scratched for hours.

She now knows that she should have quickly washed her skin with cool water and soap, and then coated it with a good vegetable oil such as almond to dilute the peppermint oil remaining on her skin.

reach of curious little hands. Drinking even a small bottle of essential oil could necessitate a trip to the emergency room.

That said, essential oils make good, convenient medicines for external use: massage oils, bath oils, herbal steams. Most recipes call for only a few drops; don't exceed these amounts. Green says you need add only two to five drops of essential oil to a child's bath. For steam inhalation, two or three drops in the pot is enough.

Massage oils. Because essential oils should not be applied directly to the skin, make massage oil by diluting essential oil in a carrier oil such as almond, apricot, or olive oil. To adapt a massage-oil recipe designed for adults for your kids, reduce the amount of essential oil by one-third to one-half. For example, a typical formula may contain ten to twelve drops of essential oil per fluid ounce of carrier oil. For a child or a pregnant woman, use only three to five drops in an ounce of carrier oil.

To test for skin sensitivity, apply a small amount of massage oil to a healthy patch of your child's skin; wait about an hour and check for reactions before applying to larger areas.

Infused oils. These oils, not to be confused with essential oils, are made just like teas, except you don't want to drink them. Fresh or dried herbs are chopped and then placed in a container and covered with a high-quality vegetable oil, such as olive or sweet almond. The jar is sealed and the herbs steeped in the oil for about two weeks. These oils can be applied directly to the skin. We find that an infused oil of St.-John's-wort is useful for kids' skin injuries, sprains, and strains; it's also good for ear infections and muscle aches.

Salves. These solid products, also called balms, are made from oils (including herbal infused oils), herbs, and a little beeswax. Salves help heal chapped lips, diaper rash, psoriasis, scrapes, bumps, bug bites, scabs, and many other skin irritations that kids are prone to. However, for skin problems that ooze or worsen under moist conditions—burns, moist diaper rashes, or weepy cases of eczema—don't apply a salve.

Poultices. This simple preparation involves applying herbs directly to the skin. If you're using fresh plants (say your child gets stung by a bee),

WHAT ARE FLOWER ESSENCES?

Back in the 1930s, London physician Edward Bach developed a number of flower remedies to help ease the minor emotional disturbances he believed contributed to disease. He created remedies from thirty-eight different flowering plants.

Preparation of the essences follows a specific process to produce dilute infusions of these flowers. Some practitioners explain the essences' actions as being not biochemical (as with herbs and drugs) but vibrational or energetic, as may be the case with homeopathy. And like homeopathy, these dilute remedies are safe.

One we have found useful is Rescue Remedy. It is made with essences of five flowers: star of Bethlehem, rock rose, cherry plum, impatiens, and clematis. When one of our children becomes upset due to injury or illness, we put four drops under her tongue, and then give ourselves a dose. It seems to help, especially with emotional trauma.

Although we can't back up our experiences with scientific studies, many practitioners (including some doctors and dentists) as well as patients testify to the effectiveness of flower essences. For essences made in your area, see the Resource Directory.

you just chop, bruise or even chew the leaves, flowers, or root, then apply directly to the skin. Many common weeds, such as chickweed, plantain, and burdock make good first-aid poultices. Dried herbs can also be used.

Compresses. These are simply cloths dampened in a freshly made infusion or decoction, then applied to an affected area. Depending on the herb and the complaint, you may want to use a hot or cold compress; for some conditions, it helps to alternate. Herbalists commonly use cool comfrey-tea compresses to help heal twisted ankles. A hot compress of burdock leaves on the throat can ease the pain of swollen glands.

Plasters and pastes. Perhaps you've made a paste of baking soda and water for bee stings. Just as easy is a paste made with one part dried, powdered herb, one part flour, and one part hot water or apple cider vinegar. Mustard powder makes a classic herb plaster for coughs, believed to stimulate circulation and draw immune cells to inflamed areas such as the lungs.

Figuring Doses for Children

How much, how often? When you get a prescription from a doctor, the answers are clear. When you're using herbs for your children's minor ailments, you get to do the math yourself.

There are three general guidelines to follow. First, start with the lowest dose in the range and work up. This is important because illness can alter the way kids respond to medicines.

Second, frequency and consistency of dosage are the keys to success. One large dose a day will not be nearly as effective as three to four smaller doses per day.

And third, your child's age and size are important. Although herbal products are generally not recommended for children under the age of six months, in some instances babies can take very gentle herbs in low doses. We'll give you more specific information about herbs for infants and toddlers in the chapters on various conditions.

When you are buying an herbal product, first confirm that all the herbs in the formula are appropriate for children. Then, to administer it to your child, follow the label directions. If the

---

WHAT IS HOMEOPATHY?

Homeopathic remedies are unlike herbal remedies, although the same plants are used. We mention homeopathy here because we find that people often confuse it with herbalism.

In homeopathy, a substance that causes an illness in large doses is greatly diluted and used to treat that illness's particular constellation of symptoms. For instance, a child with a blistery skin rash (say, chicken pox or poison ivy) might take a homeopathic preparation called Rhus tox, after the Latin name for poison ivy, *Rhus toxicodendron*. Rhus tox uses an extremely diluted tincture of poison ivy to stimulate the body's own healing response to symptoms similar to those called forth by actual exposure to the plant.

We can only offer a very simplified explanation for homeopathy within the confines of this book. Although neither of us has deeply studied this complicated discipline, health practitioners whom we respect believe in its healing power. Our general conclusion is that homeopathy is intriguing and can create valid medical results with few side effects, but we're not experts. For best results, we suggest that you work with a trained homeopath.

become more permeable, so fluid moves into tissues. The visible effect on your child is swelling, or if the airways are involved, difficult breathing.

Other useful terms to know:

Adaptogens are a particular type of tonic. They enhance the body's ability to cope with stress, strengthening the immune system and the endocrine system, including the adrenal glands, and helping these two systems to work together to maintain health.

Analgesics relieve pain. Some work topically, others internally.

Bitters are bitter-tasting herbs such as dandelion leaf that stimulate digestion and absorption of nutrients. They work best taken twenty minutes before a meal.

Calmatives and **sedatives** either calm or sedate—bringing relaxation to frazzled, wound-up kids, or sleep to those who are being kept up by coughs, ear infections, or other illnesses. Some herbs are calmatives in small doses, but have a stronger action in larger doses.

Carminatives dispel gas from the intestines, relieving gas and the cramps that sometimes accompany it. Mint and fennel are good examples.

Demulcents soothe inflamed mucous membranes and digestive tissues, protecting them from further irritation. Demulcent herbs are usually sticky or slippery when moist; oatmeal and slippery elm are two examples.

Digestives promote or aid digestion, some by adding helpful enzymes (papaya), others by stimulating the production of the body's own digestive juices (ginger).

Diuretics increase urine output by acting on the kidneys. They generally do this more gently than chemical diuretics, however, prompting some herbalists to rename them "aquaretics."

Expectorants help the body to expel mucus from the respiratory tract. They do this by stimulating bronchial secretions that thin the mucus, or

by making the mucus itself less sticky.

Laxatives operate in a number of ways to encourage bowel movements. Emollients make the stool softer; bulk laxatives swell when combined with water, encouraging the smooth-muscle contractions that move waste products out of the body. Stimulant laxatives, or cathartics, directly affect the bowels to produce contractions.

There are more action types and subcategories for medicinal herbs, but these are the most common ones. For definitions for other terms commonly used in alternative or complementary medicine, see the Glossary at the end of this book.

The Pediatric Herbal

Aloe vera

Also known as: Cape aloes
Latin binomial: *Aloe vera, Aloe* spp.
Part used: Gel from inside leaves
Main actions: Emollient, laxative, digestive, demulcent, wound healing
Typical uses: For children, externally as an emollient and to soothe burns; for adults, internally as a laxative.
Preparations: Gel or juice
Contraindications: Pregnant women and those with undiagnosed abdominal pain should not use aloe internally; no one should use it internally for more than ten days.
Of interest: Almost anyone can keep an aloe plant alive in the kitchen, where it's handy for minor burns and sunburns. Just break off a leaf, split it lengthwise, and apply the gel.

Arnica

Latin binomial: *Arnica cordifolia, A. montana, Arnica* spp.

Part used: Flowers

Main actions: Topical analgesic and anti-inflammatory

Typical uses: Sports injuries, muscle strains, bruises, and minor bumps

Preparations: Infused oil, salves, homeopathic remedies

Contraindications: Not for children's use internally or on open wounds. Safety during pregnancy is not known (homeopathic internal use is fine).

Of interest: Sunny once hit her shinbone hard on a log in the forest, fell down, and landed smack dab in an arnica patch. She rubbed the flowers directly on the contusion and received almost instant relief.

ASTRAGALUS

Also known as: Huang-qi

Latin binomial: *Astragalus membranaceus*

Part used: Root

Main actions: Adaptogenic, anti-inflammatory, antiviral, antibacterial; tones and stimulates immune system

Typical uses: To prevent colds and flu; to build immune system in children who are prone to illness. Can be used daily as an immune tonic for up to one month.

Preparations: Tea, soups, capsules, extracts

Contraindications: Not suggested during pregnancy; not for use during fevers.

Of interest: This herb is often used as a food in Traditional Chinese Medicine.

Kids' taste rating: Great

BLACK WALNUT

Latin binomial: *Juglans nigra*

Part used: Green outer hull of nut shell

Main actions: Antiparasitic, laxative

Typical uses: In formulas to fight parasites

Preparations: Capsules

Contraindications: Safety in pregnancy is unknown. Not for use for more than a few weeks at a time.

Of interest: All forms of this herb stain clothing.

Kids' taste rating: Really bad. Best given in capsules.

BONESET

Also known as: Sweat plant

Latin binomial: *Eupatorium perfoliatum*

Parts used: Flowers, leaves; must be used dried to evaporate a chemical called tremerol, which can cause vomiting if the fresh plant is used.

Main actions: Promotes sweating; antispasmodic; suppresses coughs.

Typical uses: Early stages of colds and flu

Preparations: Tea, glycerites, capsules, tincture

Contraindications: Not for use by children under one year or pregnant women. Large doses can cause vomiting or diarrhea. Modern research suggests its use for no more than seven days.

Of interest: Boneset was tremendously popular at the turn of the century as a cold, fever, and malaria remedy. (Joe Pye weed, *Eupatorium purpureum*, is closely related.)

Kids' taste rating: "Tastes a little bitter."

BURDOCK

Also known as: Beggar's buttons, gobo root, "those dumb stickers"

Latin binomial: *Arctium lappa*

Parts used: Root, seeds, leaves

Main actions: Liver and lymphatic tonic, diuretic, promotes sweating

Typical uses: Skin irritations, eczema, psoriasis, boils; root also can be used as food.

Preparations: In stir-fry meals, tinctures, capsules, glycerites; externally as a salve or skin wash, poultices, compresses

Contraindications: May have a slight estrogenic effect. Avoid during pregnancy.

Of interest: Burdock's huge leaves make great costumes; its burr balls have caused at least one herbalist to cut her long hair as the only method of removal. It will jubilantly grow to cover moist, shady areas.

Kids' taste rating: "Kinda tastes like dirt, but not bad dirt."

CALENDULA

Also known as: Flat-leafed marigold

Latin binomial: *Calendula officinalis*

Part used: Flowers

Main actions: Anti-inflammatory, analgesic, antibacterial, skin regenerator

Typical uses: Externally for strains, sprains, eczema, minor skin ulcers, bug bites

Preparations: Teas, tinctures, glycerites, infused oil

Contraindications: None known

Of interest: Do not confuse with curly-leafed marigolds (*Tagetes* spp.). Adults can use calendula tincture as an antibacterial, analgesic throat gargle.

Kids' taste rating: Fine

CALIFORNIA POPPY

Latin binomial: *Eschscholtzia californica*

Parts used: Stems, leaves, flowers

Main actions: Calmative in small doses, sedative in larger doses, antianxiety, antispasmodic

Typical uses: Children's nighttime formulas

Preparations: Tinctures

Contraindications: Not for use with MAO-inhibitor antidepressants, or during pregnancy.

Of interest: This bright orange poppy is only distantly related to the opium poppy. California's state flower grows rampantly in warmer climates.

Kids' taste rating: "This is the yucky one."

CATNIP

Latin binomial: *Nepeta cataria*

Parts used: Stems, leaves, flowers

Main actions: Calmative, nerve tonic, antispasmodic, digestive aid; promotes sweating

Typical uses: Colic, sleeplessness, minor infantile fevers

Preparations: Tea, glycerite, capsules

Contraindications: Pregnancy, due to mild uterine stimulating effects

Of interest: Historically consumed by nursing mothers to ease babies' colic

Kids' taste rating: Kind of bitter

CAYENNE

Also known as: Red pepper, capsicum

Latin binomial: *Capsicum annuum* var. *frutescens*

Part used: Fruit

Preparations: As a spice in food; capsules; ointment, salves, and creams for external use

Main actions: Anti-inflammatory, antioxidant, mucous-membrane tonic, topical analgesic

Typical uses: Internally: warming, circulatory stimulant; headache easer. Externally: pain reliever.

Contraindications: Children under two years

Of interest: Cayenne contains salicylic acid and capsaicin, making it a pain-relieving topical treatment for inflammatory skin and joint conditions. Look for a commercially prepared capsaicin-extract cream.

Kids' taste rating: Too spicy!

CHAMOMILE

Also known as: Manzanilla

Latin binomial: *Matricaria recutita, M. chamomila*

Part used: Flowers

Main actions: Antispasmodic, anti-inflammatory, nervine, digestive aid

Typical uses: Inflammation, allergies, children's calming formulas, nausea

Preparations: Tea, glycerite, tinctures, essential oil

Contraindications: Those with daisy-family (*Asteraceae*) allergies may also have allergies to chamomile.

Of interest: Wild chamomile (*Matricaria matricariodes*), also known as pineapple weed, is useful for the same complaints.

Kids' taste rating: Great

CHERRY BARK

Also known as: Wild cherry

Latin binomial: *Prunus serotina, P. virginiana*

Part used: Bark

Main actions: Inhibits coughing; antidiarrheal, mild sedative

Typical uses: Dry, irritable coughs such as bronchitis

Preparations: Tea, syrup, glycerites, tinctures

Contraindications: Do not use in high doses or longer than one week without a break.

Of interest: Cherry bark should be harvested in the fall.

Kids' taste rating: Fair; tea is tolerable if sweetened.

CLEAVERS

Also known as: Bedstraw, tangleweed

Latin binomial: *Galium aparine*

Parts used: Leaves, flowers, stems

Main actions: Blood cleanser, demulcent, tonic for lymphatic system

Typical uses: Tonsillitis, minor bladder and stomach irritations, immune tonic formulas

Preparations: Tea, glycerites, tinctures. Rarely found in tablets or capsules.

Contraindications: None known

Of interest: Fresh, moist cleavers are far superior to the dried plant, although the dried aboveground parts retain medicinal action. Strain any preparations well; the plant's tiny barbs can irritate the throat.

Kids' taste rating: Fine

CLOVE

Latin binomial: *Syzygium aromaticum* (formerly *Eugenia caryophyllata*)

Parts used: Flower bud

Main actions: Analgesic

Typical uses: Spice, dilute amounts in teething oil

Preparations: Essential oil

Contraindications: Do not place undiluted oil on infants' gums or throat. Dilute two to four drops of essential oil in one teaspoon of almond, safflower, or canola oil.

Of interest: In the courts of ancient China, people held cloves in their mouths to freshen the breath. This trick works today as a traveler's quick toothache remedy.

Kids' taste rating: Great, if it's not too strong.

COMFREY

Also known as: Boneknit
Latin binomial: *Symphytum officinale*
Parts used: Leaves, root
Main actions: Demulcent, emollient, anti-inflammatory, stimulates healing

Typical uses: Topically to relieve inflammation and speed healing of bone breaks and muscle tears

Preparations: Poultices, compresses, extracts

Contraindications: Current research suggests that comfrey, particularly the root, should not be used internally because of compounds that may cause liver damage. Extracts that are free of these compounds are now available; look for the words "pyrrolizidine-free" on the label.

Of interest: Comfrey is rich in allantoin and other substances that stimulate cell growth and tissue repair. For external use, we love comfrey. We *adore* comfrey. It should be a primary ingredient in any skin-soothing salve you make or purchase.

CRAMP BARK

Also known as: Guelder rose
Latin binomial: *Viburnum opulus*
Parts used: Bark, root bark
Main actions: Antispasmodic
Typical uses: Headaches, muscular cramps, menstrual cramps; any kind of muscle spasm, including coughs
Preparations: Tea, extracts, capsules
Contraindications: Not for use by patients with kidney stones.
Of interest: Related species, black haw (*Viburnum prunifolium*), has similar effects.

Kids' taste rating: Not great

DANDELION

Latin binomial: *Taraxacum officinale*
Parts used: Root, leaves
Main actions: Diuretic, bile duct activator, mild laxative, mineral supplement
Typical uses: Bladder irritations, liver disorders (including hepatitis and jaundice), anemia
Preparations: Tea, capsules, vinegars, extracts
Contraindications: Not for use with acute gallbladder problems
Of interest: Prescription diuretics often deplete the body's potassium stores. Dandelion reliably increases urine output, but also supplies potassium.

Kids' taste rating: Bitter

ECHINACEA

Also known as: Purple coneflower, coneflower, snake root
Latin binomial: *Echinacea purpurea, E. angustifolia, Echinacea* spp.

HERBAL JUICESICLES

Herbal juicesicles are a delicious way to introduce herb teas to children who enjoy cold foods. If your child refuses to eat them during a respiratory infection, don't worry; she may instinctively know that cold foods aren't the right medicine for her at that time. Here's how to make these cold treats.

Using the standard tea proportions of 1 teaspoon of dried herb per cup of water, prepare 1 cup of good-tasting medicinal tea. Gently simmer until the liquid is reduced by half. Add 1/2 cup unsweetened organic juice to tea, stir, pour into ice-cube trays, and put in freezer. When partly solid, insert a wooden tongue depressor or plastic spoon.

Parts used: Root, leaves, flowers, seeds

Main actions: Immune stimulant, antibacterial, anti-inflammatory, antiviral

Typical uses: Preventive for colds, flu, sore throats, and coughs; immune support during illness. Most effective if used immediately at first signs of illness.

Preparations: Teas, tinctures, glycerites, capsules

Contraindications: Not for use during immune disorders such as lupus, tuberculosis, multiple sclerosis, and HIV infection. Rarely, patients with asthma, eczema, or hay fever have shown allergic reactions to echinacea.

Of interest: The number-one-selling herb in Europe and North America, echinacea was historically used to treat snakebite. Please purchase only cultivated sources.

Kids' taste rating: "It's tingly, but tastes okay."

ELDER

Latin binomial: *Sambucus nigra, S. racemosa, Sambucus* spp.

Parts used: Flowers, berries

Main actions: Antiviral, promotes sweating

Typical uses: Flu, colds, fevers

Preparations: Tea, glycerites, tinctures, syrup

Contraindications: Do not eat or harvest red elderberries ("Don't eat red, or you'll be dead" is the herbalists' creed). Seeds of all elderberries are somewhat toxic; strain them out. Eat the raw berries sparingly or cook them to reduce hydrocyanic acid content.

Of interest: Although studies show elderberries are antiviral, traditional fever remedies used the flowers in combination with herbs such as peppermint and yarrow.

Kids' taste rating: Syrup is delicious; other forms are tolerable.

ELECAMPANE

Latin binomial: *Inula helenium*
Part used: Root
Main actions: Expectorant, demulcent, antibacterial, anti-inflammatory
Typical uses: Irritable coughs with deep or stubborn mucus, bronchitis, asthma
Preparations: Capsules, tea
Contraindications: Not for use during pregnancy or nursing. Large doses can cause vomiting.
Of interest: To disguise this herb's bitter taste, use licorice root or elderberry.

Kids' taste rating: Bitter

EPHEDRA

Also known as: Ma huang
Latin binomial: *Ephedra sinica, Ephedra* spp.
Parts used: Stems, leaves, flowers
Main actions: Stimulant, bronchodilator, antihistamine
Typical uses: Allergies, sinusitis, minor lung irritations with wet mucus, asthma
Preparations: Tea, tinctures, tablets, capsules.
Contraindications: Hypertension, MAO-inhibiting antidepressants, pregnancy, nursing; children under seven.
Of interest: Ephedra is controversial due to abuse by dieters and those searching for an herbal "high." While we believe it is a valuable herb when used correctly, it may make sensitive children too jittery. Mormon tea (*Ephedra nevadensis*) is a useful, but less potent species which may be more appropriate for your child.

Kids' taste rating: Okay if tea is brewed for fewer than ten minutes.

EUCALYPTUS

Also known as: Gum tree, blue gum tree
Latin binomial: *Eucalyptus globulus*
Parts used: Leaves, essential oil
Main actions: Bronchodilator, antibacterial, expectorant
Typical uses: Coughs due to colds
Preparations: Steams, salves, chest rubs
Contraindications: Essential oil is NOT for internal use. Do not use oil near nose or eyes on small children. Not for patients with liver, gallbladder, or digestive disorders.
Of interest: Eucalyptus is a primary ingredient in over-the-counter chest rubs. Be sure to dilute the essential oil with a vegetable oil before using on children's skin.

Kids' taste rating: Tea is rarely used internally in North America.

EYEBRIGHT

Latin binomial: *Euphrasia officinalis*
Parts used: Stems, leaves, flowers
Main actions: Mucus drying; anti-inflammatory for eyes
Typical uses: Allergies, colds, pinkeye
Preparations: Externally: infusion. Internally: tinctures, glycerites, capsules
Contraindications: None known
Of interest: Know the source of the herb in products you buy; in some regions, eyebright is being overharvested. For a recipe for an eyebright eyewash, see page 107.

Kids' taste rating: Fine

FENNEL

Latin binomial: *Foeniculum vulgare*
Parts used: Whole plant, especially seeds

Main actions: Antispasmodic, digestive, carminative

Typical uses: Stomachaches, gas, colic, cramps from diarrhea, and to promote milk flow in nursing mothers

Preparations: Tea, glycerite, tinctures, capsules

Contraindications: None

Of interest: Many nursing mothers attest to fennel's ability to increase milk supply. We use fennel seeds regularly to improve the flavor of bitter teas. Added to pizza or tomato sauces, these seeds help reduce digestive gas.

Kids' taste rating: Tastes like licorice

FEVERFEW

Latin binomial: *Tanacetum parthenium*

Parts used: Leaves, flowers

Main actions: Analgesic, antispasmodic, anti-allergenic, anti-inflammatory

Typical uses: Migraine prevention, headache relief

Preparations: Tea, glycerite, tincture, tablets, capsule

Contraindications: Feverfew's use during pregnancy has not been studied.

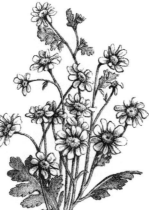

Of interest: Studies show that one raw leaf per day, or an equivalent dose in capsules, reduces occurrence of migraines. We've also found that feverfew helps with muscle aches and growing pains.

Kids' taste rating: Very bitter as tea. Best as a glycerite or tablet.

FLAXSEED

Also known as: Linseed

Latin binomial: *Linum usitatissimum, Linum* spp.

Parts used: Seed, oil

Main actions: Seed: demulcent, bulk laxative. Oil: helps the body control inflammatory responses such as allergies.

Typical uses: Seed: constipation, digestive aid for acid stomach, bath infusion for soothing irritated skin. Oil: acne, allergies, ear infections, eczema, hyperactivity; many other uses.

Preparations: Seeds and oil: culinary uses. Oil: capsules.

Contraindications: Seed: not for use with diverticulitis. Oil: do not confuse edible flaxseed oil with the denatured linseed oil used for woodworking; the latter is poisonous.

Of interest: Flaxseed oil contains high levels of anti-inflammatory omega-3 essential fatty acids, which provide its benefits. Always keep flaxseed oil and seeds refrigerated.

Kids' taste rating: From yuck to delicious.

GARLIC

Also known as: "Stinking rose"

Latin binomial: *Allium sativum*

Part used: Cloves of bulb

Main actions: Antimicrobial, antiviral, immune support.

Typical uses: Coughs, colds, flu, minor infections, preventive during cold/flu season

Preparations: Raw cloves, capsules, tablets, liquid extracts

Contraindications: Large quantities can irritate the mouth or stomach; use sparingly for children under two.

Of interest: One of the most researched herbs

on the planet. Some sources suggest that nursing mothers avoid ingesting it in large quantities. Anecdotal reports suggest removing garlic and onions from a mother's diet if her infant suffers from colic.

Kids' taste rating: Usually tolerated

GINGER

Latin binomial: *Zingiber officinale*
Part used: Rhizome but commonly called root
Main actions: Antinausea, digestive aid, anti-inflammatory, warming, antiviral
Typical uses: Nausea, digestive cramping, inflammation such as arthritis, muscle aches, headaches
Preparations: Culinary uses, tea, glycerites, tinctures
Contraindications: Childhood fevers, gallstones

Of interest: A delicious, safe anti-inflammatory herb. Effective against morning sickness, motion sickness, and post-operative nausea.

Kids' taste rating: Great, especially with a bit of sweetener.

GINKGO

Latin binomial: *Ginkgo biloba*
Parts used: Leaves, roasted seeds
Main actions: Antioxidant, short-term memory tonic, brain circulation booster
Typical uses: Altitude sickness, anti-allergenic
Preparations: Tea, capsules, extracts, standardized products
Contraindications: Not for use with MAO-inhibiting antidepressants. Raw seeds are toxic.
Of interest: Ginkgo leaf is used in antidepres-

WHERE'S THE GOLDENSEAL?

There are a few well-known medicinal herbs we have chosen not to recommend, for the following reasons.

Goldenseal (*Hydrastis canadensis.*). This plant, a powerful alternative to antibiotics, has been severely overharvested in the wild. This may be because it once had an erroneous reputation for being able to cleanse the body of the residues of recreational drugs. Should you stumble upon some wild goldenseal, please leave it growing. Purchase goldenseal products only if the label clearly states they are derived from cultivated plants.

Osha (*Ligusticum porteri, L. canbyi*). Like goldenseal, this plant has been nearly depleted

in many areas. Osha has a long traditional use in respiratory tract infections, but many good herbal alternatives exist: pleurisy root, horehound, mullein, elderberry, thyme, sage, and astragalus. Use these to give osha time to recover from overharvesting.

Ginseng (*Panax ginseng, P. quinquefolius*). The roots of these plants are well-known adaptogens that also provide immune support. While they are often used to combat stress, low energy, and chronic fatigue in adults, they are generally not considered appropriate or necessary for children. Instead, we recommend Siberian ginseng (*Eleutherococcus senticosus*), which has some of the same effects.

sant herbal formulas and for soft tissue injuries and eye problems.

HAWTHORN

Latin binomial: *Crataegus oxycanthus, Crataegus* spp.
Parts used: Berries, leaves, flowers
Main actions: Nervine, anti-inflammatory, cardiovascular tonic
Typical uses: Hyperactivity, tension, minor heart arrhythmias, hypertension, skin repair, gum disease
Preparations: Tea, syrup, extracts, capsules, tablets
Contraindications: May increase the effects of prescription heart medications such as digitalis.
Of interest: Hawthorn berries can help stimulate tissue repair in sprains, strains, and tears; the herb is also a good addition to calming formulas such as those for attention-deficit and hyperactivity disorder.

Kids' taste rating: Delicious

HOPS

Latin binomial: *Humulus lupulus*
Part used: Flowers (called strobiles)
Main actions: Sedative, antispasmodic, nervine, analgesic, antibacterial, digestive, estrogenic, promotes milk flow
Typical uses: Restlessness, pain, hyperactivity, headaches
Preparations: Capsules, extracts
Contraindications: This herb should probably not be taken by those with estrogen-dependent disorders; it is definitely not for use by

pregnant women. Not for long-term use.
Of interest: Nursing mothers may drink non-alcoholic dark or bitter beer for the hops' milk-promoting effect.

Kids' taste rating: Bitter

HOREHOUND

Latin binomial: *Marrubium vulgare*
Parts used: Leaves, flowers
Main actions: Expectorant, mild diuretic, promotes sweating
Typical uses: Coughs with loose, rattling mucus in the lungs
Preparations: Tea, glycerite, syrup, lozenges
Contraindications: Pregnancy, heart disease, hypertension. Huge amounts could be laxative or cause heart-rhythm irregularities.
Of interest: Horehound's expectorant qualities were known to the ancient Greeks; Dioscorides (A.D. 40–90) recommended it for asthma and coughs.

Kids' taste rating: Bitter; disguise taste with licorice and a little orange peel.

HORSETAIL

Also known as: Shavegrass
Latin binomial: *Equisetum arvense*
Parts used: Stems, leaves, flowers
Main actions: Diuretic, wound healing, lung tonic
Typical uses: Bedwetting, broken bones, wounds
Preparations: Tea, extracts, poultices
Contraindications: Kidney or heart disease. Not to be used raw for more than seven days because it depletes thiamine (vitamin B1). Avoid during pregnancy.
Of interest: Horsetail is a potent source of

naturally occurring silica and calcium, and makes an excellent poultice for injuries.

Kids' taste rating: Fine

HYSSOP

Latin binomial: *Hyssopus officinalis*
Parts used: Leaves, flowers
Main actions: Expectorant, promotes sweating; antibacterial, antispasmodic, nerve tonic, uterine muscle stimulant
Typical uses: Lung tonic for spasmodic coughing, antifungal for athlete's foot and *Candida* infections.
Preparations: Tea, extracts, capsules
Contraindications: Pregnancy
Of interest: Research is being conducted on hyssop's activity against retroviruses such as HIV. It combines well with elderberry and lemon grass to ease mild childhood fevers.

Kids' taste rating: Fair to yucky

KAVA-KAVA

Also known as: Kava
Latin binomial: *Piper methysticum*
Part used: Root
Main actions: Calmative in small doses, sedative in large doses; antispasmodic, analgesic
Typical uses: Tension, anxiety, hyperactivity, and urinary, intestinal, or menstrual cramps
Preparations: Extracts, capsules, tablets
Contraindications: Avoid if using prescription sedatives or alcohol, if pregnant or nursing.
Of interest: Revered plant of South Pacific cultures. It appears to be nonaddictive, but long-term use can create medical problems.

Kids' taste rating: "It tastes funny; it tingles."

LAVENDER

Latin binomial: *Lavandula officinalis*, *Lavandula* spp.
Part used: Flowers
Main actions: Nervine, anti-inflammatory
Typical uses: In aromatherapy for headache, tight muscles; diluted essential oil for skin injuries and burns
Preparations: Flowers in tea, tinctures, and glycerites; essential oil for topical uses
Contraindications: Essential oil is not for internal use in children.
Of interest: Sunny's little boy describes lavender's scent like this: "It's kind of like praying. You can't see it, but you know it's there."

Kids' taste rating: Tea smells better than it tastes.

LEMON BALM

Also known as: Melissa, balm, sweet melissa
Latin binomial: *Melissa officinalis*
Parts used: Leaves, flowers
Main actions: Antispasmodic, antibacterial, antiviral, promotes sweating, carminative, nervine,
Typical uses: Gas, cramping, excitability, minor anxiety, respiratory illness, mild fevers, herpes virus (Types I and II, as both a preventive and topical soother of sores)
Preparations: Tea, glycerite, tincture, baths, essential oil
Contraindications: None known
Of interest: We find this an essential herb for our children's herbal medicine chests because it has so many uses.

Kids' taste rating: Delicious

LICORICE

Also known as: "The Great Harmonizer" for its synergistic action with many herbs, and the ability of its flavor to mask the taste of more bitter plants

Latin binomial: *Glycyrrhiza glabra*

Part used: Root

Main actions: Demulcent, anti-inflammatory, antiviral

Typical uses: Stress, premenstrual syndrome, inflammatory bowel disease, psoriasis, eczema, ulcers, hepatitis, herpes, raw throats, hay fever, constipation

Preparations: Tea, powdered root in capsules or tablets, liquid extracts; also used externally in creams and compresses.

Contraindications: Hypertension, kidney or liver disease, pregnancy, breastfeeding, diabetes. Because it can cause retention of water and sodium do not use internally for more than six weeks.

Of interest: Many kids like to chew on the long, dried roots to ease sore throats.

Kids' taste rating: Sunny estimates that three out of four kids love the sweet, anise-like taste of licorice; one in four hates it.

LOBELIA

Also known as: Pukewort, Indian tobacco

Latin binomial: *Lobelia inflata*

Parts used: Stems, leaves, and flowers

Main actions: Expectorant, sedative

Typical uses: Asthma, coughs associated with lots of lower respiratory mucus

Preparations: Tea, tincture, capsules

Contraindications: Lobelia can cause vomiting, which has been a part of some historical treatments for getting rid of deep coughs. This practice, called emesis therapy, is rarely used today, thank goodness. Not for use during pregnancy.

Of interest: Combines well with licorice root. Lobelia was used internally and smoked by many Native Americans for coughs. The Mesquakie tribe used it as a "love charm" to restore harmony to bickering couples.

Kids' taste rating: Yuck

MALVA

Also known as: Cheeseweed, mallow

Latin binomial: *Malva neglecta, Malva* spp.

Parts used: Whole plant, especially root

Main actions: Demulcent, anti-inflammatory

Typical uses: Stomachaches, urinary tract irritations, diarrhea, skin inflammations

Preparations: Tea, tinctures, capsules, poultices

Contraindications: None known

Of interest: Malva's green, immature fruits, which resemble tiny wheels of cheese, can be eaten raw. Most people consider this edible and medicinal plant a weed. Virtually interchangeable with marshmallow root.

Kids' taste rating: Leaf tastes better than root.

MARSHMALLOW

Latin binomial: *Althea* spp.

Parts used: Flowers, leaves, and especially root

Main actions: Demulcent, immune support

Typical uses: Sore throats, digestive upsets, diarrhea, urinary inflammations

Preparations: Teas, liquid extracts, capsules

Contraindications: Take several hours apart from any other medications

Of interest: It's hard to believe this is the

source of the original marshmallow. Hundreds of years ago, *Althea* root was roasted, caramelized with sugar, and used to relieve stomachaches. Now, synthetic marshmallows *give* kids stomachaches.

Kids' taste rating: Yuck

MEADOWSWEET

Also known as: Spiraea
Latin binomial: *Filipendula ulmaria* (formerly *Spiraea ulmaria*)
Parts used: Aerial parts
Main actions: Pain relief
Typical uses: Headaches, muscle aches, fever
Preparations: Tea, extracts, capsules
Contraindications: Contains salicylates; avoid use during viral infections. See cautions under "willow."
Of interest: The word aspirin comes from *Spiraea*.

Kids' taste rating: Tea is very bitter.

MILK THISTLE

Latin binomial: *Silybum marianum*
Parts used: Seeds
Main actions: Liver protective and tonic, anti-inflammatory, digestive aid
Typical uses: Liver tonic, liver support during allergies, food intolerance or other chronic health challenges, hepatitis, jaundice
Preparations: Tinctures, capsules, standardized products, roasted seeds
Contraindications: None recognized
Of interest: Seeds are quite tasty: roast for two minutes in a cast-iron pan and cool. Grind as needed for a nutritious superfood.

Kids' taste rating: Okay

MULLEIN

Also known as: Toilet-paper plant, gordolobo
Latin binomial: *Verbascum thapsus, Verbascum* spp.
Parts used: Leaves, flowers
Main actions: Leaf: demulcent, expectorant, antispasmodic. Flower: analgesic

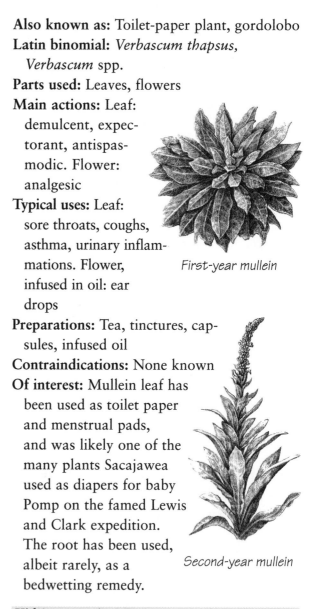

First-year mullein

Typical uses: Leaf: sore throats, coughs, asthma, urinary inflammations. Flower, infused in oil: ear drops
Preparations: Tea, tinctures, capsules, infused oil
Contraindications: None known
Of interest: Mullein leaf has been used as toilet paper and menstrual pads, and was likely one of the many plants Sacajawea used as diapers for baby Pomp on the famed Lewis and Clark expedition. The root has been used, albeit rarely, as a bedwetting remedy.

Second-year mullein

Kids' taste rating: Fine

NETTLE

Also known as: Stinging nettle
Latin binomial: *Urtica dioica*
Part used: Leaves
Main actions: Antihistaminic, blood building
Typical uses: Allergies, anemia

Preparations: Steamed, fresh greens as a food; tea, capsules

Contraindications: Severe allergies, especially those resulting in anaphylactic shock

Of interest: Stinging nettles do sting! Avoid touching the plants; wear long sleeves and long pants on any nettle-gathering trip. Use gloves or plastic bags over your hands when gathering; snip the young leaves or stalks with clippers. Deactivate the sting by drying or steaming the leaves.

Kids' taste rating: Not bad

OATS

Also known as: Wild oats

Latin binomial: *Avena sativa, A. fatua*

Parts used: Fresh, green seeds with white "milk"

Main actions: Nervine, digestive aid, emollient

Typical uses: Internally: hyperactivity, nervous conditions, digestive upsets. Externally: itchy skin

Preparations: Foods containing oats; baths, tea, extracts

Contraindications: None known except gluten allergies

Of interest: Oatmeal supplies many of the same benefits as wild oats and makes a great breakfast for extra-active kids; try adding nuts or other sources of protein.

Kids' taste rating: Great

ORANGE PEEL

Also known as: Bitter orange, sour orange

Latin binomial: *Citrus aurantium*

Part used: Peel

Main actions: Digestive aid

Typical uses: Nausea, digestive formulas

Preparations: Tea, glycerite, tinctures

Contraindications: Citrus allergies. Children have had severe reactions to eating large amounts of fresh orange peel and seeds. For the non-allergic, one or two square inches of the dried peel are safe in teas.

Of interest: Use only dried orange peel; fresh peel contains large amounts of essential oils, which may irritate mucous membranes. Wash the orange thoroughly before peeling; better yet, buy organic if you can.

Kids' taste rating: Good

OREGON GRAPEROOT

Also known as: Holly grape, barberry

Latin binomial: *Berberis aquifolium, B. nervosa, Mahonia* spp.

Parts used: Root, root bark

Main actions: Antibacterial, antiparasitic, digestive, liver tonic

Typical uses: Internally: colds with greenish nasal discharge, bacterial infections, sinusitis, minor lung inflammations, intestinal parasites, coughs. Externally: eczema

Preparations: Tea, tincture, glycerite, skin wash

Contraindications: Not for use in children under age one or during pregnancy.

Of interest: Oregon graperoot is a good alternative to the overharvested goldenseal (*Hydrastis canadensis*).

Kids' taste rating: Terrible

PAPAYA

Latin binomial: *Carica papaya*

Parts used: Leaves, fruit, seeds

Main actions: Digestive aid

during pregnancy (a cup of tea per day maximum, for no more than one week).

Of interest: Easy to grow in most gardens, but don't confuse sage with sagebrush (*Artemisia* spp.).

Kids' taste rating: Varies from yummy to yucky. Best as tea with honey and lemon, but beware of steeping more than five minutes.

St.-John's-wort

Also known as: St.-Joan's-wort; Klamath weed

Latin binomial: *Hypericum perforatum*

Parts used: Flowering tops (the top of the plant including the flowers and about four inches of stem and leaves)

Main actions: Antidepressive, wound healing, nerve tonic, antiviral

Typical uses: Alternative to prescription antidepressants in mild or moderate depression; in massage oils and salves for sprains, strains, and minor injuries

Preparations: Tea, glycerite, tincture, capsule, tablet, infused oil, salves

Contraindications: Never substitute for prescription antidepressants without a doctor's supervision; toxic interactions also occur with some prescription antidepressants. Not suggested for pregnancy.

Of interest: If you want to grow St.-John's-wort, check with your local weed-control agency first. This species is considered a noxious weed in a number of states.

Kids' taste rating: "Makes my mouth pucker."

Shiitake mushroom

Latin binomial: *Lentinus edodes*

Parts used: Fresh or dried mushroom

Main actions: Immune tonic, antiviral

Typical uses: Colds, flu, recovery from chronic illness, immune-system enhancement

Preparations: Tinctures, capsules, and as food

Contraindications: None known.

Of interest: These delicious mushrooms are becoming more widely available both dried and fresh. You can easily add them to soups or side dishes.

Kids' taste rating: Great, if they like mushrooms.

Siberian ginseng

Also known as: Eleuthero

Latin binomial: *Eleutherococcus senticosus*

Part used: Root

Main actions: Adaptogen, immune support, antiviral

Typical uses: Boosting energy, stress, recovery from physical exhaustion or illness

Preparations: Tea, tinctures, glycerites, capsules

Contraindications: None known, although many herbalists err on the side of caution and say to avoid it during pregnancy. Limit children's use to two weeks, then take a one-week break.

Of interest: This plant is not a true ginseng of the *Panax* genus, but for both adults and children it is a superb tonic for supporting the body during physical or mental stress.

Kids' taste rating: Fine

Skullcap

Also known as: Scute

Latin binomial: *Scutellaria lateriflora*

Parts used: Stems, leaves, and flowers

Main actions: Nervine, sedative, antiviral

Typical uses: Hyperactivity, nerve formulas

Preparations: Tea, extracts

Contraindications: None known

Of interest: The majority of antiviral research has centered on *Scutellaria baicalensis,* which has similar actions and constituents.

Kids' taste rating: Very bitter

SLIPPERY ELM

Latin binomial: *Ulmus fulva*

Parts used: Inner bark

Main actions: Demulcent, astringent

Typical uses: Internally for sore throats, coughs, urinary tract irritation, diarrhea; externally for inflamed skin, wounds, burns.

Preparations: Tea, powdered bark, extracts, tablets; externally as a poultice

Contraindications: None known

Of interest: Wild sources of slippery elm bark are dwindling; purchase products made from cultivated trees only.

Kids' taste rating: Yuck

TEA TREE

Latin binomial: *Melaleuca alternifolia*

Parts used: Leaves and flowers

Main actions: Antifungal, antiseptic

Typical uses: Externally for fungal and bacterial skin infections, including nail fungus

Preparations: Essential oil

Contraindications: Dilute for external use on small children, starting with one to two drops of tea tree oil per teaspoon of other oil, such as almond or olive. Do not give internally; store securely.

Of interest: Indigenous to swampy areas of New South Wales in Australia.

THYME, LEMON THYME

Latin binomial: *Thymus vulgaris, Thymus × citriodorus*

Parts used: Stems, flowers, leaves

Main actions: Antispasmodic, expectorant, antimicrobial

Typical uses: Anti-inflammatory, cough remedy

Preparations: Tea, glycerites, tinctures, capsules, essential oil

Contraindications: None known

Of interest: Sunny's kids call it "tiny thyme" to help them remember the name of the miniature leaves. This herb has excellent antibacterial properties; two drops of essential oil in an eight-ounce spray bottle of distilled water makes a natural antiseptic spray. Add two drops of lavender essential oil for a cooling, inspiring scent.

Kids' taste rating: Good.

TURMERIC

Latin binomial: *Curcuma longa*

Parts used: Rhizome

Main actions: Antioxidant, anti-inflammatory, cholesterol-lowering

Typical uses: Allergies, arthritis, injured or swollen joints

Preparations: Capsules

Contraindications: Do not use during pregnancy, or if your child has gallbladder or liver disease, or ulcers.

Of interest: Not widely used for children but shows promise for allergies and other inflammatory conditions.

Kids' taste rating: Superyuck! Give only in capsule form.

USNEA

Also known as: Old man's beard
Latin binomial: *Usnea* spp.
Part used: Lichen
Main actions: Antibacterial, particularly against staph and strep; antifungal, antiparasitic
Typical uses: Coughs, bacterial infections
Preparations: Tinctures, salves
Contraindications: None known
Of interest: If you're going to wildcraft usnea, learn from a botanist how to identify it, since a similar lichen, *Letharia vulpina,* is toxic. Usnea is one of the few herbs for children that does not extract well into glycerine.

Kids' taste rating: Fine

UVA-URSI

Also known as: Bearberry, kinnikinnick
Latin binomial: *Arctostaphylos uva-ursi*
Part used: Leaves
Main actions: Urinary antiseptic, astringent
Typical uses: Internally: minor bladder inflammations. Externally: itchy or inflamed skin.
Preparations Tea, capsules, tinctures
Contraindications: Not for use during pregnancy, kidney disease
Of interest: A strong infusion of uva-ursi can be used on a tissue-tightening compress for a new mother's post-delivery hemorrhoids. It has also been used as a tonic astringent for bedwetters.

Kids' taste rating: Fair

VALERIAN

Also known as: Garden heliotrope
Latin binomial: *Valeriana officinalis, V. dioica, Valeriana* spp.
Parts used: Root
Main actions: Sedative, antispasmodic
Typical uses: Insomnia, anxiety, hyperactivity
Preparations: Glycerite, tincture, tea, capsules
Contraindications: Some experts caution against use during pregnancy
Of interest: For about 5 percent of the population, valerian sometimes has a slightly stimulating effect.

Kids' taste rating: "Ick—smells like dirty socks!"

VERVAIN

Also known as: Blue vervain, verbena
Latin binomial: *Verbena hastata, Verbena* spp.
Parts used: Stems, leaves, flowers
Main actions: Nervine, sweat-promoting, bitter, diuretic
Typical uses: Hyperactivity, minor fevers, pain relief during ear infections
Preparations: Tea, extracts, capsules
Contraindications: Not for use during pregnancy.
Of interest: This safe, calming herb is not often used in kids due to its bitter taste. Not to be confused with lemon verbena (*Aloysia triphylla*).

Kids' taste rating: Very bitter

VIOLA

Also known as: Johnny-jump-up, pansy, heartsease
Latin binomial: *Viola tricolor*
Parts used: Flowers, leaves
Main actions: Analgesic, demulcent

Typical uses: Internally for stomachaches, scratchy throat; internally and externally for skin inflammations including cradle cap.

Preparations: tea, topical oil

Contraindications: None known

Of interest: The first flower that blooms in Sunny's Montana garden, this cheery little plant reproduces prolifically. The edible flowers also make great decorations for salads and cakes.

Kids' taste rating: Delicious

WILD YAM

Latin binomial: *Dioscorea villosa*

Parts used: Rhizome

Main actions: Antispasmodic, anti-inflammatory

Typical uses: Minor muscle spasms that come with tension headaches; intestinal gas pains

Preparations: Tea, tinctures, capsules

Contraindications: Inappropriate for use in some hormonal disorders. Many herbalists caution against using wild yam during pregnancy. Limit use with children to one week.

Of interest: Chemicals in wild yam gave drug researchers their start on creating birth-control pills. The root is rough on electric coffee grinders; Sunny has broken two with this plant! You can buy it in powdered form or in white cakes of powder from Chinese herb stores.

Kids' taste rating: Not great

WILLOW

Also known as: White willow

Latin binomial: *Salix alba, Salix* spp.

Part used: Bark

Main actions: Analgesic, anti-inflammatory, fever-reducing

Typical uses: Headaches, pain relief

Preparations: Capsules, tablets

Contraindications: Not for use during viral infections

Of interest: Contains naturally occurring salicylates, the compound from which aspirin is derived. Life-threatening Reye's syndrome is associated with the use of aspirin during viral infections, so many natural health-care practitioners advise parents to avoid giving their children willow during viral infections. However, no documented cases associating Reye's syndrome with the use of willow have been reported.

Kids' taste rating: Very bitter

YARROW

Latin binomial: *Achillea millefolium*

Parts used: Flowers, leaves

Main actions: Anti-inflammatory, promotes sweating, stops minor bleeding

Typical uses: Internally: fever, colds, and flu. Externally: baths for inflamed skin conditions such as chicken pox, poison ivy and/or oak

Preparations: Internally: capsules, extracts. Externally: in baths.

Contraindications: Pregnancy, daisy-family (*Asteraceae*) allergies

Of interest: Named for Achilles, the Greek warrior who traveled days to gather yarrow. He used this plant to slow the flow of his wounded soldiers' blood.

Kids' taste rating: Bitter

Chapter 4

KEEPING KIDS HEALTHY

In many ways, our grandparents knew best. The keys to keeping children healthy are a good diet, a clean environment, exercise, ample sleep, and a strong immune system. Although these things sound simple, sometimes they're difficult to follow. We'd like to pass along our basic techniques for keeping our children strong and healthy. None of them is original; in fact, you may find some of your own grandmother's wisdom here.

If possible, breastfeed your babies for at least the first six months. A newborn's immature immune system is vulnerable to infections. Breast milk helps this system by providing antibodies, white blood cells, and other immune chemicals. Nursing particularly protects your baby from respiratory and gastrointestinal infections.

Breastfeeding for longer than six months decreases your baby's risk of allergies later in life, possibly because sensitization to the cow's milk in formulas may trigger sensitization to other substances. Such allergies and intolerances can contribute to problems such as asthma, eczema, and recurrent middle-ear and sinus infections.

In terms of when to start feeding babies solid foods—cereal grains and cooked, pureed fruits and vegetables—the American Academy of Pediatrics says to begin feeding these foods at about four months for bottle-fed babies, six months for breast-fed babies. Introduce only one food at a time. Before trying the next food, wait at least three days and watch for signs of intolerance (cramps, gas, diarrhea, constipation, skin rash). Foods to save until after the age of twelve months include those that commonly cause food allergies: cow's milk, eggs, nuts, peanuts, strawberries, chocolate, tomatoes, and shellfish. Check with your health practitioner for more detailed guidelines for your infant's diet.

Make sure the whole family eats well. Base meals on whole foods, including vegetables (especially the green leafies), grains, and fruits. Start getting your infant used to more exotic grains and vegetables from about twelve months onward, as soon as he's eating a variety of foods and before he closes his mind to experimentation. Infants and toddlers aren't as picky about their food as preschoolers.

Whenever possible, buy produce and meats that are free of pesticides and antibiotics, and look for the phrase "Certified Organic" to assure purity. Avoid junk foods; their high sugar content can reduce the ability of your child's white blood cells to digest and destroy bacteria. That means greater chance of infection and lower resistance to illness.

PROTEIN AND FAT: WHAT'S ENOUGH, WHAT'S TOO MUCH?

Parents often worry about their children getting enough protein, specifically animal protein. Proteins are essential for normal growth. Kids' requirements are relatively high. But because Americans tend to have plenty of food available, kids rarely become deficient in protein. Childhood obesity is a much greater risk, and the animal proteins that are easiest to obtain and prepare are often high in cholesterol and saturated fats. Below is a chart of daily protein-intake recommendations for children.

Compared to children in many other countries, American kids have higher intakes of saturated fats and cholesterol and higher blood-cholesterol levels. Autopsy studies of young people killed in accidents show that atherosclerosis begins in childhood and adolescence. The American Academy of Pediatrics recommends no restrictions on fat and cholesterol for infants under the age of two years. For kids between the ages of three and eighteen years, however, the Academy recommends maintaining total fat intake between 20 and 30 percent of total calories and keeping saturated fat below 10 percent of total calories. Bridling fat intake is one way to reduce the chances of obesity, another risk factor for heart disease and other chronic illnesses.

AGE	GRAMS OF PROTEIN PER DAY
0–6 months	13*
6–12 months	14
1–3 years	16
4–6 years	24
7–10 years	28
11–14 years, males	45
11–14 years, females	46
15–18 years, males	59
15–18 years, females	44

* Infants get all the protein (and other essential nutrients) they need from breast milk. Commercial formulas closely match breast milk's protein amounts.

TWO NUTRIENTS TO WATCH: VITAMIN A, CALCIUM

We understand: Just when you think you're making sure your child gets the right amount of vitamins, minerals, and other goodies, along comes some news story about a supplement you've never heard of. We'd like to focus instead on two old favorites: Vitamin A and calcium—plus calcium's partner, magnesium.

Vitamin A and its carotene constituents are essential for growth and development, eyesight, immune function, and maintenance of healthy skin and mucous membranes. Carotenes include beta-carotene, lutein, and lycopene. The body converts some of these compounds, particularly beta-carotene, to vitamin A.

Carotenes are also good antioxidants and play a protective role against cancer and atherosclerosis. Vitamin A aids in fighting infections, particularly viral infections. Carotenes are not associated with toxicity from overdose, but vitamin A can be toxic in large doses.

Vitamin A is found mostly in animal products, including butter, whole milk, fortified reduced-fat milk, liver, and kidneys. Carotenes are present in some animal foods (salmon, egg yolks, milk, poultry), but mostly in plants, either dark green, leafy ones (dandelion root and leaves, parsley, collard greens, nettle leaves, kale, spinach, mustard greens, broccoli, alfalfa) or those colored yellow, orange, or red (carrots, sweet potatoes, mangoes, orange squash, cantaloupe, apricots, tomatoes, sweet peppers, pink grapefruit, and guava). While cooking destroys vitamin C, carotene-containing foods must be well-cooked, pureed, or chewed thoroughly to release the goodies. Also, you need to eat these foods with a little fat (olive oil does nicely) to ensure proper absorption.

Calcium got more headlines in stories about older people than in those about children until researchers realized that it's during prime bone-building years that calcium intake is most crucial. If you have a health practitioner worth her salt, she will quiz you about your child's calcium intake. Peak bone

HOW MUCH CALCIUM DOES YOUR CHILD NEED?

AGE	RECOMMENDED DAILY INTAKE
Under six months	400 mg. Infants this age should be on a diet of breast milk or formula rich in calcium.
6–12 months	600 mg
1–5 years	800 mg
6–10 years	800–1200 mg
11–24 years	1200–1500 mg

mass during childhood and adolescence predicts the risk of osteoporosis. Girls achieve about 90 percent of their total bone mass by the age of 17. Calcium also plays a part in regulating blood pressure, muscle growth, muscle contraction, and nerve transmission.

One study of premenopausal women found that high current intake of calcium had no significant impact on bone mass, but that high intake during childhood had a positive effect on bone mass. In other words, if your daughter makes strong bones now, she lowers her risk for osteoporosis in old age. Likewise, your son will lower his chances of bone fragility and fractures as an old man. Plus, it always makes sense to eat well for good health now.

You can also support your child's calcium intake by avoiding the following calcium stealers: carbonated beverages, excess protein, refined sugar, and caffeine.

What about magnesium? Also important for bone formation and maintenance, magnesium works hand-in-hand with calcium. The data on children's requirements are scarce. A study on calcium and magnesium balance in nine- to fourteen-year-old children found two things: 1) higher calcium intakes (about 1,350 mg/d) benefited children during puberty, but not before; and 2) the RDA for magnesium was not enough to meet the needs of all children.

The general rule of thumb is to make sure your child receives half as much magnesium as calcium each day. Some researchers suggest that children receive 3 to 6 mg of magnesium per pound of body weight per day. For example, a 50-pound child will need between 150 to 300 mg of magnesium daily. Start with the lower dose, because magnesium sometimes acts as a laxative.

HOW MUCH MAGNESIUM DOES YOUR CHILD NEED?

AGE	RECOMMENDED DAILY ALLOWANCE OF MAGNESIUM IN MG
0–6 months	40
7–12 months	60
1–3 years	80
4–6 years	120
7–10 years	170
11–14 years, males	270
11–14 years, females	280
15–18 years, males	400
15–18 years, females	300

CALCIUM-RICH FOODS

Many experts recommend that you and your child get your daily calcium from foods rather than supplements. Usually three or four servings of calcium-rich foods will do it. Here are some possibilities.

FOOD	CALCIUM (MG PER 3-OUNCE SERVING)
Kelp*	1,093
Cheddar cheese	750
Kale, collard, turnip greens	250
Almonds*	234
Dandelion leaves*	187
Brazil nuts	186
Goat's milk and buttermilk	121
Sesame seeds	110
Sunflower seeds	120
Goat's milk	129
Cottage cheese	94
Oysters, molasses,* brewer's yeast*	210
Yogurt, tofu*	128
Calcium-fortified orange juice	112

	CALCIUM (MG PER CUP)
Nonfat yogurt	450
Calcium-enriched rice and soy milk	300
Whole milk	295
Cottage cheese	125

(* also a magnesium source)

Fortified rice or soy milks are generally lower in fat than cow's' milk and may not provide sufficient calories for a child under two.

Find quality child care. Kids in day care have an increased exposure to infections and consequently a higher rate of illnesses such as colds, coughs, sore throats, middle-ear infections, and diarrhea. Minimizing the number of children to whom your child is exposed can help. Try for day care that has a maximum of six to ten children per room. One study found that children in day care centers had an increased risk of diarrhea, but that children in smaller "family-style" day care, with fewer children enrolled, did not.

Keep cigarette smoke away from your child. In the United States, cigarette smoking ranks as the number-one preventable cause of death. Passive smoke (breathing the smoke from someone else's cigarette) is the third leading cause of preventable death and a major preventable cause of children's illness. Parental smoking rings up $4.6 billion per year in children's medical expenses.

Every year, smoking contributes to low birth weight, sudden infant death syndrome, viral bronchiolitis, acute middle-ear infections, asthma, and fire-related injuries. A recent study found that a mother who smokes nearly quadruples her child's risk for infection with *Neisseria meningitidis,* a bacteria that can cause blood infection and meningitis. Both smoking and passive smoking also cause hardening of the arteries.

Enough statistics. All you really need to know is that cigarette smoke has a huge effect on your child's health—a negative effect.

Keep your home and surroundings toxin free. Avoid using pesticides. Whenever possible, find alternatives friendlier to human and general environmental health. Keep paints and varnishes tightly sealed and far from reach. Store harsh cleansers out of harm's way, or better yet, use old-fashioned vinegar, baking soda, and citrus instead. If you live in an area where the ground is known to contain radon, an odorless, colorless gas that causes lung cancer, you may want to call your state health department to find out about testing. In addition, shop for unscented, biodegradable detergents and cleansers. Environmental illness and chemical sensitivities are on the rise, and many seem related to exposure to synthetic, petrochemical-based house products, paints, and varnishes.

Protect your child's skin from sunburn. Whether sun exposure is beneficial or harmful depends upon the amount, the time of day, the season, and the altitude at which you live. Small doses of sunlight—in the range of fifteen to thirty minutes a day—improve well-being, stimulate the body's production of vitamin D, and regulate certain hormones. Larger amounts can cause painful sunburn and lead to premature aging and skin cancer. For a few years, many of us thought liberal use of sunscreens was the answer.

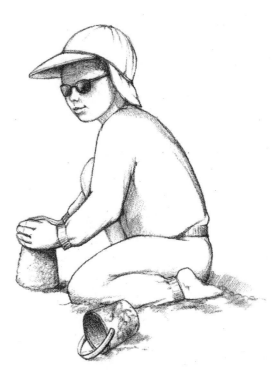

A savvy sandcastle architect covers up to prevent sunburn.

Recently, however, research has linked sunscreen use with an increase in skin cancers such as melanoma. Sunscreens don't completely block the cancer-causing effects of sunlight, and perhaps they encourage people to stay outside longer than they otherwise would.

What's a parent to do? Certainly not keep the kids indoors all day. They can't make proper mud pies or ride bikes in the house. And at some point you'd all go insane. Instead, try to schedule outdoor time for mornings or late afternoons, making midday a time for indoor projects.

Infants, especially those under six months, should be kept out of bright sunlight because they have thinner, less pigmented skin. Also, many sunscreen ingredients can irritate babies' skin. Although some UV waves will pass through fabric, it's still wise to cover babies' bodies with clothing and their wee heads with wee bonnets. Find a stroller with a good hood or rig one out of baby blankets.

Older children can follow your example, so cover up with hats, sunglasses, long sleeves, and pants. Most T-shirt fabric has an SPF of about 10. We're believers in sunscreen and sun-protecting lip balm that blocks both UVA and UVB wavelengths. Experts recommend that fair-skinned kids use a product with an SPF of 30 or greater.

Worried about your kids getting enough vitamin D? Though sunscreens do block the sun enough to prevent this key vitamin's formation, a mere ten to fifteen minutes of unprotected exposure a day produces all the vitamin D that a body needs. Our eyes absorb sunlight, and we suspect that enough UV sneaks in through clothing and in areas where sunscreen wasn't applied or has been washed off to make this a non-issue. We also think the risk of skin cancer down the line far outweighs the risk of children becoming deficient in vitamin D.

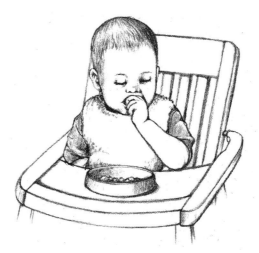

Introduce your child to a wide range of grains and vegetables from one year onward, before the dreaded "picky eater" phase.

Teach your child good hygiene skills. Here, we're talking mostly about washing hands before eating, after going to the bathroom, after sneezing into their hands, or blowing their noses. It's also nice if children don't cough in people's faces and know how to use (and dispose of) tissues for drippy noses.

Get up and move. You can set a good example for your child by demonstrating that exercise has a place in your daily routine. We're not suggesting that you encourage your small child to jog or lift weights; excessive exercise can injure a developing musculoskeletal system. Gentler activities that better suit small children include working alongside you in the garden, tossing a ball, dancing, playing tag or hopscotch, splashing with you in the pool, and walking. Walks sometimes work best if you have a mission that piques your child's interest—hunting for rocks, watching birds, counting crickets. Once they reach first or second grade, many kids start to enjoy bicycling, skiing, swimming, hiking, and team sports such as soccer, baseball, and basketball. The possibilities are endless.

Make sure your child gets enough rest and reduce stress. We know that this is easier said than done, especially with the hectic lives that parents of young children lead. Try to avoid over-scheduling. This requires that you learn to say no to things; try standing before the mirror and practicing. If "no" seems too harsh, try saying, "Sorry, but that doesn't work for me." Offer no explanations; a polite person won't ask for them. If your child is in school, try to leave some afternoons free of lessons or other organized activities.

You know how much sleep your child needs. Stand firm about lights out. We also hold sacred the last half-hour of the day for reading, talking, and snuggling. It's a nice way to end the day, to smooth any rough edges or arguments that occurred earlier.

Give your child lots of TLC. Slow down and hold your children as if they are the most precious gifts you have ever received. Ashley

---

IMMUNE-BOOSTING SOUP

For ages: 2 years and up
Yields: 6–8 servings

During the winter illness season, you can use this basic recipe as an immune-building base. Experiment. See what's in your pantry. Add foods your children like. We find our kids will consume more soup if we add whole wheat pasta or nuts to it.

1 large onion, chopped
     (antibacterial, antiviral)

3 cloves garlic, minced
     (antibacterial, antiviral

2 tablespoons olive oil

4 or 5 astragalus sticks
     (immune stimulant, antiviral)

1 cup celery, chopped
     (fiber and vitamin source)

1 cup green beans, chopped
     (fiber and vitamin source)

2 cups carrots or other
   root vegetables, chopped
     (rehydrating, potassium source)

2 large potatoes, chopped
     (potassium source)

4 dried or 2 fresh shiitake mushrooms
     (immune stimulant)

Basil, parsley, tarragon, or
   other culinary herbs to taste
     (antibacterial)

1 pound tofu, cut into small cubes
     (protein source)

1 to 2 tablespoons white miso
     (alkaline, rehydrating)

1 cup whole wheat pasta
     (fiber source)

8 cups water

Sauté onion and garlic in oil in a large stockpot until softened. Add water and bring to a boil. Add vegetables and astragalus. Simmer, covered, 30 minutes. Add tofu and simmer an additional 20 minutes; add herbs and pasta and simmer 10 more minutes. Remove from heat. Remove astragalus sticks and stir in miso to taste. Depending on your child's tolerance for spiciness, you may want to add hot pepper sauce, fresh ground pepper, or additional fresh garlic.

Montague, Ph.D. writes in his book, *Touching,* "Affectionate tactile stimulation is clearly, then, a primary need, a need which must be satisfied if the infant is to develop as a healthy human being." Certainly this holds true for all ages of childhood and adulthood, too.

Show your child your spiritual side. In his book, *Words of Wisdom,* Larry Dossey, M.D., tells how prayer has affected his medical practice. He discusses study after study that shows prayer helps heal. We are not suggesting that you pray to any particular deity, nor that you do anything that rubs against your spiritual grain. You will demonstrate your attitudes by the way you interact with fellow humans, animals, plants, and the environment at large.

Nurture intimate connections. The more contact you and your children have with friends and family, the healthier you'll be—mentally, spiritually, and physically. Studies have shown that people with fragile social webs fall ill more easily than those who love bountifully.

Pay attention to your life and that of your child. In a way, we're back to spirituality again, or one aspect of it. One way to express your love and augment your child's *joie de vivre* is to live as much as possible in the present moment. If you're an adult, this is harder than it sounds, especially if you tend to engage the world in high gear; we, too, often succumb to this sort of mania. But children need parents to listen to them, to take in their world with all possible senses, to really *be* with them.

Start small. See if you can attend to your child completely for fifteen-minute intervals. This means you watch your child's hands sculpt the bird, smell the clay, hear talk about how this bird will sing lullabies, taste the grape she feeds you. While this is happening, try to set aside thoughts about the phone call you needed to return, the pile of laundry on the floor, the uncooked dinner. These things can wait, for a little while anyway. Your child will not. He will grow up, whether or not you pay attention. If you let him, your child can teach you to live more in the moment.

Recommended Reading

Garth, M. *Starbright: Meditations for Children.* New York: Harper Collins, 1991.

Mendell, E. *Parents' Nutrition Bible.* Carson, CA: Hay House, 1992.

Murray, M. *Encyclopedia of Nutritional Supplements.* Rocklin, CA: Prima, 1996.

Tamborlane, W. V. *The Yale Guide to Children's Nutrition.* New Haven, CT: Yale University Press, 1997.

Chapter 5

FIRST AID

Living is sometimes a hazardous enterprise. Everything that benefits our kids—every tool, toy, appliance, medicine, means of locomotion—carries certain risks. It's almost as if some higher power said, "Sure, go ahead, invent scissors. They'll make cutting easier. But look out—those sharp edges could also slice off a fingertip, and those pointy tips could poke out an eye."

So what do we do? Never let our children use scissors? Have them chew the construction paper instead? Avoid art projects and the fun they bring kids?

Of course not. We teach children about safety and take reasonable precautions instead of worrying a lot and trying to enforce all kinds of limitations. However, parents must be prepared for the inevitable accident, and part of that preparation is learning first aid. When the whirlwind of a crisis descends, consulting a book will be the last thing on your mind—if you can even find the book. Better to learn basic first aid before your family needs it. When you know what to do in a crisis, you can stay calm, reassure your child, and take action to help him.

Children can learn to take care of themselves, friends, and siblings, too, if they are taught. In the average household, enough owies and boo-boos occur to provide good training. In Linda's home, when one of the children accidentally injures another, Linda comforts the hurt child while instructing the other on the care of the wound. As a result, her kids know all about cleaning wounds and applying ice packs, salves, and bandages. And there's less yelling.

Everyone in the family should know where the household first-aid kit is kept, what it contains, and how to use the supplies. Babysitters, grandparents, and anyone else who visits often should know, too. We think it's also wise to keep a full kit in the car, and smaller ones in your purse, backpack, and bike pack. You can make your own herbal first-aid kit (see next page) or purchase one and add herbal remedies to it.

Near each telephone in your house, post emergency phone numbers. In most areas of the United States, dialing 911 will put you in touch with a dispatcher who will send emergency medical help without further calls. Children as young as three years can learn to dial 911, just as they can learn their name, address, and phone number. Practice dialing with your child (with your finger on the receiver button to prevent a real call) and rehearse the information your child is likely to be asked.

Also post the numbers for your doctor, the poison control center, neighbors, and immediate family members near the phone. Finally, add your

BASIC HERBAL FIRST-AID KIT

☐ Adhesive bandage strips

☐ Sterile gauze pads (4" x 4")

☐ Roller gauze

☐ Adhesive tape

☐ Sterile cotton balls

☐ Cotton swabs

☐ Sterile eye patches

☐ Antiseptic wipes or solution

☐ Antibiotic ointment

☐ Packet of tissues

☐ Elastic (ACE) bandage for sprains

☐ Soap

☐ Syrup of ipecac (keep out of reach of small children)

☐ Index card with pediatrician's phone numbers, insurance numbers

☐ Tweezers

☐ Blunt scissors

☐ Triangular cloth to use as a sling and a big safety pin to hold it in place

☐ Flashlight with fresh batteries

☐ Change for pay phone

☐ Index card reminding you how to use remedies

☐ Black tea bags

☐ Saline eye drops

☐ Echinacea extract or glycerite

☐ Echinacea salve

☐ Oregon graperoot extract

☐ Ginger extract or crystallized ginger chunks

☐ Valerian extract

☐ Peppermint essential oil inhaler or lozenges

☐ Lavender essential oil or aloe vera gel

☐ Comfrey/calendula salve

☐ Rescue Remedy flower essence

own address and phone number. If your babysitter must make an emergency call, she may need this information, especially if she knows your house so well that she only remembers it as "the blue one on the corner."

Skin Injuries

Scratches and Scrapes

Skinned knees and scraped elbows seem to accompany children everywhere. For such injuries, a good washing with lots of tepid water and mild soap usually is the only first aid needed. Skin cleansers containing grapefruit-seed extract have broad antimicrobial activity against bacteria such as strep, staph, and tetanus. Dishwashing detergent works well, too, because it cuts the grease that may be contained in minor road rash from cycling mishaps or other falls.

If the wound contains debris such as tiny stones or bits of grass, try gently removing them with a clean, damp washcloth, sterile gauze, or tweezers. Some children become very upset if anyone tries to touch the wound. Sometimes it helps to tell the child that leaving the wound alone will cause infection, more pain, scars, and, in the case of falls on asphalt, permanent gritty tattoos.

Some children would rather remove the debris themselves and can do so successfully; others will give it a try and then let the parent finish the job. If your child seems old enough to try cleaning the wound, there's no harm in giving her a chance. Preschoolers and up can participate if willing. If neither parent nor child can remove the debris, it's time to call the doctor, who can administer local anesthesia and clean the injury thoroughly without causing further pain or injury.

NATURAL REMEDIES FOR SPLINTERS

To draw out a splinter, try placing honey or sticky pine resin over it, cover with a bandage, and wait from one hour to two days. You may be surprised how quickly these ingredients work to pull splinters out.

The pine-resin technique comes in particularly handy if you're out in the wilds without your first-aid kit. Just find a pine tree and scrape up some of the sticky stuff that oozes from various spots on the trunk. Alcohol—rubbing alcohol, drinking alcohol, or a tincture—will remove the sticky resin once the splinter's out.

Here's another way to draw splinters out if you're not out in the wilds, but at home. Cut a slice of raw potato or steam a cabbage leaf until it's limp, and apply a small section to the splinter area, bandaging it in place if necessary. Before bedtime, replace this with a another piece, bandage, and leave on overnight. By morning, the splinter probably will be gone.

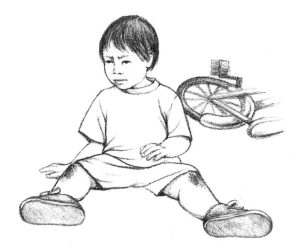

Scrapes and road rash on knees and elbows can benefit from herbal salves that help keep scabs soft.

Minor scrapes usually don't require commercial antibiotic ointments to prevent infections. Salves help keep the wound moist, however, which improves healing. If infection is a concern, you can apply echinacea tincture or glycerite to the injured skin. When wounds on the knees or elbows scab over, herbal ointment and salves can keep the scabs soft so they don't break open and bleed when the child bends the joint. The herbs in them can also speed healing and prevent infection.

Wounds generally heal faster when left open to the air, so don't cover them with a bandage unless your child is headed to school or plans to excavate the backyard. In those cases, taping on a gauze dressing will keep out some of the dirt and keep in the salves.

Cuts

First cover the wound with sterile gauze or clean cloth and apply direct, steady pressure until the bleeding stops. If the dressing soaks through, place a fresh one on top of the bloody one—rather than removing it—and keep pressing. Once the bleeding has stopped or slowed to an ooze, wash the cut with plenty of clean water and mild soap. If you have povidone-iodine, a skin cleanser widely used in hospitals, dilute it one part to ten with warm tap water before applying.

For small cuts, stop the bleeding with styptic herbs applied directly to the wound. Powdered yarrow leaf or flower, rose petals, horsetail, bistort root, and wild geranium root stanch minor bleeding when applied directly to the wound. Use the powder dry or mix with a little water to form a paste. Cayenne powder from your spice shelf can stop bleeding, too, and it hardly stings when applied to a minor wound.

Some parents swear by hydrogen peroxide to clean cuts, but it is only weakly antimicrobial and can interfere with blood-clot formation. Herbal tinctures, which contain alcohol, sting briefly when

WHEN TO CALL A DOCTOR ABOUT A CUT

Ten to fifteen minutes of steady pressure against the wound doesn't stop the bleeding

The edges of the cut are ragged, or the laceration exceeds 1/2 inch and tends to separate when the child moves

The cut goes all the way through the skin to the fat layer or deeper

The wound crosses a joint

The face, hands, or feet are damaged; a hand surgeon or plastic surgeon may be needed

A foreign body remains in the wound

Infection occurs, as indicated by redness, heat, swelling, yellow drainage, and/or foul smell

applied to open wounds, and straight rubbing alcohol can actually damage tissue. Use tinctures to disinfect wounds only if nothing else is available. Although glycerites made with antimicrobial herbs don't sting, they're somewhat messy to use.

Puncture Wounds

When a sharp, narrow object such as a nail or a big splinter punctures the skin, infection becomes a concern. Bacteria penetrate the skin along with the object, and because such wounds don't bleed much, the body can't flush out the microbes. Such wounds tend to heal quickly, too, sometimes sealing in the infection. And in this oxygen-free environment, the tetanus bacteria can come alive.

Tetanus bacteria are everywhere: in soil, air, animal feces, and on skin; the spores can live for hundreds of years in soil, resisting heat, cold, and drought. In living flesh, they may remain dormant for months, resisting antiseptics and other treatment. They cannot grow in the presence of oxygen, but given an airless wound, tetanus spores can become active, multiply, and produce a toxin that interferes with nerve function, leading to muscle spasms, pain, seizures and sometimes difficulty breathing. The most common symptom is a stiff jaw—"lockjaw"—caused by muscle spasms. Sorry to scare you, but tetanus infection can be fatal.

To reduce the risk of infection with tetanus or less worrisome microbes, wash the puncture wound thoroughly, and remove any debris from the wound. Then soak the area for fifteen minutes in water as hot as your child can stand. If it helps your child, soak the wound for five minutes in hot water and one minute in cold water; repeat three times. This technique also stimulates circulation of immune cells to the area. If desired, add diluted povidone iodine or diluted grapefruit-seed extract to the warm water. For the first day, bandage the wound to protect it from dirt.

Note: In the case of puncture wounds, don't apply herbs that hasten wound closure, such as comfrey, plantain, or aloe. Rapid closure seals in microbes that cause infection. Instead, chose herbs with antimicrobial properties until the wound seals itself, and then use cell-repairing herbs to help the scar heal.

A Word About Tetanus Shots

Although dirty wounds and punctures are the most typical sites for tetanus infection, even minor scratches or burns can allow tetanus bacteria to enter the body. Consequently, many doctors recommend getting a tetanus booster after skin trauma if ten years or more have elapsed since the last tetanus vaccination (or, in the case of dirty cuts, if five years have elapsed). If a child has never been immunized and has a dirty wound, the doctor may also recommend a shot of tetanus antibodies, which provide immediate protection against the microbe.

If your child has a puncture wound or a burn that exposes her to a potential tetanus situation, we suggest you take her to a doctor for a vaccination, regardless of your opinion about other immunizations. Risks from tetanus vaccinations are minor, and risks from actually getting tetanus are huge. Keep a record at home of your child's vaccinations so that he doesn't get more shots than necessary.

Are there herbs that kill tetanus bacteria? Maybe, but we wouldn't bet our children's lives on it.

WHEN TO CALL A DOCTOR ABOUT A PUNCTURE WOUND

The head, chest, or abdomen is punctured

The puncture seems to penetrate a joint

The object that caused the injury was dirty or rusty, went through the shoe, or remains lodged in the wound

Debris remains in the wound

The wound is ragged, with skin flaps

Your child isn't up to date on tetanus shots

Signs of infection develop: redness, warmth, swelling, pus, increased pain, or foul smell. Red stripes on the skin that radiate from the injury may indicate a serious infection.

As Healing Progresses

Herbal poultices or compresses can promote the healing of skin wounds. They're simple to make, effective to use, and the ingredients are easy to find.

Plantain. During the spring and summer, fresh plantain leaves serve well as a backyard bandage; this so-called weed grows nearly everywhere.

Sunny has used plantain for years to help heal scratches and owies. Scientific research backs up plantain's traditional use, showing that it contains antimicrobial and anti-inflammatory chemicals. It also contains allantoin, a substance that helps "knit" cells back together.

Learn to identify plantain correctly, and look for it around your yard. To use plantain as a poultice, grab a couple of fresh leaves whenever your child has a minor scratch. Wash the leaves, mash them into a moist blob with a grinder or mortar and pestle, apply to the injury, and cover with an adhesive bandage.

Aloe vera gel penetrates injured tissues to reduce pain and inflammation and enhance the healing of burns and wounds. Studies have shown it hastens wound healing. Besides containing allantoin, aloe is rich in salicylic acid, a "natural aspirin" that reduces pain, fever, and inflammation. To use the herb fresh, slice a leaf lengthwise and scrape out the gooey inner gel and apply it to the skin. Commercial preparations are equally effective if they contain pure aloe vera gel and little or nothing else.

Calendula, commonly known as pot marigold, is anti-inflammatory, astringent, antiseptic, cooling, and inhibits bleeding. It also stimulates new skin growth. Use this herb fresh or dried by making a tea from the flowers. Prepare a compress by dunking a clean cloth into the warm tea. Wring it out, and place the cloth over the wound. Even the most sensitive skin usually tolerates this gentle yet powerful healing herb.

Comfrey. This herb, which also contains allantoin, makes a good fresh poultice for skin wounds that are beginning to heal. Bruise the fresh leaves and tape them over the wound or wrap wet comfrey leaves in a warm, moist bandanna and bandage the cut with it. Comfrey powder or salve can be can be applied to wounds to encourage healing. When the skin has started to heal, apply comfrey salve daily.

Caution: Rare cases of liver toxicity are associated with taking comfrey by mouth, so we advise you to use it externally only.

Cayenne. Well known for reducing pain, cayenne helps wounds heal. In comparison to common over-the-counter and prescription antibiotic creams and aloe vera gel, cayenne produces the fastest rate of skin regrowth. Look for commercial creams containing cayenne's most active analgesic compound, capsaicin.

Vitamin E oil. If you want to apply vitamin E oil to prevent scarring, wait until the wound has healed, because the oil can interfere with scab formation. Then pop a vitamin E capsule open with a pin, apply a few drops to the wound two or three times a day, and cover with an adhesive bandage. Apply the oil for up to two months.

If Infection Threatens

Tea tree oil destroys a wide range of infectious microbes. It's particularly useful for treating or preventing fungal and bacterial skin infections. Use twice a day. Tea tree oil can generally be used undiluted, but try a test patch for about an hour and watch for irritation. Discontinue use if your child's skin becomes sore or inflamed. According to case reports, some people develop skin rashes with tea tree oil use. If this happens, stop using it.

Thyme. This herb's volatile oils can destroy bacteria, and some viruses, fungi, and parasites. We make a thyme tea and wash the affected area with it twice a day. The essential oil is very potent, so we don't recommend you use it undiluted; the tea is quite strong enough. If you like thyme essential oil, however, place one or two drops in a tablespoon of carrier oil.

Echinacea fights infection when taken internally and applied externally. Taken by mouth, it stimulates the body's immune system against infection. Applied to the skin, it helps wounds and burns heal more quickly. Almost any form of echinacea will do—tincture, powder, or tea.

Burns

Burns can result from exposure to the sun, fire, hot substances, electricity, radiation, friction (as in rug burns), and chemicals. During fires and explosions, inhaling hot air, smoke, or toxic fumes can damage the respiratory tract.

Regardless of the cause of the burn, skin damage is measured by degrees. In first-degree burns, the skin is red and painful. Blistering characterizes second-degree burns. Third-degree burns destroy nerves and tissue; therefore, they're painless. The skin appears white or charred.

If your child receives a first- or second-degree burn from a heat source, immediately immerse the injured area in cold water or apply a cold compress. Continue for ten minutes or until the pain stops. Don't put straight ice directly on the skin. If your child has burned her mouth, she can suck on ice cubes to relieve her pain.

Exposure to lye, acids, drain cleaners, and other chemicals can cause burns. Treat such burns immediately by removing chemical-splashed clothing and rinsing the skin with lots of cool water, preferably in the shower. Then identify the chemical and call poison control or 911.

Do not break the blisters of a second-degree burn or apply ointments or butter. Instead, keep the burned area clean by gently washing it twice a day with water and mild soap. The blisters will eventually break and drain on their own, usually after several days. At this point, parents can carefully trim away the dead skin.

If your child receives a third-degree burn, call 911 or an alternate number for emergency medical services. While awaiting help, elevate burned extremities to prevent swelling, and cut away clothing unless it has adhered to the burn. Loosely cover the wound with sterile gauze or clean cloths such as linen or muslin. Do not put anything else on the burn, and do not immerse the wound in water.

Natural Remedies for Minor Burns

For minor burns, our favorite remedies are lavender essential oil and aloe vera gel. Both are

WHEN TO CALL A DOCTOR ABOUT A BURN

Call 911 if:
Your child has a third-degree burn.

Take your child to the emergency room (or call 911 if you can't get him there) if:
The burn, although less severe than a third-degree burn, covers a large area

Electrical shock, explosion, or an extremely hot source caused the burn

See the doctor immediately if:
The burn involves the face, eyes, respiratory passages, hands, feet, or genitals

Go to the doctor's office if:
Signs of infection develop

time-tested; research has confirmed aloe vera's efficacy. Simply apply lavender essential oil (if your child is an infant or has sensitive skin, dilute by adding one to two drops to one teaspoon of vegetable oil) or commercial aloe vera gel. Or, if you have an aloe plant, break off a spine, split it and apply the gel that oozes out directly to the burn.

Vinegar is a time-tested remedy for sunburn. Apple cider vinegar works just fine, if you don't mind your child smelling like a pickle; distilled vinegar has less scent. We dilute the vinegar half and half with water and apply to the burn as often as the child allows; keep away from the eyes to avoid stinging. Some children will cheerfully apply the mix themselves if given a spray bottle.

Tea, both green and black, contains tannic acid, which helps cool sunburn. Tea also is rich in antioxidants. Exposure to the sun's ultraviolet rays produces free radicals in the skin, but the antioxidants in tea may mop them up before they damage tissue. To use, brew strong tea and let it cool. Apply to the burn with a compress or in a bath.

As Healing Progresses

Calendula gel is both soothing and anti-inflammatory, and helps relieve minor burns.

Gotu kola extracts, used both internally and externally, help heal burns and decrease scarring. Sunny likes gotu kola for sunburn, especially the fresh leaves.

Witch hazel has long been used in folk medicine to heal wounds and decrease inflammation. Because it possesses antioxidant and astringent properties, it may also help with sunburn. Apply the witch hazel liquid, available at drug stores, with a spray bottle or clean cotton ball.

Bloody Noses

When they don't result from a blow to the face, nosebleeds are typically caused by dry air, nasal irritation from a cold, blowing the nose too hard, nose picking, or a foreign body lodged in the nose.

To stop a nosebleed, pinch the nostrils together tightly for ten minutes. Have your child sit up and lean forward so less blood runs down the back of her throat. Give her a basin in case blood does drain into her mouth, then encourage her to spit it out. If the bleeding continues or if a small object could be lodged in the nose, take your child to the doctor.

Natural Remedies for Bloody Noses

Increasing the moisture available to the nose's delicate membranes helps prevent nosebleeds that occur when the tissues dry, crack, and bleed. One way to accomplish this is to encourage your child to drink more water so the membranes receive more moisture. This is especially important before, during, and after hard exercise, such as a basketball or soccer game, because heavy breathing draws increased air through the nose.

Adding humidity to your child's bedroom, especially in a dry climate or during winter, also helps reduce nosebleeds. Children may also

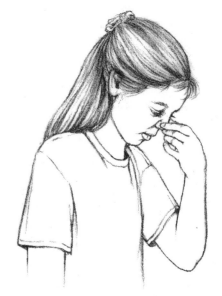

To stop a nosebleed, have your child sit up, lean forward, and pinch nostrils together.

benefit from using nasal saline drops or sprays that both moisten the membranes and break up excess mucus. Although commercial preparations are available, you can easily make a salt solution at home. Dissolve 1/4 teaspoon of salt in one cup of warm water. Many drugstores carry small, empty, plastic squirt bottles designed to hold nasal saline. Make the solution fresh daily.

One of Linda's children is prone to winter nosebleeds. Before bedtime, he applies a product that contains coconut oil, beeswax, and vitamin E to the mucous membrane that covers the septum—the cartilage that runs down the center of the nose—where most bleeding occurs. Comfrey salve will also work.

Dietary Considerations

Sometimes a boost in dietary nutrients can reduce the frequency of nosebleeds. Foods rich in vitamin C and bioflavonoids help strengthen the small-caliber blood vessels involved in nosebleeds. Citrus fruits, rose hips, cantaloupe, apricots, broccoli, buckwheat sprouts, squash, and other yellow/orange foods contain high levels of natural bioflavonoids. The white pulp inside orange peels is an excellent source of vitamin C, although most kids won't eat it. Stinging nettle, a common herb, is rich in vitamin C and carotenes to help strengthen mucous membranes.

If nosebleeds continue even when the child eats a high-C diet, you can try supplementing her meals with commercial preparations of vitamin C and bioflavonoids. Follow the manufacturer's recommendations, but begin each supplement at a low dose and work up gradually. If diarrhea develops, decrease the dose by half.

If all these measures fail to substantially reduce or eliminate nosebleeds, consult your health-care practitioner.

Muscle Cramps, Strains, and Sprains

Cramps

Cramps—painful muscle spasms—occur suddenly. Most muscle cramps that occur during or after exertion are caused by dehydration, so make sure that your child drinks enough water, particularly during hot weather and strenuous activity.

If your child gets a muscle cramp, reassure him that this painful sensation won't last long. When the cramp eases, help him stretch the affected muscle and gently massage the area.

Heat relaxes muscles. Although a hot-water bottle can help, moist heat is best. You can apply a wet towel that is as hot as your child can stand. Or let him soak in a warm bath to ease a cramp. Strengthen the healing powers of the bath by adding teas of sage, calendula, arnica, or mint to the water. We make about two cups of very strong tea from any of these herbs, or a mixture, and pour it into the tub. Serve him mineral-rich herb teas, too, such as dandelion, nettles, or horsetail. Calcium supplements may help.

Strains and Sprains

Muscle strains, or pulled muscles, result from injury or overuse; tenderness, stiffness, and sometimes slight swelling follow. Muscle injuries in small children typically result from blunt trauma, such as when soft tissue collides with pavement. Older children and teens are more likely to develop muscle strains during athletic activities.

Sprains, another sports injury, are more serious. In a sprain, a ligament tears where it joins the bone, near a joint. Rapid swelling, localized pain and tenderness, limited movement of the joint, and sometimes bruising signal a true sprain. Kids get sprains less often than teens and adults do.

Use the RICE method to manage mild sprains and strains at home: Rest, Ice, Compression, and Elevation.

Rest means just that. This sounds easy, unless the patient happens to be a bouncy preschooler. Encourage your child to sit and read with you or listen to music or a story on tape. A normally active young child who stays still or refuses to move may signal an injury serious enough to warrant a trip to the doctor.

Ice. Apply a bag of frozen vegetables (peas conform nicely), a commercial cold pack, or a plastic bag of ice wrapped in a damp cloth to protect the skin. The day of the injury, ice the area three or four times, for twenty to thirty minutes each time. For the next six to ten days, continue ice compresses once or twice a day, more often if needed.

But don't take this guideline on how often to ice as a hard-and-fast rule. Experiment and see what technique works for you and your child, or ask your doctor.

Compression. Wrap the injured limb with an elastic bandage, but only as snugly as, say, a nylon sock. Wrapping a bandage too tight cuts off circulation and increases swelling below the injury. Remove and rewrap the bandage at least twice a day.

Elevation. This requires raising the injured area above the heart. Find an activity your child can do while lying down, then prop the hurt extremity on pillows.

Broken Bones, Dislocations, and Serious Sprains

Kids with broken or fractured bones, dislocated joints, and serious sprains belong in the emergency room. Their injuries require full evaluation and expert treatment.

Young children fracture bones more often than adolescents and adults, in part because their bendable bones tend to buckle or to break only on one side, resulting in "green-stick" fractures. Although kids' fractures heal quickly,

such injuries may damage the growth plate, the band of actively dividing cells at either end of the long bones, preventing the bone from reaching full growth.

While You Await Medical Help

If a bone has pierced the skin, cover the wound with a sterile dressing. If a bone appears misaligned, don't try to straighten it. Do not move the child unless absolutely necessary, especially if you suspect injury to the spine. If you suspect less severe fracture or dislocation, and you know how to do so, splint the injured area before attempting to move the child. (To learn

WHEN TO CALL A DOCTOR ABOUT BONE INJURIES

Call 911 for an ambulance if:

A bone area is deformed

Bone protrudes from a wound

Take your child to see a doctor immediately if:

The child has intense pain, especially over a bone

Bruising and swelling are significant

The arm or leg is numb below the site of the injury

The injured body part won't move normally or bear weight

Call a doctor if:

The injury is moderate

You have doubts about treating it

how to splint bone breaks or move an injured person safely, we recommend taking a first-aid course.)

Supporting Healing with Natural Remedies

Once your child has received medical or surgical treatment for a serious injury, herbal remedies can ease her pain and hasten healing.

Feverfew. While most of the research on feverfew has examined its effects against migraine, Sunny finds it effective in relieving children's pain of any type, including muscle spasms. It tastes bitter, so choose capsules or glycerites. Use three to four times daily, following package dosage instructions.

Kava kava. Studies show that this herb eases pain, inflammation, and cramping. Its traditional use, however, is for calming anxiety and lifting the spirits. All these properties make kava a good remedy for musculoskeletal injuries. See Chapter 21, Sleep, for recommendations on using kava for kids.

Turmeric. Studies have shown that curcumin, the active ingredient in turmeric, relieves inflammation as well as hydrocortisone, but without toxicity. Turmeric is a relative of ginger. For a child of 50 pounds, half a capsule one to three times daily can be helpful. Turmeric is generally considered safe, except for pregnant women.

Protein-digesting enzymes, or proteases, help relieve inflammation by disposing of some byproducts of inflammation and inhibiting the formation of others. One study in adults with injuries such as bruises, muscle strains, and ligament tears found that bromelain decreased swelling, pain, and tenderness. Check your health-food store for bromelain capsules and follow package instructions for children's dosage. Pineapple is rich in bromelain.

Licorice decreases inflammation in a way similar to the body's own corticosteroids. A typical anti-inflammatory serving for a five-year-old child would be one cup of licorice tea twice daily for one week.

Pain-Relieving Herbal Rubs

Children—especially injured kids—need plenty of tender touch. A warm herbal rub promotes relaxation and healing and generally makes a child feel better.

St.-John's-wort oil, a pain reliever and anti-inflammatory, is a good choice for sprained ankles and muscle soreness. It once gave Sunny

---

ST.-JOHN'S-WORT OIL

This recipe is especially designed for cooks who hate to measure.

1 pint jar, clean, with a tight lid
About 1¾ cup extra virgin olive oil
A bunch of fresh St.-John's-wort flowering tops, as much as you can cram in the jar

Directions: "Flowering tops" refers to the top 4 inches of the plants. Cut the stems into 1-inch long pieces; stuff as much of the herb into the jar as possible. Fill the jar with olive oil and cover. Place the jar in a warm, dark place for 2 to 4 weeks, shaking daily. Strain the bright red oil through several layers of tightly woven cloth. Label the oil and store in the refrigerator up to a year.

Caution: This oil is for external use only. Use may cause increased risk of sunburn, so keep affected areas away from sun. Keep out of reach of small children.

almost instant relief from a throbbing, twisted ankle. We also use it as massage oil when our kids have trouble sleeping or growing pains.

Arnica oil. In Germany, physicians prescribe arnica infused oil regularly for bruises, muscle aches, and joint dislocations. It relieves pain and swelling and works against bruises. Use it externally only, and never on open wounds.

Cayenne. When capsaicin, the active ingredient in cayenne, is first applied to the skin, it activates pain nerves, then renders them unresponsive, thus relieving local pain. Studies have found repeated application of ointments or creams containing capsaicin effective in reducing serious pain. If you use a rub containing cayenne, follow the manufacturer's recommendations.

FLOWER ESSENCES FOR TRAUMA

Rescue Remedy is a Bach flower remedy that eases feelings of panic and stress. It's available in liquid extract or ointment forms. Although we can't cite studies or explain how the remedy works, when we give our children about 4 drops under the tongue after a physical or emotional trauma, they calm down right away. We usually take a dose ourselves too.

Linda once sustained a major head bonk while playing a game of tag. Afterward, she felt nauseated, dizzy, and disoriented. A dropperful of Rescue Remedy cleared her head instantly. Her head still hurt, mind you, but she felt able to cope, even ready to laugh about the incident.

Supplements for Healing

The healing of bone injuries increases the body's demand for calcium and magnesium, so give your child foods high in these healing minerals. If he is over two years old, you may want to give him a daily supplement of 800 mg of calcium and 400 mg of magnesium for two weeks. Then decrease the dose to 500 mg of calcium and 250 mg of magnesium for another month.

Finally, you may want to see a chiropractor. Many specialize in treating children's injuries in a gentle, painless way. If your child limps due to a leg injury or has been on crutches, a chiropractic adjustment may help set him straight again. If the back, neck, or pelvis was injured, however, check first with an orthopedist or neurologist.

Head Injuries

Although common, most childhood head bonks are not serious. Because the scalp has a rich blood supply, it bleeds heavily when cut, making the injury appear much worse than it really is. Bleeding under the skin may create hematomas, thick bruises that are better known as "eggs." As bruising settles with gravity, black eyes may develop a few days later. Although all of this is alarming, only one to two percent of head injuries involve skull fracture. Head bonks rarely require X rays. Serious head injury, such as can arise in an automobile accident, is another matter and deserves a full neurologic evaluation at the hospital. Pediatricians do see a lot of head injuries in toddlers who fall down stairs while in walkers.

After a minor head bonk, wash cuts and scrapes and apply gentle, steady pressure to stop bleeding. Use cold compresses to reduce swelling. Observe your child. If she is soon up and running, you can probably rule out serious head injury.

For more worrisome accidents, keep a close eye on your child for twenty-four hours. If he vomits, give him only clear liquids until he feels better. Repeated vomiting is a sign of serious injury. Although headaches commonly accompany head trauma, don't give pain medications because they can mask your child's true reaction to the injury.

WHEN TO CALL A DOCTOR ABOUT A HEAD INJURY

Call a doctor immediately if:

Your infant under 12 months has sustained a significant blow to the head

Your child's pupils are not of equal size

Your child loses consciousness, even momentarily, becomes confused, loses memory, or has a seizure

Blood-tinged or watery fluid seeps from the child's nose or ears

Your child walks unsteadily or develops slurred speech, blurred or double vision, or arm weakness

Your child complains of severe pain in the head or neck

Your child becomes very sleepy or difficult to arouse

Your child cries inconsolably for more than twenty to thirty minutes, especially if you suspect the tears come from pain rather than fear

Your child vomits more than three times within two hours of the injury

Ten to fifteen minutes of steady pressure doesn't stop bleeding from a scalp cut

Encourage your child to lie still and rest. To minimize swelling, apply a bag of ice (or frozen peas) to the injury for ten to twenty minutes. Your child may feel sleepy—that's normal—but keep her awake for the first hour after the injury to check her level of consciousness. After that, let her sleep but check her periodically. During the first night after the injury, awaken the child twice—once before you go to bed, and again about four hours later. If the child hit her head just before bedtime, awaken her every one to two hours for the first few hours to check her level of consciousness. If you wake your child and she can tell you the names of her pets and siblings, and other pertinent details, her consciousness level is okay. For infants, behavior is what matters most. If something's wrong, you'll probably know it.

Dental Trauma

If a blow to the mouth results in mild bleeding from the gums and slightly loose teeth, it counts as a minor injury, and healing usually occurs within three days. Sucking on ice or popsicles may ease the pain. If your child's tooth is very loose (displaced by more than one-eighth of an inch) or painful, or if it later becomes discolored or sensitive to cold or heat, call your dentist.

If your child's tooth is knocked out, it's an emergency. Find the tooth and, holding it by the crown, gently rinse it with water. Reinsert the tooth into its socket and instruct your child to bite down on a wad of gauze or cloth until you get to the dentist's office or hospital emergency room. Alternately, wrap the tooth in a wet clean cloth or soak it in a cup of water, milk, or contact-lens wetting solution. Head for the dentist's office or hospital emergency room.

As Healing Progresses

After your child is treated by the dentist or

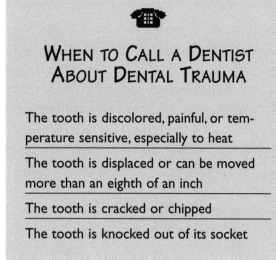

WHEN TO CALL A DENTIST ABOUT DENTAL TRAUMA

The tooth is discolored, painful, or temperature sensitive, especially to heat

The tooth is displaced or can be moved more than an eighth of an inch

The tooth is cracked or chipped

The tooth is knocked out of its socket

emergency-room staff, help reduce the pain with drops of clove essential oil, an old-time herbal remedy still used in dentists' offices today. It relieves pain and disinfects the area around the hurt tooth. Clove essential oil is sold in health-food stores. To use on your child's sensitive gums, dilute one to two drops in a teaspoon of vegetable oil. Moisten a cotton swab with this mix and apply directly to the injured area. In another half hour, reapply with a fresh cotton swab.

Eye Injuries

Black eyes are simply bruises around the eyes. Often caused by a direct blow to the eye or a head trauma, they usually heal within a couple of weeks without treatment. If your child receives a blow to the eye without the skin tearing or other complications, use an ice pack for the first twenty-four hours and then apply warm compresses.

Foreign Object in the Eye

When your child get something in his eye, the automatic response is to rub it. Stop him from rubbing the eye, even though you know it hurts and burns and you see tearing, rapid blinking, and increased sensitivity to light. To remove the object, first try rinsing the eye. While your child lies on his side with the injured eye down, flush with copious running water. A younger child may be more comfortable putting his face in a bowl of clean, warm water and blinking. If rinsing doesn't remove a foreign object (and if your child can cooperate), gently lift his eyelids and ask him to look the opposite direction. In other words, he looks up while you peer under the lower lid. Once you locate the object on the eye or eyelid, gently wipe it away with a water-moistened clean cloth, tissue, or cotton swab. Never use dry cotton or tweezers. If the object is embedded in the eye, have your child close both eyes, loosely cover them with sterile dressings or clean cloths, and take him to the hospital.

If a chemical has splashed into your child's eye, rinse with running water for at least ten to fifteen minutes before going to the hospital.

WHEN TO CALL A DOCTOR ABOUT A BLACK EYE

Get a doctor's advice immediately if:
The skin is split open

An object moving at high speed (a baseball, for example) caused the black eye

The offending object may have left fibers or fragments in the eye or eyelids

Your child's pupils are not of equal size

Your child's eye continues to tear excessively or later becomes pink and produces a yellowish discharge

Your child complains of persistent eye pain or double, blurred, or decreased vision

(For instructions on making an herbal eyewash, see Chapter 9, Colds, page 109.)

WHEN TO CALL A DOCTOR ABOUT A FOREIGN OBJECT IN THE EYE

The foreign object is embedded

You can't remove a mobile foreign body

You remove the debris from the eye, but your child continues to have pain, redness, tearing, and increased sensitivity to light

You remove the object, but your child later develops eye redness and discharge

As Healing Progresses

No herb can substitute for professional medical care for injured eyes. After a child receives that care, however, herbs support healing.

Black tea. A plain old black tea bag moistened with cool water makes a splendid remedy for black eyes. The tannins in the tea shrink swollen tissue and cause dilated blood vessels to contract, relieving inflammation. Since caffeine can be absorbed by the skin, you may prefer the decaffeinated tea. Other astringent herbs that would work equally well include raspberry leaves (also available in teabags), yarrow leaves, comfrey leaves, chickweed, plantain, or cabbage leaves. To use, moisten and mash the herbs; wrap in a clean, cool, damp cloth; and apply over the injured area for fifteen minutes. Keep the eye closed while this simple poultice is in place.

Eyebright provides our favorite treatment for mild eye irritation. Its astringent, soothing, and antiseptic properties reduce redness and irritation from dust, pollens, minor infections, and allergies. You can apply an eyebright tea bag or poultice, or wash the eye with a well-strained, cooled infusion.

Insect Bites and Stings

Every region has its own biting insects, and some of these bugs can live practically anywhere. Mosquitoes, chiggers, lice, bedbugs, fleas, and flies can raise a welt with their bites, but they're

WHEN TO GET MEDICAL HELP FOR STINGS

Call 911 for an ambulance if your child shows the following symptoms:
Difficulty swallowing or breathing

Sudden and severe swelling of the lips, face, eyes, or tongue

Collapse

Go to the emergency room if your child develops:
Severe local pain and swelling

Itching all over (not just at the sting site) or hives

Severe stomach cramps, nausea, vomiting, or diarrhea

A week to twelve days after the sting, your child develops fever, malaise, swelling, hives, muscle aches, and joint pain (These are signs of serum sickness.)

Call a doctor if:
The sting is inside the mouth or throat

The child received ten or more stings

not poisonous. Wash the bite with soap and water. If the bite burns or itches, apply a cold compress of mashed plantain leaves.

Stinging insects include fire ants, honeybees, hornets, yellow jackets, and wasps. All but the honeybee can sting repeatedly. The honeybee stings only once, leaving its stinger in your child's skin, after which the bee dies. To remove the stinger, gently scrape it out with your fingernail or a credit card; squeezing it out with fingernails or tweezers may release more venom. Then apply a cold compress.

An insect bite or sting on the tongue can cause it to swell and interfere with breathing. Multiple stings (ten or more) can produce nausea, vomiting, diarrhea, fever, and headache. These symptoms result not from allergy, but from the volume of venom. Allergy to bee or other insect venom can cause severe reactions within half an hour: wheezing, difficulty breathing, chest tightness,

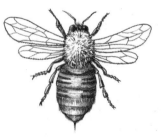

If a honeybee stings your child, you'll probably need to remove the stinger.

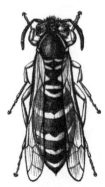

Yellowjackets are wasps, not bees. They won't leave a stinger, but can sting repeatedly.

HERBAL INSECT REPELLENT

If you're bound and determined to avoid products made with DEET, a strong chemical repellant, try this effective herbal substitute.

1 part eucalyptus essential oil

3 parts citronella essential oil

1 part lavender essential oil

8 parts almond oil

1 part pennyroyal essential oil (optional; do not use if pregnant)

Blend the oils and store in a bottle. Try a test patch on your child's skin for an hour; if irritation develops, discontinue. Because the essential oils evaporate quickly, reapply the oil every 45 minutes.

and hives. If this happens, call an ambulance or place your child in the car and head for the emergency room. If your child has a history of bee-venom allergy and is stung, administer the epinephrine shot you probably already have.

A rare, delayed allergic reaction to bee stings is called serum sickness. Call your doctor if, seven to twelve days after the sting, your child develops fever, malaise, hives, muscle aches, and joint pain and swelling. Serum sickness requires immediate medical attention.

Home Remedies

You can neutralize bee stings, which are acidic, with an alkaline substance such as baking soda. For wasp stings, which are alkaline, use vinegar or lemon juice. In a real pinch, you can use urine.

Just rubbing the sting with an ice cube helps relieve pain temporarily. Because chlorophyll has a soothing, pain-relieving action, you can also rub on almost any green (nonpoisonous) plant.

WHEN TO CALL A DOCTOR ABOUT A TICK BITE

Your doctor will probably want to examine your child if:

You can't remove the tick or only got part

Days to weeks later, your child develops an infection around the bite, fever, aches, malaise, or swollen lymph nodes

Your child develops a rash that looks like a bull's-eye: enlarging rings with whitish skin on the inside and a larger red ring around it

The bite later shows signs of infection or ulceration

Plantain leaves can be made into a poultice to ease the discomfort of insect bites. Witch hazel bark, twigs, and leaves (or the fluid concentrate) can be used in a poultice for bites, stings, and mild burns. You can also apply essential oil of lavender directly to insect bites and stings. The same goes for aloe vera gel.

Tick Bites

Ticks, which belong to the spider family, burrow into the skin to suck blood. Although most ticks are benign, some transmit illness such as tick fever, Rocky Mountain spotted fever, and Lyme disease.

Should you find a tick embedded in your child's skin, grasp it as close to the skin as possible (tweezers work well) and pull steadily until the tick releases its grip. Avoid using undue force, otherwise you may shear the tick's body from its head. The remaining head or mouth parts can later cause infection. So can fluids from the tick's body if it gets squashed or punctured during the removal.

Avoid once-popular tick-removing techniques such as holding a flame to the tick or suffocating it by covering it with petroleum jelly or heavy oil. The first method is dangerous to the child; the second generally fails because ticks breathe only a few times each hour.

After you dispose of the tick, wash the bite thoroughly with soap and water and apply an antiseptic tincture such as echinacea, calendula, or Oregon graperoot. Give your child an extract of both echinacea and Oregon graperoot three times a day to protect against infection. You may want to use an antibiotic skin ointment, too.

Spider and Scorpion Bites

Most spider bites aren't serious. The ones that *are* include those from brown recluse spiders (tan with a dark violin-shaped mark on the back), black widow spiders (black or brown with a red hourglass shape on the underside), or scorpions (lobster-like with a stinger on a flexible tail). These bites can produce serious illness, especially in children.

Other spider bites should be treated like insect bites unless the child shows signs of a serious reaction (see box on page 70).

Snake Bites

Only five percent of snake species worldwide are venomous; some snakes bite without injecting venom. Poisonous American snakes include cottonmouths, copperheads, rattlesnakes, and coral snakes. Reactions to their bites vary depending upon the type of snake and the amount of venom injected. Signs and symptoms include pain, swelling, and a bruise-like discoloration near the bite, as well as general weakness, dizziness, chills, nausea, vomiting, respiratory distress, and shock.

If your child is bitten by a snake, call 911 immediately and wash the wound. Ideally, have someone else call for help while you tend your child. If you don't have access to a phone, carry your child to help.

WHEN TO CALL A DOCTOR FOR A SPIDER OR SCORPION BITE

Call an emergency room for instructions or go directly to one if: You're sure a brown recluse spider, black widow spider, or scorpion bit your child

You didn't see the spider but your child develops the following reactions: Severe pain or numbness around the bite, skin discoloration or rash, muscle rigidity, malaise, difficulty breathing, headache and dizziness, and nausea and vomiting

If you recognize the spider involved, tell the emergency operator so hospital staff can prepare the correct antivenin. Otherwise, try to capture or kill the spider for later identification if possible, but don't get bitten yourself.

The hospital staff will need to know the type of snake in order to prepare the correct antivenin. This, of course, presumes that you or your child got a look at the snake. Many emergency texts suggest killing the snake for later identification, but our advice is to memorize the snake's appearance if you see it. Killing it may delay seeking help and cause further endangerment.

While You Await Help

As with venomous spider bites, your primary goal is to slow the spread of venom through the blood vessels and lymphatic system. Have your child lie still with the bitten area below the level of the heart. Remove constricting jewelry or clothing and keep the child warm and calm.

Unless advised otherwise by a medical profes-

sional, do not give your child pain medication, particularly aspirin. Many anti-inflammatories inhibit blood clotting, thus aggravating problems created by the venom.

Do not apply a tourniquet or a cold compress. Both impair circulation and increase tissue damage. If you must wait more than a half hour for medical help, you can apply a gently constrictive band close to the bite, between it and the heart. The band should be just tight enough to block the flow of lymph and blood within superficial vessels. Make sure you can slip a finger under the band. If you can't, loosen it.

Many myths surround first-aid for snakebite. Here are some facts: do *not* cut open the bite wound, as this can cause more harm than good. Do *not* bother with the suction cups in snakebite kits—most aren't strong enough to draw the venom backward through the puncture.

Herbal Care for Snake Bites

Herbs can complement emergency medical care or help while you're waiting, but they can't substitute for such care. Several tribes of Native Americans have used echinacea against snake bites and other venomous bites. Snake and spider venom contain an enzyme that breaks down cell connections, causing the venom to spread. Research shows that echinacea interferes with this enzyme and suggests it may slow the spread of the venom. If one of our children was bitten by a snake, we would apply echinacea extract directly to the wound and give her one full dropperful by mouth every 15 minutes while on the way to the hospital.

Animal Bites

Pets can make valuable additions to family life. They also carry risks, particularly the risk of aggression against humans, warranted or not. The domestic animals most likely to bite are cats and dogs. Rodents such as mice, rats, guinea pigs, gerbils, and hamsters can nip. Aside from your child's emotional trauma at being bitten, the main concern is preventing bacterial infection at the bite wound. Prevention goes a long way here. Teach your child not to try to catch, harass, or pet wild animals or unknown domesticated animals. Make sure your pets receive appropriate vaccinations, including rabies shots.

For mild bites and cat scratches, wash the area with plenty of soap and running water. Seek medical help for bites that break the skin, particularly those resulting in deep cuts, lacerations, or puncture wounds. Bites to the hand or head are particularly dangerous. If the animal is unknown to you, contact the police or animal control officers to capture the animal and quarantine it. If the wound is bleeding, raise the injured area above the heart and apply direct, steady pressure. Once the bleeding slows, vigorously wash the bite with soap and water.

If any possibility exists that the animal was rabid, follow washing with a five-minute soak in rubbing alcohol (which burns, but can kill the rabies virus). Sunny has been through the rabies-shot series; it's really not that bad. The injections are given in an arm or buttock, not in the stomach, as some believe.

Human Bites

Human bite wounds are more likely to become infected than bites from other animals because of the different bacteria contained in the human mouth. Wash the skin with soap containing grapefruit seed extract or with infusions of antibacterial herbs such as echinacea, Oregon graperoot, coptis root, baptisia root, yarrow, calendula, chaparral, walnut leaves, or chamomile. Human bites to the hand require immediate medical attention.

Poisoning

When a child ingests or inhales a toxin, it's an emergency. If you think your child ate or inhaled something that could be poisonous, call 911 to reach your local Poison Control Center, emergency medical services, or the hospital. The staff person will want to know your child's name, age, weight, current symptoms, and your best estimate of what was swallowed or inhaled, how much, and how long ago.

Do not try to neutralize the poison or induce vomiting unless a health professional tells you to do so. Depending on the type of toxin, vomiting can cause further damage. If your doctor or the Poison Control Center staff says to induce vomiting, follow their instructions. Syrup of ipecac is often recommended to induce vomiting, but if you don't have any, the staff person can recommend a substitute such as dishwashing detergent. Drive to the hospital with a basin into which your child can vomit.

For Further Reading

Barkin, R., ed. *Emergency Pediatrics: A Guide to Ambulatory Care.* St. Louis: Mosby, 1990.

Fuentes, R. and C. Lowe. *The Family First-Aid Guide.* New York: Berkley, 1994.

Handal, K. A. *The American Red Cross First-Aid & Safety Handbook.* New York: Little, Brown and Co., 1992.

McGuffin, M., et al, eds. *American Herbal Product Association's Botanical Safety Handbook.* Boca Raton: CRC Press, 1997.

Rose, J. *Jeanne Rose's Modern Herbal.* New York: Perigee, 1987.

Schmitt, B. D. *Your Child's Health* (2nd ed.). NY: Bantam, 1991.

Scott, J. *Natural Medicine for Children.* New York: Avon, 1990.

Chapter 6

About Antibiotics

There's a reason they're called "miracle drugs"—antibiotics save lives. Their name is indicative of how they work: they go to war against living organisms that infect your child, often vanquishing diseases caused by bacteria such as staph and strep. But antibiotics are not always used wisely. These medicines can't kill viruses, yet they are often prescribed for viral illnesses. In 1992, doctors in the United States wrote twelve million antibiotic prescriptions for bronchitis, colds, and other upper respiratory infections—a group of illnesses primarily caused by viruses.

Why the unwarranted prescriptions? For one, in pediatric practice, doctors can't always determine the source of an infection. It could be viral, it could be bacterial; it could be both. For example, take ear infections, the number-one pediatric diagnosis and the number-one reason for giving antibiotics to American children. Precise diagnosis is tricky. The doctor needs a good look at the eardrum, but in infants, the age group most at risk, the slant and narrowness of the ear canal and the resistance that little ones typically mount to having a scope stuck in an ear makes for a challenging examination.

In addition, ear wax may block a child's ear canal. Maybe the physician tries, but can't remove enough ear wax to get a good look at the eardrum. Doctor, child, and parent are, by now, sweaty and grouchy from the exertion of the failed ear exam. Possibly the physician hasn't the heart to further torment the child. Nevertheless, the child is sick. What's a doctor to do?

Or maybe the eardrum looks just a bit red. The cause could be an early bacterial infection—or viral inflammation, fever, or the fussing provoked by the ear exam itself.

Best-case scenario: the doctor gets a good look at the eardrum; it's clearly infected. But what's causing the infection? Bacteria, probably. Doctors who want to know for sure can tap the eardrum with a needle and withdraw fluid for culture. But this infrequently performed procedure isn't wildly popular among kids or parents, either.

The fact remains that the child is sick, unhappy, and in pain. In a perfect world, the physician sends the family home after instructing the parent to phone the next day, or, if the child hasn't improved, to return to the doctor's office. But will the parent follow through? Perhaps the physician doesn't know the family well (likely in a world of HMOs) and can't be sure. Maybe the mother looks like she's at the end of her rope—a fraying rope. Maybe she looks like she just needs to see this child getting better—right away.

Neither doctors nor parents want to be responsible for letting the child's illness worsen—perhaps even causing death—by not starting antibiotic treatment quickly or aggressively enough. Sometimes parents plead for an antibiotic. Often, physicians perceive or imagine that the parent wants antibiotics. Squeezed by these various pressures, the doctor writes the prescription. It seems both safe and expedient.

Why is a policy of "when in doubt, prescribe antibiotics" a bad thing for children? There are several reasons.

Bacterial resistance. Studies note an alarming rise in bacteria that routine antibiotics no longer destroy. To survive, bacteria mutate upon exposure to antibiotics; the more medication, the more bacteria change. When the bacteria have changed so much that the antibiotic is useless, doctors must prescribe newer, and usually more expensive, drugs to treat common infections.

Some bacterial strains now survive all antibiotics. Others have become resistant to frequently prescribed antibiotics. For instance, some strains of *Streptococcus pneumonia,* which can cause middle-ear infections, sinusitis, and pneumonia, have become resistant to penicillin. In some day-care centers, the number of children infected with penicillin-resistant strep runs as high as 29 percent. If antibiotics become ineffective against such bacterial infections, the very young and the very old will suffer most.

Countries that have mounted campaigns to decrease antibiotic use report declines in bacterial resistance. A small study in a Nebraska day-care center found that a decrease in antibiotic use by the children led to a striking decrease (from 53 to 7 percent) in infection with resistant strains.

Side effects. Adverse reactions to antibiotics vary, depending upon the individual and the type of drug. Most antibiotics cause side effects in some individuals; the ones caused by run-of-the-mill drugs for pediatric infections are relatively benign (e.g., diarrhea) and go away once the medication is stopped. The most common drug allergies are to the penicillins, including amoxicillin and ampicillin. These allergies can manifest in symptoms ranging from a rash to anaphylaxis, a potentially deadly allergic reaction marked by swelling, spasm of the airways, and low blood pressure. The antibiotics that are reserved for resistant bacteria and serious infections can have such side effects as kidney damage, auditory nerve injury, and decrease in certain types of blood cells.

Other effects. While antibiotics wipe out the bacteria that cause disease, they also destroy the bacteria that normally inhabit the intestines, vagina, urethra, and upper respiratory tract. These good "bugs" have many benefits, including maintaining the health of mucous membranes. Without them, undesirable organisms, such as other disease-causing bacteria and fungi, can take hold. This means that babies taking antibiotics run an increased risk of diaper rash and oral thrush. Girls, particularly after they begin menses, can develop vaginal yeast infections. Some health practitioners also believe that frequent antibiotic use contributes to food allergies and intolerances, because out-of-control undesirable organisms can inflame the digestive system, allowing larger food molecules to enter the bloodstream.

Recurrence. Some, but not all, studies indicate that when kids take antibiotics early in the course of a bacterial infection, they face a greater chance of getting the infection again.

What Parents Can Do

Boost your child's immunity. Discourage bacterial infections by adopting a healthy lifestyle and following the prevention strategies. Use herbs and other complementary medicines to support your child's natural immunity; sometimes, your child may be able to fight off an infection without antibiotics.

Work with your physician. Respect antibiotics as powerful medicines; don't demand them from your doctor. If your child has a viral illness, antibiotics won't do a lick of good and can even cause problems. Educate yourself about common viral illnesses, learn how to treat them at home, and be aware of warning signs that you need a health practitioner's support.

If your doctor or physician's assistant gets out her prescription pad, you can ask if she believes antibiotics are really necessary. If she says, "Not really," or "It's too soon to tell," you may take the prescription with you and wait to fill it until the culture results are available, or until you see if your child improves on his own. Ask your doctor how long to wait and what symptoms to watch for.

Be patient. Healing takes time—both your time away from work and your child's time away from school. When parents demand broad-spectrum antibiotics for convenience, no one, particularly the sick child, benefits. Employers must understand the need for time off or the flexibility to work from home when a child is sick.

What Doctors Can Do

Doctors can prescribe antibiotics only for bacterial infections. This means they have to do their best to identify the focus of the infection and possibly take cultures to confirm a bacterial cause.

Sometimes children recover just as rapidly from less severe bacterial infections without antibiotics. We wish American doctors would follow the lead of European countries that prescribe antibiotics more conservatively, reserving them for children overwhelmed with bacterial infection.

Doctors can also prescribe shorter courses of antibiotics as some in the United States and many in Europe already do. Studies have compared shortened courses (usually three to five days) to the standard ten-day treatment for the three most common bacterial illnesses: middle ear infection, sinusitis, and strep throat. Results have been generally positive, although there are pros and cons. Your doctor should be willing to answer your questions if she prescribes a short course of antibiotics for your child.

Health maintenance organizations and individual clinics should do whatever is necessary to make sure that physicians have enough time with each patient, both for proper diagnosis and to educate parents about antibiotic use and home remedies. One study actually showed that patients with respiratory infections gleaned greater satisfaction from communication with their physician than from receipt of an antibiotic prescription.

So When *Should* Your Child Take Antibiotics?

When an infection becomes too widespread or too virulent for your child to fight off or when complications threaten, antibiotics may be the wisest course. Trust your physician, fill the prescription, and make sure your child takes all of the pills for as long as she is supposed to. If she doesn't, she risks a rebound infection, as the challenged bacteria mount a strengthened response. Failure to complete a course of antibiotics gives bacteria a better chance to become resistant—it's like letting these bugs practice.

Please don't think of antibiotics as a sign that you have failed. They are a gift, a potent medicine that can do good when used wisely. While your child is taking antibiotics, continue to support her immune function with rest and good nutrition.

Use gentle, immune-boosting herbs that will help her body fight the bacterial invaders.

Care for your child's digestive system by replacing the normal intestinal bacteria. This simple measure can reduce his chances of antibiotic-related diarrhea. Give your child *Bifidobacterium bifidus* if he is under age two; *Lactobacillus acidophilus* bacteria if he is two or older. Follow dosage instructions on the label, or use Clark's rule to convert adult dosages to one appropriate for your child's weight if children's doses aren't listed.

Stay in touch with your physician, especially if your child suffers antibiotic side effects or does not get better. When used to treat susceptible bacterial infections, antibiotics usually improve a child's condition quickly, but need more time to completely eradicate the target bacteria. If antibiotics give your child a rash, contact your doctor and try applying a salve containing burdock, plantain, comfrey, calendula, yarrow, chickweed, or other herbs. See Chapter 21, Skin Problems, for instructions on making a salve.

ECHINACEA AND ANTIBIOTICS—TOGETHER?

Can these two powerful infection fighters work together? They certainly can. Germany has a very extensive system for testing and prescribing herbs, and according to the German Standard License for the use of echinacea:

"The use of Echinacea root preparations, when prescribed medically, does not exclude the simultaneous administration of antibiotics or chemotherapeutic agents; their application in the appropriate condition is indeed essential."

Chapter 7

ALLERGIES AND INTOLERANCES

A family doctor Linda knows, when asked how her practice was going, sighed and said, "Ah, the sniffling, sneezing, and wheezing masses." But respiratory symptoms are only the most visible effects of allergies. These inflammatory reactions can involve almost every bodily system. Airborne substances provoke allergic reactions, but so can the food your child eats and things he merely touches. According to estimates by the American Academy of Allergy, Asthma and Immunology, about one-fifth of all Americans, including children, are affected by some type of allergy.

Kids haven't always been so sniffly, sneezy, and itchy: A Swedish study of more than 7,000 schoolchildren revealed that, between 1979 and 1991, the number of cases of asthma, hay fever, and eczema nearly doubled. These three allergic reactions are covered in later chapters. In this one, we'll explain the fundamentals of allergies and then focus on food intolerances.

What exactly is an allergic reaction? It happens when a person's immune system responds adversely to a substance that doesn't trouble other individuals. While a normal immune-system response helps the body protect itself, an allergic immune response unnecessarily inflames tissues.

When the immune system reacts to such a foreign substance, blood vessels dilate, mucus production rises, and membranes swell, triggering symptoms such as runny nose, sneezing, wheezing, watery eyes, rashes, and gastrointestinal upsets. Depending upon the type of immune response, allergic reactions can occur immediately or over a period of days. The results of this overreaction to ordinary and benign substances can be annoying—or life-threatening. Repeated reactions of this kind can tax the immune system, impairing its ability to combat infection.

When your child has allergic symptoms within a few hours of exposure to an allergen, such as bee venom, it's easy to pinpoint the cause. It can be more difficult to diagnose an allergy that causes a less dramatic reaction three or four days after

POSSIBLE SYMPTOMS OF ALLERGIES OR INTOLERANCES

Other ailments can also cause these symptoms. Any time your child manifests them, call your doctor; don't try to diagnose the cause yourself.

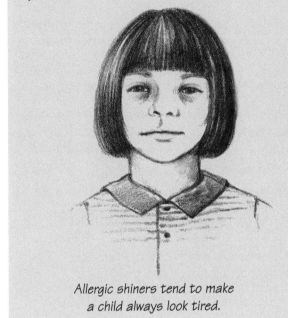

Allergic shiners tend to make a child always look tired.

Allergic "shiners"—dark circles and creases under the eyes

Puffy, watery, itchy eyes and runny nose

Chronically swollen glands, especially in the neck

Sneezing

Wheezing

Recurrent headaches or migraines

Skin rashes such as hives and eczema

Recurrent episodes of gastrointestinal distress—stomachache, gas, diarrhea, sometimes constipation

Bedwetting and incontinence

Chronic or recurring infections of the ears, bladder, sinuses, or other body systems

Hyperactivity or poor concentration

Anxiety, irritability, depression, or insomnia

---

exposure. Poison ivy and some food intolerances create such delayed reactions.

In sensitive people, substances in certain foods can mimic allergy-like symptoms, either because they contain a class of inflammatory chemicals called histamines, or because they provoke the body's cells to release such chemicals. Known offenders include sausage, sauerkraut, tuna, wine, spinach, tomatoes, strawberries, chocolate, bananas, papayas, alcohol, some nuts and shellfish, cabbage, cheese, citrus, and potatoes.

Many health practitioners believe subtle allergic reactions that standard diagnostic tests can't detect underlie a host of chronic illnesses. They particularly focus on food intolerances; standard allergy tests pick up only about 15 percent of these reactions to common foods. Here's an example of how even a mild allergic response can create disease elsewhere in the body.

A child is allergic to milk. His immune response leads to inflammation of the upper respiratory tract. Boggy mucous membranes and excess secretions block his middle ear's drainage duct. Mucus and bacteria become trapped in the middle ear and infection ensues. Treating the ear infection with antibiotics may cure the symptoms, but because the child continues to drink milk, the ear infection is likely to recur. When a patient has recurrent health problems, holistic practitioners often investigate allergies as a possible underlying cause.

Why Do Allergies Happen?

Why are kids so allergic now? No one knows exactly. A number of causes are probably involved, preventing scientists from casting blame on any one thing. For instance, a child's genetic heritage has some influence; allergic disorders tend to run in families. Yet, some kids with allergies have no family history of such ailments.

Many health professionals point an accusing finger at our chemically altered world. Chemicals

---

ALLERGIES: DEFINING THE TERMS

If you're on a quest to track down the cause of your child's allergies, you may need a guide to the medical lingo as well as the mechanism involved.

Allergen refers to any substance capable of triggering an allergic response in certain people. Pollen, mold, animal dander, dust, dust mites, medications, certain food and environmental chemicals are among the things that can cause allergies in certain people.

Anaphylaxis is a whole-body response to an allergen or toxin. It usually occurs soon after exposure. The skin may break out in hives. Mucous membranes swell and the airways constrict, making breathing difficult. Dilation of blood vessels causes blood pressure to plummet. Swift injection of epinephrine can put the brakes on the process. For example, parents who know that their child is allergic to stings should carry an epinephrine injection kit.

Antibodies are part of that immune-system response. There are five major known types of these protein-based substances. One type of antibody, immunoglobulin E or IgE, encourages particular cells to release histamine—the stuff that causes itchy eyes and runny noses.

People with allergies have high levels of this antibody.

Antigen refers to any substance that the body's immune system identifies as foreign— a virus, bacteria, cancer cells. Pollen is an antigen only to those individuals who are allergic to it. The immune system usually mounts a response to the invader.

Hypersensitivity is a term used interchangeably with allergy.

Intolerance is a broader term that can include allergies, but typically refers to more subtle reactions to a substance. Often health practitioners use this label when diagnostic tests do not reveal an allergy, but a certain food seems to cause symptoms. Intolerance can also have a narrower meaning. For instance, many people suffer from lactose intolerance because their intestines no longer make enough lactase, the enzyme that digests lactose, or milk sugar. These folks typically experience digestive upset after drinking milk or eating ice cream, but can tolerate buttermilk, yogurt, and cheese—products in which bacteria have already broken down the milk sugar. People with true milk allergy respond poorly to all dairy products, because their immune systems react to the protein in milk.

pollute our air, water, soil, and food. Preservatives and artificial colors and flavors lace processed foods. Artificial scents and colors infuse the detergents we use to wash our clothes and skin. Homes made of fabricated wood products, carpets, drapes, and upholstery can give off noxious gases. Even medications for children may contain artificial colors and sweeteners. Although the human body can cope with such substances in small amounts, an overload may tax our defenses and result in allergies.

Dietary imbalances probably also fit into the allergy puzzle. Many parents have lost sight of the importance of a balanced diet in maintaining health. Highly processed milk and cheese foods, fast foods, and take-out meals have replaced home food preparation. The result is an emphasis on relatively few foods—wheat, corn, and tomato, for instance. These culprits often turn up on lists of foods that cause allergies. When an individual eats a limited number of foods frequently, the likelihood that they will become intolerant to these foods goes up.

The "Leaky Gut" Theory

Another theory about the origin of allergies suggests that the intestines normally have a built-in filtering system to allow only small molecules—vitamins, minerals, and other nutrients from digested foods—to cross from the digestive system into the bloodstream. This process works efficiently when it includes healthy bowel bacteria, a good layer of mucus, and intact mucous membranes and capillaries.

Frequent assault by various stressors disrupts this protective barrier. Culprits include poor digestion, imbalanced bacterial flora, overuse of anti-inflammatory drugs such as aspirin or ibuprofen, frequent use of antibiotics, chronic constipation, current or past parasites, and intestinal infection. All these factors can inflame the intestines and make them more permeable, allowing larger molecules from poorly digested foods to squeeze through the lining. When these molecules, usually proteins, enter the bloodstream, the body perceives them as invaders—antigens—and mounts an immune reaction. The symptoms of this reaction can manifest soon after eating, or several days later, making diagnosis difficult. Repeated exposure to these molecules creates an oversensitized immune system, one that can become so embattled it can't rally properly when faced with infection.

Intestinal immaturity can lead to incomplete digestion of foods. Newborns have leakier guts (or, in medical language, greater intestinal permeability) than older children. Their more porous intestines allow the absorption of beneficial antibodies and other immune goodies from breast milk, and thus provide protection from infection. The downside is that infants who sample solid foods too soon also absorb incompletely digested fragments into the bloodstream, increasing the risk of developing food allergies.

Reducing Allergic Disorders

On a positive note, limiting exposure to allergens and other sensitizing substances often reduces the occurrence of allergic disorders. In one study of 444 newborns with family histories of allergies, parents agreed to follow a preventive regimen. The infants were breastfed for the first six months, and the parents used soy milk supplements when breast milk was unavailable. Parents eliminated household dust and banned smoking indoors. After four years, researchers found that only 18 percent of these children had allergic disorders such as hay fever, asthma, and eczema, compared to 32 percent of children in a control group.

In another study, 279 infants at risk for allergic disease were first breastfed, then weaned to a hypoallergenic diet. Their parents kept them away from cigarette smoke, and the children did not attend day care till age two years or older. When the children were three years old, allergy incidence was less than a third as high as in a group of children that received no preventive interventions.

Testing for Allergies

So it's easy to prevent your child's allergic symptoms, right? Not necessarily. In order to help your child avoid an allergen, you have to identify it first. A number of tests exist for allergies; some are very expensive, and others virtually free. But some tests can detect only certain types of allergies, because they only screen for certain types of antibodies.

To diagnose a classic, antibody-provoking allergy, you'll need to see a medical practitioner qualified to perform allergy testing. A naturopathic or medical doctor with a specialty in clinical ecology or environmental sensitivities may be your best bet. Ask which tests will most likely get to the bottom of your child's problems. Chances are, you'll have more than one option; your health practitioner can tell you the pros and cons of each.

Elimination/Provocation Testing

Many holistic practitioners view this test as the "gold standard" for uncovering food intolerances. It isn't the kind of test you simply go to the doctor's office and receive, however. It requires substantial dedication by parents, and can take several weeks.

The first part, the elimination diet, involves removing a number of potential problem foods from the family's diet. Common culprits include milk and other dairy products, processed meats, wheat, corn, citrus, peanuts, chocolate, and eggs.

Parents also need to look out for these foods as ingredients in—unfortunately—everything from tomato sauce to fruit leather.

How long does your child need to stay off potential problem foods? Experts cite time periods varying from a minimum of one week to up to a month. Previously ingested food takes about four days to move out of the intestinal tract. Withdrawal reactions such as malaise, headache, increased appetite, and irritability sometimes occur in these first days. Assuming the problem food has been eliminated, allergy symptoms often disappear by the fifth or sixth day. To minimize the effect on the family's diet, we suggest removing one food at time, for a week at a time.

The second part, provocation testing, entails reintroducing these foods, again one at a time, and observing and recording reactions. If you don't see new allergy symptoms, you can restore the food to your child's menu. If, on the other hand, that food produces reactions, a child shouldn't eat it for at least six months. How long should you wait between each test of a suspect food? Recommendations vary from one to four days.

After time allows your child's immune system to rest and his intestines to heal, tolerance for a food sometimes returns. This means he can eat it again, as long as consumption isn't frequent.

Even those with mild health problems may need assistance in orchestrating an elimination/provocation test. A nutritionist or naturopathic doctor should be able to help.

The elimination/provocation test requires that families temporarily change eating, shopping, and cooking habits. But the commitment can pay off by pinpointing food allergies, even subtle ones. People who complete elimination diets know which foods make them ill. They also know which ones merely make them feel less well. Armed with this knowledge, older children and adults can make conscious choices to enjoy problem foods and suffer the consequences, or avoid them in search of better health.

We know that an elimination diet is initially difficult. But we believe that if your child with ear infections, asthma, or chronic colds recovers or improves significantly because you did something as simple as eliminating one kind of grain from her diet, you'll count the work as effort well spent. Studies have shown that low-allergen diets also reduce symptoms in colicky infants and in children with attention deficit disorder and migraines. For more information on elimination/provocation testing and rotation diets, consult the books in the Recommended Reading List at the end of this chapter.

Caution: Children or adults with chronic illness, severe food allergies, or any history of anaphylactic reactions should attempt an elimination diet only under a physician's supervision. In these cases, food reintroductions are performed in a medical setting. This way, a trained professional is on hand in case of severe allergic reactions.

Conventional Treatment

The number one strategy behind any treatment is avoiding the allergen. Chapter 14, Hay Fever, and Chapter 15, Asthma, contain tips on diminishing exposure to airborne allergens. The next steps in conventional treatment for allergies involve immunotherapy or drugs to alleviate symptoms. Drug choices depend upon the symptoms and include antihistamines to decrease hives, runny nose, and itchy, watery eyes; decongestants to reduce stuffy nose; bronchodilators to open the airways in the case of asthma; and corticosteroids to decrease inflammation. Corticosteroids can be applied topically to hives, used intranasally for hay fever or asthma, or taken orally. Oral use of these drugs is usually limited to serious allergic reactions, widespread hives, or

recalcitrant asthma. That's because, although these drugs powerfully suppress inflammation, they also suppress immune function in general. Side effects include increased susceptibility to infection, acne, elevated blood sugar, behavior disturbances, and other problems.

In immunotherapy, also called allergy shots, tiny but increasing amounts of a known allergen are injected into the skin. Over time, the dose increases to a certain maximum. The theory is that the body slowly comes to accept this substance and stops reacting to it. The process can take years and is usually quite expensive.

Natural Treatments

A good holistic practitioner with training in nutrition and allergies can help you identify and eliminate allergens and correct any underlying factors such as poor digestion. Several of your child's body systems may need nutritional and herbal support. Continued exposure to histamines and other inflammatory substances can tax the immune system, exhaust the liver's detoxifying powers, and overwork the adrenal glands' anti-inflammatory capabilities. Herbs and other nutritional supplements can help heal these systems, in addition to relieving allergic symptoms.

Herbs to Ease Allergic Symptoms

Eyebright has anti-inflammatory and astringent actions and works remarkably well to decrease excess eye and nose secretions. Eyebright makes a bland, grassy-tasting tea. It is also available in glycerite, tincture, and capsule forms.

Bayberry contains tannins, the same astringents found in black and green tea. It helps dry excess respiratory secretions. If your child's throat is dry and scratchy, choose a different herb to avoid additional irritation; but for sneezing and runny nose, bayberry tea or capsules can be helpful.

Nettles may seem like the strangest herb in the world to use for allergies. Why, you may ask, would we recommend giving your child an herb that causes skin welts upon contact? Because only fresh stinging nettles cause skin reactions. Once they are dried or steamed, nettle leaves actually have an antihistaminic effect, and are a safe and effective allergy fighter. Nettle capsules, tea, or extracts can be taken at the first sneezy, drippy signs of hay fever season. Nettles tone boggy respiratory tissue and relieve minor allergic irritations, especially those affecting the nose and eyes. Start with one half capsule or one half cup of tea per day for a 50-pound child. If well tolerated, increase to one dose three times per day during allergy season.

Rose hips are the reddish seed cases left after the petals fall. They make great-tasting herbal teas, syrups, and glycerites; they're also among the highest sources of natural vitamin C and bioflavonoids on the North American continent. These nutrients have natural antihistamine and immune-boosting properties.

You can harvest rose hips in the fall, right after the first frost, when the plump red seed pods start to shrivel and begin to look a bit like red raisins but are still moist. Rose hips at this stage taste delicious; you can eat some on the spot and take the rest home to dry and make into syrup or glycerite.

Ephedra (*Ephedra sinensis*) and **Mormon tea** (*Ephedra nevadensis*). Ephedra, also known as ma huang, works powerfully to open the airways, making it a time-honored treatment for asthma and moist, congested conditions such as drippy allergic reactions. Like its synthetic counterpart pseudoephedrine (the active ingredient in Sudafed), it also decongests swollen mucous membranes. But ephedra is quite strong and not generally considered appropriate for small children, although naturopathic physicians and other holistic practitioners use it for kids with asthma. Mormon tea, on the other hand, is a much gen-tler species of the same plant family as ephedra. It contains less of the active alkaloid ephedrine, making it generally less effective, but safer for children's use.

Neither species extracts well into glycerine; your choices include tea and capsules. To decrease seasonal allergy symptoms, you may wish to serve your child over seven years old a quarter cup of Mormon tea (or a quarter capsule).

Cautions: Use good judgment, dose lightly, and do not serve ephedra or Mormon tea to children on a daily basis. Do not use either herb while pregnant or nursing. Ephedra stimulates the cardiovascular system, causing increases in blood pressure and heart rate; people with high blood pressure or heart disease should not take it. Ephedra also stimulates the central nervous systems. Sensitive children may have trouble sleeping if they take a dose after 3 or 4 P.M. Those taking certain antidepressants (the MAO inhibitors such as Nardil, Parnate, etc.) should not use either species.

If your child has asthma due to allergies, do not substitute ephedra or Mormon tea for your child's prescription asthma drug, and don't add the herbs to his regimen without professional guidance. If you go ahead on your own, you may harm your child. For more information on asthma, consult Chapter 15.

Herbs to Support Immune and Adrenal Health

In addition to our standby herb for immune health, echinacea, we also recommend the following immune-boosting plant medicines.

Reishi. A medicinal mushroom, this valuable plant is rich in immune-stimulating polysaccharides and liver-protecting compounds. Chinese and Japanese practitioners use it as an anti-inflammatory, antiasthma herb and to nourish weakened immune systems.

To support the immune system before and during allergy season, try reishi capsules or alcohol extracts. The standard dose for a 50-pound child is one 500-mg capsule per day. You can also apply Clark's rule to the dosage instructions on the bottle. A tonic dose is one dose per day, six days per week, for six weeks. Herbal experts consider reishi very safe, though your child may find it slightly sedating.

Astragalus. This immune-supporting herb is adaptogenic, meaning it can support the body through a number of different stresses, including illness. Like reishi, you can give it to your child as a tonic during allergy seasons—one dose a day, six days per week for six weeks. You can also cook with astragalus root, use a decoction, or follow package instructions on a bottle of capsules or extract.

Caution: Traditional Chinese Medicine practitioners often suggest that children with fevers not take astragalus. Because other astragalus species have been associated with adverse effects, make sure you purchase *Astragalus membranaceus.* Do not harvest wild species of American astragalus.

Licorice root has significant anti-inflammatory activity; it produces cortisone-like effects without the drawbacks of prescription cortisone drugs. An adaptogen, licorice also nourishes the adrenal glands. It makes a good addition to any allergy blend and is generally useful for all types of mucous membrane irritation, including coughs, runny nose, and stomachaches.

Caution: Licorice can create problems for children who already take prescription cortisone drugs to control hay fever or asthma; consult your pediatrician before using licorice if your child takes such medications. Do not use if your child has high blood pressure. Do not use for more than six consecutive weeks nor during pregnancy.

Chamomile has nerve settling, antihistaminic abilities, tastes good, and is a soothing addition to any tea blend. Chamomile contains several anti-inflammatory chemicals and is used worldwide as a daily tonic. The dried chamomile flowers should smell fresh and fruity when you buy them. Several noted herbalists have found that chamomile tea can be used topically as a skin wash for hives.

Caution: If your child has severe allergies to members of the daisy family, it may be prudent to avoid chamomile tea as well.

Herbs to Promote Healthy Liver Function

The liver has several functions, among them detoxifying chemicals in the blood. Improving liver function can help restore overall health.

Dandelion root makes a nontoxic addition to any allergy formula. The bitter taste stimulates the liver and gallbladder to produce bile and increases the hydrochloric acid output of the stomach. The end result is stronger digestion. Eating slightly bitter dark-green, leafy vegetables such as dandelion leaves, chicory, or kale also stimulates this same digestive capability.

Milk thistle is the most researched herb in the liver-tonic category. Holistic practitioners use the seeds to heal the liver when it has been overburdened from any kind of toxin, including food allergens. You can give your child this safe herb in a tonic dose during allergy season—one dose per day, six days per week for six weeks. Take a one-week break before launching another six-week program. To calculate dosage for your child, use Clark's rule for the adult dosage on the package.

Turmeric is a member of the ginger family. This bright yellow, resinous herb is used in curry powders and other seasonings. Turmeric and at least one of its active ingredients, curcumin, have potent anti-inflammatory action. In one study, curcumin was as effective as the anti-inflammatory drug phenylbutazone for decreasing pain after surgery.

Natural health-care providers see turmeric as the up-and-coming herb for treating allergic reactions. However, turmeric does not make a good glycerite, so your child will need to take it in capsules. A 50-pound child may start with 1/2 capsule per day, gradually working up to one capsule twice daily during allergy season. You can purchase turmeric powder at the grocery store and fill your own capsules, or open a manufactured capsule and discard half the contents. Or you can just cook with a lot of turmeric in curries and other piquant sauces. Be careful—turmeric stains!

Caution: Avoid medicinal doses of this herb if your child has gallbladder disease or an ulcer, or if you are pregnant. The amounts used to season foods are safe.

Nutritional Supplements for Allergies

Vitamin C and bioflavonoids have antihistamine effects and can help bolster the immune system against infections. One particularly helpful flavonoid is **quercetin**. Research suggests that it blocks several pathways of inflammation, including histamine reactions, and generally protects the intestines from insult, including that produced by food allergens. Quercetin is abundant in onions and garlic. Supplements are also available; follow package directions for children's doses.

Probiotic refers to supplements of beneficial digestive bacteria such as *Lactobacillus acidophilus* and *Bifidobacterium bifidus*. These supplements may minimize food allergies by promoting a healthy intestinal barrier, alleviating inflammation, and boosting digestion. Some research suggests that supplementation can reverse increases in intestinal permeability caused by cow's milk. In a study of infants with cow's milk allergy and eczema, those who took an acidophilus supplement for one month had a significant decrease in intestinal inflammation compared to those who didn't.

Digestive enzymes can be added to your child's diet during allergic symptoms to improve the

---

STEPS THAT MAY PREVENT ALLERGIES

If possible, breastfeed your babies for a minimum of six months to decrease their chances of developing food allergies, eczema, and asthma.

If your solely breastfed infant shows signs of allergies, something you're eating may be causing the symptoms. Cow's milk is one common culprit. For further guidance, consult your health-care practitioner. You can also contact the La Leche League for the name of a local lactation adviser (1-800-LA-LECHE).

Delay the introduction of solid foods until your bottle-fed baby is at least four months old or your breastfed baby is six months old. Talk to your naturopath or pediatrician about guidelines for introducing solid foods, starting with easily digestible, hypoallergenic foods.

Try becoming a semi-vegetarian family during flare-ups of hay fever, asthma, or eczema. Animal fats, except those from fish, are high in arachidonic acid, which encourages the production of inflammatory substances. One small study showed that when asthmatic sufferers adopted a vegan diet (no meat, eggs, or dairy products), 71 percent had relief after four months. After one year, 92 percent showed improvement.

body's breakdown of foods. Look for tablets containing bromelain, papain, protease (a protein-digesting enzyme), and amylase (starch-digesting enzyme).

Essential fatty acids feed chemical pathways that help reduce inflammation. Flaxseed oil is rich in beneficial omega-3 fatty acids; it's also inexpensive. You can grind the seeds, use flax flour, or take flaxseed oil. Kids can take flaxseed oil by the teaspoonful, in capsules, or blended into dips, salsas, bread spreads, and salad dressings. Cold-water fish such as salmon, mackerel, herring, sardines, anchovies, and bluefin also contain benefical omega-3 fatty acids. Borage, black currant, and evening primrose oils contain omega-6 fatty acids that can also reduce inflammation.

Recommended Reading

Barkett, V. M. *Diagnosing Your Own Food Allergies.* New York: Vantage Press, 1992.

McNichol, J. *Your Child's Food Allergies: Detecting and Treating Hyperactivity, Congestion, Irritability and Other Symptoms Caused by Common Food Allergies.* New York: John Wiley & Sons, 1992.

Rapp, D. *Is This Your Child? Discovering and Treating Unrecognized Allergies in Children and Adults.* New York: William Morrow, 1991.

Rona, Z. R. *Childhood Illness and the Allergy Connection.* Rocklin, CA: Prima, 1997.

ALLERGY-EASE GLYCERITE

For ages: 1 year and up
Yields: 2½ cups, or ten 2-ounce tincture bottles (enough to last several children through an allergy season)

*1/4 cup nettle leaves
        (antihistamine)*

*1/8 cup dandelion root
        (liver support)*

*1/8 cup astragalus root
        (immune and adrenal support)*

*1/8 cup wild oat seed
        (nerve support)*

*1 tablespoon lemon grass leaves
        (antiviral, flavoring)*

*1 teaspoon dried, chopped ginger
        (anti-inflammatory)*

2½ cups vegetable glycerine

1½ cups distilled water

Chop all herbs into a coarse powder in a clean coffee grinder. Blend well and pour into a 2-quart jar with a tight-fitting lid. Mix water and glycerine and pour over herbs. Shake well to moisten all herbs thoroughly. Tighten lid. Store in a cool, dark area, shaking daily to mix the herbs. If necessary, use a canning weight to keep the herbs from rising above the level of the liquid.

After two weeks or more, strain twice through a clean, dry cloth. Pour into about twenty 1-ounce or ten 2-ounce clean, brown-glass dropper bottles. Label. Store refrigerated for up to 1 year.

Dosage: For a 50-pound child, start with 10 to 15 drops, up to four times per day.

Chapter 8

FEVERS

Fever is not a disease, but rather a symptom of an illness. We have devoted a chapter to fevers for three reasons. First, childhood fevers scare grown-ups. Second, fever is maligned and misunderstood. Finally, controversy surrounding the management of fever causes anxiety for parents, because they're not completely sure what to do when their child has one.

It may help parents to remember that fever is only one part of the picture of an illness. In fact, for children under eight years of age, and especially for infants, the severity of a fever is an unreliable indicator of the severity of the child's illness. For example, infants and toddlers can be very sick with a low or even subnormal temperature. Conversely, children three to eight years old can be running about quite cheerfully with a fairly impressive fever. The important thing is *how your child is acting,* not the thermometer reading.

We unashamedly admit to feeling afraid when, upon caressing our sick child, we detect a burning hot forehead. We think this anxiety is normal. The first time Linda's son became sick with fever, she flashed back to scenes of the pediatric emergency room from her internship days. Her panicked brain jumped to a somewhat drastic conclusion: meningitis. She imagined her son in a fetal position, draped in blue surgical cloths, the small of his back orange from the antiseptic solution, a long needle poised to tap his spinal fluid.

But Linda's son soon recovered. He just had a run-of-the mill viral infection. This is not to say

that kids with serious illnesses don't get fevers. In this chapter, we'll help you sort out ordinary fevers from the more serious ones that require immediate medical care.

Defining Fever

First, let's define normal body temperature. Most people say 98.6°F (37°C) is normal, but this does not account for individual variations or the fact that kids tend to run a bit hotter than adults. Think of anything between 97° and 99.4°F (36° and 37.4°C) as normal. Recent exercise, consumption of hot food, over-bundling, hot weather, or an overheated room can drive body temperature up a degree or two. Body temperature also varies during the course of the day, and, with teenaged girls, the menstrual cycle.

Fevers usually hit their highest point in the late afternoon. Conversely, kids often have their lowest temperature of the day early in the morning. So don't panic at 4 P.M. when your child's fever rises slightly; this does not necessarily forebode a raging fever. On the other hand, if your child has a low-grade fever on awakening, you may want to keep him home.

How to Take Your Child's Temperature

When we use temperatures in this chapter, we're referring to oral temperatures. To convert thermometer readings from other parts of the body to oral measurements:

Rectal thermometer: SUBTRACT one degree

Axillary (armpit) thermometer: ADD one degree

In-the-ear thermometer: Congratulations; you paid big bucks for accuracy!

Types of thermometers include glass (rectal ones have a rounded tip, oral ones are more elongated) and digital. The digital thermometers are accurate, easier to read, and won't break off in a child's mouth or rectum. Temperature-sensitive strips or pacifiers are not very accurate. Nor do hands make for good thermometers. Usually we overestimate the warmth.

Rectal temperatures are the most accurate measurements in children under five years old. Drawbacks include the possibility of injuring the rectum and upsetting your child. Here's how to do it. Clean the thermometer with cool water or alcohol and put a dab of petroleum jelly on the end. Turn your child on his belly. Talk to him in a soothing voice and tell him what you're doing and why. Talk to him even if you think he's too young to understand your words. Part his buttocks. Insert the thermometer one inch into the rectum; this should not hurt. If it does, stop. Hold in place three minutes or until the silver stops rising (for a glass thermometer) or when the digital thermometer gives you a final reading. Do not leave your child during this time. Remove and read the thermometer.

Oral temperatures work well in older, cooperative children. Make sure your child hasn't had a hot or cold beverage just beforehand, and stay with him while he holds the thermometer under his tongue. Leave it in for three minutes or until the silver stops rising (for a glass thermometer), or until the digital thermometer gives you a final reading.

Axillary temperatures are easy and convenient, but less accurate than the other two methods. If you want a general idea of your child's temperature without upsetting him, it's the way to go.

TEMPERATURE READINGS FROM DIFFERENT TYPES OF THERMOMETERS

THERMOMETER TYPE	NORMAL RANGE	FEVER READING	COMMENTS
Rectal	98–100.4°F (36.6–38°C)	100.5°F (38.1°C) or above	Most accurate for children under 5 years
Oral	97–99.4°F (36–37.4°C)	99.5°F (37.5°C) or above	Best for children 5 and up
Axillary (armpit)	96–98.4°F (35.5–36.8°C)	98.5°F (37°C) or above	Less accurate than oral or rectal methods
In-the-ear	97–99.4°F (36–37.4°C)	99.5°F (37.5°C) or above	Highest accuracy but costly
Thermal strips or pacifiers	—	—	Avoid use due to inaccuracy

Make sure his skin is dry. If your child is small enough, hold him on your lap and slide the thermometer into his armpit. Gently hug him to hold his arm down for four minutes (or whenever the digital thermometer lets you know it's done). If he's old enough to do this himself, stay with him till the signal.

Ear temperatures can be measured quickly and accurately with an electronic thermometer. Most physicians' offices use them. If you can afford one, great. Just be sure first to stabilize your child's head to avoid damaging the ear canal.

How Fever Happens

Infections most commonly launch fever, especially in children. Other triggers include juvenile rheumatoid arthritis, transfusion reactions, tumors, inflammatory reactions caused by trauma, medications (including some antibiotics, antihistamines, or an overdose of aspirin), immunizations, and dehydration. Most physicians do not believe that teething directly causes significant fever, but we've seen it happen.

When infectious "bugs" stimulate white blood cells in a specific way, they release a substance called endogenous pyrogen, which signals the brain's hypothalamus to raise the body's thermostat setting. In turn, the body heats up by increasing its metabolic rate, shivering, or seeking warm environments. It also minimizes heat loss by restricting blood flow to the skin, giving it a pale appearance. Once body temperature rises, the skin flushes and sweats. A fever sufferer may lose appetite and feel lethargic, achy, and sleepy. When these phenomena happen to our children, we just tuck them into bed and let them sleep.

A basic fever, one due to minor bacterial or viral illness, can be an expression of the immune system working at its best. Given that most animals (vertebrates, anyway) mount a fever in response to illness, it's likely that humans have preserved this evolutionary response because it improves survival. Some research supports this theory; animal studies show when fever is blocked, survival rates from infection decline.

Fever increases the amount of interferon (a natural antitviral and anticancer substance) in the blood. A mild fever also increases the white blood cells that kill cells infected with viruses, fungi, and cancer, and improves the ability of certain white blood cells to destroy bacteria and infected cells. Fever also impairs the replication of many bacteria and viruses.

Bottom line: A moderate fever is a friend, but not one you want to spend a lot of time with. So it makes sense to avoid suppressing moderate fevers with drugs, while continuing to monitor your child for dramatic increases in temperature and worsening of any other symptoms.

Can Fever Do Harm?

Any time body temperature rises, salt and water are lost via sweating and stores of energy and vitamins, especially the water-soluble ones, are burned up. During moderate fevers, we can compensate for these losses by drinking appropriate fluids, ingesting nutritious foods, or taking vitamin supplements. Replacing water-soluble vitamins (chiefly C and Bs) makes sense. However, during fevers, the body makes some minerals unavailable for a good reason—bacteria need them to thrive. In terms of energy stores, our bodies switch from burning glucose (the favorite meal of bacteria) to burning protein and fat. This means a few days of poor appetite is probably adaptive. In other words, don't cajole or coerce your children into eating during fevers if they don't feel hungry; they'll likely regain any lost weight quickly after the illness ends. You do, however, need to encourage fluids, because dehydration alone can drive up fever.

Very high fevers—above 106°F (41°C)—can harm the heart and brain. Some authorities, however, say that fever is unlikely to cause brain damage in a previously healthy child. During most infections, the brain keeps body temperature at or below 104°F (40°C). So in *most*—not all—cases, you don't need to fear that your child's temperature is going to keep rising above that point.

What About Febrile Seizures?

First, let's define them. These abnormal jerking movements occur in children between the ages of

FEVER AND CHILDREN UNDER TWO

Largely because their immune systems are immature, infants under two are more susceptible to bacterial invasion of the blood and tissues—bacteremia, pneumonia, and meningitis. Furthermore, the telltale signs and symptoms of infection are often absent in infants, not to mention the fact that they can't tell you how they feel.

For these reasons, it's hard to tell whether the illness in an infant is trivial or serious. Here's one clue: Most of these serious illnesses produce temperatures of 104°F (40°C) or higher. The exception is in babies under three months old, in whom temperature does not correlate well with severity of illness.

How commonly do symptomless infections happen? Between 2 and 10 percent of feverish infants and toddlers who have no obvious source of infection on physical exam and don't even act very sick have bacteremia. If not treated with antibiotics, about 10 percent of these children will develop serious infections such as pneumonia or meningitis.

What should you do if your child under two runs a fever? If your infant is under three months, call your doctor immediately. He or she will probably want to examine him right away. For infants between three and six months, evaluation depends upon how your child looks and acts. For babies older than six months, especially older than a year, it becomes easier and safer to adopt a policy of watchful waiting. In these older infants, fever of greater than 104°F (40°C) increases the chance of serious illness. Once your child passes infancy, you probably don't need to call your health-care provider until your child's fever exceeds 104°F (40°C) or she acts very ill.

To summarize:
Babies under three months with fevers or any sign of illness should be seen immediately. Also get help if your infant acts ill (listless, irritable, won't nurse), regardless of his temperature. Do not give fever-reducing medications without consulting your doctor.

Feverish children three to six months old should be seen by a doctor in the very near future.

If your infant is between six and twenty-four months old, the fever is under 102°F (38.8°C), and your child is not acting very sick, your doctor may be able to evaluate the situation in a phone conversation.

three months and five years in association with a fever, but without evidence of infection of the nervous system. The seizure lasts no longer than fifteen minutes (usually five minutes or less) and causes twitching all over. About 3 percent of kids get febrile seizures.

The reason some children have this susceptibility isn't well understood. Of those kids who have a first-time febrile seizure, about one-third have a recurrence. Risks for recurrence go up with younger age at the first seizure (sixteen months old or less) and a family history of febrile seizures.

Frightening as these seizures are for parents, they're benign; once they pass, the child continues to develop normally. Often, pediatricians can help parents learn to block high temperatures by giving ibuprofen or acetaminophen when fevers

---

☎
WHEN TO CALL A DOCTOR FOR FEVERS IN CHILDREN TWO YEARS AND OLDER

Your child's fever lasts more than three days

Your child refuses fluids

You suspect your child has: a middle-ear infection (irritability, poor feeding, ear pain), strep throat (throat pain, headache, stomachache, and enlarged and tender lymph nodes in the neck), sinusitis (pain over the sinuses, headache, malaise, nasal discharge that persists beyond ten days), urinary tract infection (frequent, painful urination, discomfort over the area of the bladder or kidneys)

Your child's fever reaches 103°F (39.4°C). Call your doctor just to check in. Describe the symptoms and ask about danger signals to watch for. Ask what infectious diseases are currently going around. If your doctor thinks an office visit is in order, go.

See a doctor immediately if:
Your child's temperature exceeds 104°F (40°C) or higher

Your child has a seizure or convulsion

Your child has a history of febrile seizures (unless your doctor has already given you guidelines to follow during a fever)

Your child cries inconsolably or otherwise acts extremely irritable

Your child acts lethargic or confused or won't awaken easily

Your child complains of stiff neck and/or can't touch his chin to his chest

Your child breaks out in a purple rash that resembles tiny bruises. This could be a sign of a rare but serious infection

Your child seems to be in severe pain

Your child becomes dehydrated (dry skin and lips, crying without tears, no urination within eight hours or more, listlessness)

Your child has respiratory distress (rapid breathing, sucking of the skin between the ribs and above the breastbone when breathing in, bluish tinge around the mouth, wheezing or crackling sounds with breathing)

start. For the few children who have recurrent febrile seizures, anticonvulsants or sedatives may be used.

What Should You Do if Your Child Has a Febrile Seizure?

Try to stay calm. That's a tall order, but your child needs you to be collected. Take a deep breath. Let it out. Tell yourself that the seizure won't last long (although it may seem like forever) and that your child will likely be fine afterward.

Look at your watch to time the length of the seizure. This sounds like a big demand, given the anxiety a parent naturally feels. However, you will otherwise overestimate the time, and the duration of the seizure is important information for the doctor. If it exceeds five minutes, call 911.

Turn your child on his side. This reduces his risk of gagging on or inhaling secretions.

Make sure the immediate environment is safe. Remove objects your child might hit.

Do not restrain your child.

After the seizure is over, comfort and reassure your child, then call your doctor for an immediate appointment. He or she will want to evaluate your child for any abnormalities (other than fever) that may have triggered the seizure. If the seizure lasted longer than five minutes and/or your child seems very sick, your physician may tell you to go to the emergency room right away.

Over-the-Counter Medications for Fevers

It makes sense to us that if fever helps defend against infection, giving fever-reducing medications may make things worse. In addition, some fever medications can have undesirable side effects. On the other hand, no one likes to watch a child suffer. And fever can deplete a child's energy. Here's a profile of over-the-counter medicines for reducing fever and discomfort.

Acetaminophen reduces fever and pain but not inflammation. Follow package instructions. Because of the risk of liver damage, do not dose more frequently than every four to six hours or for more than five consecutive days. There's no need to awaken your child to give her a dose; sleep will do far more good.

Ibuprofen (Children's Motrin, Pediaprofen, Advil) reduces fever, pain, and inflammation. Follow the package instructions. Do not give more often than every six hours unless your physician advises otherwise. This medicine can cause stomach upset.

Aspirin reduces fever, pain, and inflammation, but pediatricians rarely recommend it.

Use of aspirin in children during viral illness has been linked to Reye's syndrome, a disease characterized by severe liver dysfunction and brain swelling. Symptoms include effortless and repeated vomiting, then a change in the level of consciousness (lethargy, stupor, combative behavior, delirium, seizures, coma). No one knows the cause of Reye's, but it seems to be linked with aspirin use during viral illnesses. For this reason, authorities have recommended that children under twenty-one years with symptoms of viral respiratory illness or chicken pox not take aspirin. Sometimes herpes outbreaks and viral gastroenteritis (marked by vomiting and/or diarrhea) are included in the list of illnesses during which aspirin must be avoided. Unfortunately, it's often difficult to be certain of the cause of an illness when it starts. Aspirin is a component of many cold and flu over-the-counter medications, so avoiding it requires careful label reading on your part.

Fever medications can act as a screen. Here are some pros and cons to giving your child over-the-counter medication to ease a fever. Medication such as acetaminophen can help sort out whether your child feels miserable due to a fever or due to infection. Some physicians use a trial of acetaminophen as a screen. If, after the drug kicks in, the child looks and acts better, it's less likely that he has a fever or that his infection is serious.

Fever medications can make your child feel better. He may be more likely to drink fluids, nibble food, and sleep. All can help him recover.

Fever medications can mask symptoms. In other words, your child acts as though his health has improved, but it really hasn't.

Fever medications may actually prolong the illness. This opinion of some practitioners is backed by a few studies. Assuming the body's response to illness (fever, inflammation, sleepiness) is adaptive, it seems reasonable to assume that interfering with the process may do more harm than good. Here are some examples that support this theory.

- A study of adults with colds found that aspirin and acetaminophen suppressed production of antibodies and increased cold symptoms, with a trend toward longer infectiousness.

- In a study of children with chicken pox, acetaminophen prolonged itching and the time to scabbing compared to placebo treatment.

- In test-tube studies, therapeutic levels of aspirin suppressed the ability of human white blood cells to kill bacteria. Acetaminophen did not have this effect. Another study found that a host of pain relievers, including aspirin and ibuprofen, inhibited white-cell production of antibodies by up to 50 percent.

The bottom line. Use these medicines sparingly when your child is in pain or suffers discomfort from a fever over 102°F (38.8°C). Ask yourself whether you're giving the fever-reducing medicine to make your child more comfortable or to decrease your own anxiety. Non-drug approaches can go a long way toward helping your child feel better. If the situation doesn't seem urgent, you might consider a trial of herbal treatment before you pull out the acetaminophen.

Home Management of Fevers

Do give your child lots to drink. Fever increases fluid loss, and dehydration can drive up your child's temperature. Kids with fever often don't feel thirsty, or by the time they do, they're already dehydrated. So keep offering fluids. Small, frequent sips are often best, especially if the child feels nauseated. If necessary, use a plastic medicine dropper to gently insert water into your child's mouth. The type that holds several ounces is best.

If your child craves cold foods, you can make her a frozen treat of diluted juice and/or herb tea. Pour the fluid into an ice cube tray, pop in the freezer, and later let her suck the frozen cubes. To make herbsicles, insert sticks when the solution is half frozen. Good herbs to try include lemon balm, peppermint, elder flowers or berries, oat straw, or

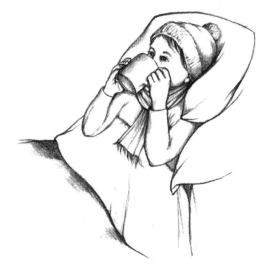

For a feverish child who feels chilled, pile on the clothing and serve warm tea or broth.

chamomile; you can also freeze diluted ginger ale or lemon water. For an unusual but tasty and nourishing frozen treat, make herbsicles out of our Immune-Boosting Soup recipe, page 51. If you don't tell your children that these ice cubes are

medicine, they may even like them and get valuable nutrition and fluids in a fun way.

Dress lightly or bundle? The answer depends upon your children's perception of temperature—follow her cues. If your child looks pale, shivers, or complains of feeling chilled (things that tend to happen in the early stages of fever), bundle her in breathable fabrics so that sweat will evaporate, but make sure she can easily remove the layers. If she's comfortable and her fever is low, dress her snugly and give warm liquids to assist the body's fever production. If she sweats and complains of heat, dress her lightly and let her throw off the covers. Older kids will take care of this themselves.

Don't push food. People with fevers generally don't have much appetite. Let your child determine when and what she eats. Just bear in mind that consumption of sugary foods could delay the natural immune response.

A Word About Roseola

Roseola infantum (aka *exanthem subitum* or pseudo-rubella) is caused by a virus, probably herpesvirus 6, which manifests different symptoms than other herpes simplex viruses. It typically occurs in children between six months and three years old. The child develops a high fever, up to 105°F (40.5°C). He may act downright playful, or he may act irritable and have swollen lymph nodes in his neck, behind his ears, and at the back of his head. After four to five days, the fever suddenly breaks. You think your child's out of the woods.

Lo and behold, a red, lacy rash appears on the child's trunk and spreads over the neck, face, arms, and legs. The rash may last a few hours or several days. The child may also have a sore throat and swollen lymph nodes, or he may feel completely fine.

Usually roseola runs a benign course (if you don't count the anxiety that it engenders in parents) and requires no treatment. Occasionally, the high fever precipitates a febrile seizure. If this happens, see your doctor. Your child probably is contagious until the rash disappears, so keep him away from siblings, friends, and schoolmates. Echinacea and other antiviral herbs can help support your child through this illness.

Herbal Remedies for Fevers

A rule of thumb that herbalists like to use during minor illness with fever is: "First, do nothing," meaning that a short period of observation ought to precede any action against the illness. Follow our guidelines above for seeking medical assistance for feverish children under the age of two, and encourage fluids. For older children, give liquids, make them comfortable, and observe closely. Is your child drinking fluids well? Urinating at least once every eight hours (ideally, every three to four hours, or wetting eight to ten diapers per day)? Does your touch console her? Is she playing normally? If the answer to these questions is yes, she's probably not seriously ill.

This observation time can also help you to decide which of the following herbs are most indicated and effective.

Boneset. We can't find much current research on this herb, but folklore, historical medical texts, and personal experience tell us it works. Consider the opinion of the Drs. John Uri Lloyd and Harvey Felter from 1898, two of the most respected herb doctors in American history: "In influenza, it relieves the pain in the limbs and back. Its popular name, 'boneset,' is derived from its well-known property of relieving the deep-seated pains in the limbs which accompany this disorder."

And that's exactly what we've found boneset best for: relieving discomfort during that achy, feverish stage of the flu. Limit a 40-pound child to three-quarters of a cup of hot boneset tea three times a day for three days; adjust the quantity for children of differing weights.

Caution: Large doses can cause vomiting, so watch the dosage here.

Echinacea. This herb's immune-enhancing, bacteria-killing, virus-fighting abilities all justify its use during children's fevers. In glycerite form, echinacea is tasty and easy to give to kids several times a day. You'll be providing much-needed fluids as well if your child will drink echinacea tea. Give your normally healthy child good-sized doses of echinacea three to five times a day.

Catnip is the classic traditional herb for babies' fevers. Again, we want to make clear that infants under three months old with a fever need to see a health-care practitioner. But if your six-month-old teething child is also running a mild fever, think about catnip tea as your remedy of choice. Although catnip stimulates cats, it has a safe and calming effect on humans.

Oregon graperoot contains large amounts of berberine, a superb infection fighter. While many herbalists consider berberine a purely antibacterial chemical, it also works as an anti-inflammatory for lowering fevers. With kids, the trick i disguising the taste of this bitter root. Try making an herbal glycerite, or look for a flavored variety in stores.

Other herbal tips for fevers. Sometimes your child just needs rest, and a dose of herbal sedatives can help. Herbs to try include chamomile and catnip for children under three years old, and skullcap, passionflower, or valerian for older kids.

Willow bark. Because we get so many questions about the safety of willow bark, let's talk a bit about it here. Willow bark, as many people know, is called the "original aspirin," even though aspirin actually borrowed its name from the botanical name of another plant, meadowsweet (*Spiraea*). Willow contains salicylic acid, which is the naturally occurring version of man-made acetylsalicylic acid, or aspirin. Because of the connection between aspirin and the serious children's illness, Reye's syndrome, willow has been a little suspect, too. According to Varro Tyler, Ph.D., Lilly Distinguished Professor of Pharmacognosy at Purdue University, a typical dose of willow bark may contain 60 to 120 mg of total salicin, yielding approximately one-fifth that of an aspirin tablet. He theorizes that it is tremendously unlikely, although not impossible, for that small amount to cause Reye's syndrome. In addition, there's not a single recorded case of willow bark—or any herb containing natural salicylates—being associated with Reye's syndrome.

However, we prefer to err on the side of caution, so we don't recommend willow or other salicylate-containing herbs during kids' fevers. And frankly, willow bark tea tastes so bad, it's hard to get ANY down a child.

Herbal water spritzes can also help send a feverish youngster off to sleep. Combine two drops of essential oil of chamomile, lavender, thyme, ylang ylang, or rose with four ounces of water in a spray bottle. These oils provide some antibacterial action along with a sense of tranquility. Spritz liberally on arms, legs, back, and chest, but keep this spray away from eyes and out of the reach of small children. It's best to use these in a warm, steamy bathroom so that your child doesn't get chilled.

THE ACHY-BRAKY SIPPING AND BATH TEA

For ages: 4 and up

Yields: 1 soak-and-sip treatment

This tea can help ease a low-grade fever of under 102°F (39°C) by inducing sweating. It is also beneficial for kids with chills or muscle aches. Do not use if your child has a fever over 102°F (39°C).

If you have access to any of these herbs fresh, double the amounts.

2 teaspoons peppermint leaves
(antiviral, helps break fevers)

2 teaspoons elder flowers
(antiviral, helps break fevers)

2 teaspoons yarrow flowers
(antibacterial, helps break fevers)

2 teaspoons boneset flowers and leaves
(helps break fevers)

4 cups hot water

Honey or maple syrup to sweeten

Combine the herbs. Use 1 teaspoon of the dried blend or 2 teaspoons of fresh blended herbs per cup of boiling water. Steep for 5 minutes, and strain. Sweeten a cup to taste for your child to drink; pour the rest in the bath. To induce sweating, serve this tea as hot as your child can comfortably drink it. We recommend serving it in a plastic mug while your sick child sits in a comfortably warm bathtub in a warm bathroom. After your child spends 10 minutes soaking and sipping, gently and slowly help him out of the tub. Watch for signs of dizziness; if they occur, allow your child to cool off a bit while still in the bathroom. Offer a glass of cool, not cold, water. Dry your child and dress him in warm clothes, warm socks, and a hat. Tuck him into bed and cover with lots of blankets; offer another cup of hot tea.

Caution: Not recommended for children with seizure disorders or a history of febrile seizures.

Chapter 9

COLDS

You know how it starts. It's a rainy Saturday morning, and your kids are corralled indoors. Your three-year-old son rubs his drippy nose, then snatches his older sister's teddy bear. A struggle ensues. You hold the coveted bear, sit a child on either side of you, and mediate a peace agreement. Your son turns his interest to drawing, sneezing into the box of markers as he begins. You hand the bear to your daughter. She nuzzles and kisses its face. You rub your tired eyes. Your spouse enters the room and you exchange a good-morning kiss. Within two to five days, you're all dripping and sneezing.

It's not the severity of common colds that makes them so troublesome; it's how often we get them and how generously we share them. For adults and children, colds are the leading cause of acute illness, doctor's office visits, and missed days from work and school. Children come down with six to eight colds a year, unless they're in day care, in which case they may get as many as a dozen. As you've probably noticed, the cold season begins about mid-September and extends until spring—in other words, most of the school year. Adults get an average of four colds a year—more if they smoke or spend a lot of time around small children.

Why are colds so catching? For starters, over 150 different types of viruses can cause colds. These viruses can slightly change their antigens, the components that the human body recognizes as foreign and against which cells direct their immune response. The strategy resembles donning disguises, so that at each invasion, the immune system must mount an entirely new response. In contrast, chicken pox is always caused by the same virus. Your child's body recognizes it, crafts a response, retains a memory for the bug, and usually remains forever immune from reinfection.

Also, the viruses that cause colds are virulent—in other words, highly contagious. They're transmitted primarily in the home, at school, and at day care centers, through direct contact with infected secretions and via droplets coughed or sneezed into the air. The amount of virus in the nose of a cold sufferer peaks on the second to fourth day of the illness, but can be carried for a couple of weeks after that—so someone with a cold can be contagious for a long time.

How Do I Know It's Just a Cold?

Most of us are well acquainted with the hallmarks of a cold: sneezing, runny and/or stuffy nose, and reddening of the outer nostrils. Scratchy throat, hoarseness, and a slight cough often accompany a cold. Infants and young children may run a low-grade fever. Colds and other viral upper respiratory infections are usually benign and self-limiting, meaning they don't do permanent damage and usually go away with or without treatment. Colds generally do *not* include high fever, body aches, extreme malaise, or significant appetite loss, symptoms more typical of influenza.

Depending upon the type of virus causing the cold, sneezing and runny nose usually peak by the second or third day. Nasal discharge usually starts out clear, but after one to three days becomes thicker and yellowish. That's because the discharge contains sloughed lining cells, white blood cells, and the bacteria that normally inhabit the upper respiratory tract. Cough frequently accompanies other cold symptoms.

Cold symptoms usually begin to subside around the third to fifth day, with complete resolution occurring between days seven and fourteen. Coughing may hang on into the third week.

Sometimes a cold results in complications. Viral infection and the body's own immune response inflame the respiratory mucous membranes. Viruses can also damage the cilia, tiny hair-like projections on the lining cells. Normally the cilia move like little whips to propel mucus toward the mouth, where it is swallowed. During a cold, excess secretions and boggy membranes can block the drainage ducts from the sinuses and the middle ear. Bacteria may invade these normally sterile areas, become trapped, and multiply, causing sinusitis and middle-ear infections. Some cold viruses can also cause conjunctivitis, or pinkeye. And some viruses that cause colds in adults can infect the tiny lower airways of children under two years of age to cause bronchiolitis. Bacteria can also infect the bronchi (larger airways) to cause bronchitis.

Conventional Treatment

No standard pharmaceuticals can shorten the course or improve the outcome of a cold. Most don't even relieve symptoms. Some, such as antihistamines, dry up infected secretions, making them even harder to expel. But the shortcomings of these products don't stop Americans from buying them, probably indicating both the power of these products' advertising and our deep-seated desire to make our children feel better.

One study done in 1994 found that more than half of American three-year-olds had received

HOW TO TELL A COLD FROM FLU

	COLD	FLU
Onset	Usually gradual	Abrupt, dramatic
Nose and sinuses	Runny nose, stuffy sinuses, sneezing	Runny nose, stuffy sinuses
Throat	Scratchy throat, hoarseness	Sore throat
Cough	Mild cough	Nagging cough
Temperature	Normal or slightly elevated	Fever
Headache	Slight	Strong
Other		Malaise, fatigue, poor appetite, body aches

Kids, Herbs, and Health

some kind of over-the-counter drug during the previous month, the most common being cough and cold medicines. Although these drugs did make the kids drowsy, they had little effect on cold symptoms. Another study published three years later looked at the management of colds by family practitioners. Over a six-month period, nearly a third of kids under age five had received a prescription, usually for various combinations of antihistamines, decongestants, and cough suppressants. None of these drugs successfully allevi-

ated cold symptoms and some may have unnecessarily exposed the children to side effects.

No antiviral drugs exist for treating the common cold. Some physicians treat colds with antibiotics, even though such treatment is without benefit. A 1996 study found that doctors in the United States prescribe antibiotics for 60 percent of their sniffling patients. The annual estimated cost of unwarranted use of antibiotics for colds runs about $37.5 million. Although some people (including physicians) believe other-

☎

WHEN TO CALL A DOCTOR ABOUT A COLD

Call a doctor for an appointment if:
Your child's cold symptoms, such as nasal discharge and sore throat, begin to worsen after three to five days or persist beyond two weeks.

You suspect your child has developed middle-ear infection. Symptoms are fever, irritability, poor feeding, lots of crying, ear pain, tugging at the earlobe, and difficulty sleeping.

You suspect your child has developed sinusitis. Signs are yellow-green nasal discharge lasting more than two weeks and accompanied by symptoms such as headache, fever, dizziness, fatigue, and malaise.

You suspect that nasal discharge has resulted from some foreign object your small child stuck up her nose (clues include discharge from only one nostril, foul smell, or a confession from your child).

Your child complains of severe sore throat, especially if nasal discharge and cough are minimal. Sore throat, headache, stomach

upset, and enlarged, tender lymph nodes in the neck may indicate strep infection.

Seek immediate medical attention if:
Your child develops signs of respiratory distress: severe cough, bluish discoloration around the lips, rapid breathing rate, wheezing, a raspy sound when taking a breath (a sign of croup), and labored breathing. In infants and toddlers, watch for skin that sucks in above the collarbone and between the ribs on each inhalation. Infants may have trouble nursing or drinking from a bottle.

Your child begins otherwise to act very ill—extreme irritability or lethargy, fever over 104°F (40°C), severe pain.

Call 911 if:
Your child develops signs of serious upper airway infection: high fever, a muffled voice, drooling, sitting with neck jutted forward to breathe.

98

What's in Over-the-Counter Cold Medications?

Analgesics such as aspirin, acetaminophen, and ibuprofen reduce pain and fever; aspirin and ibuprofen also reduce inflammation. Many over-the-counter cold remedies contain one of these drugs. And many pediatricians liberally recommend acetaminophen, but discourage aspirin use in children with respiratory viral infections and chicken pox because of its association with Reye's syndrome, a serious illness.

Acetaminophen is not an altogether benign drug. Overuse and overdose can cause liver and kidney damage. One study has found that acetaminophen and aspirin actually suppress immune response to the cold virus and increase symptoms such as nasal congestion.

Antihistamines include brompheniramine (Dimetane), chlorpheniramine (Chlor-Trimeton), and diphenhydramine (Benadryl). Most cold medicines contain antihistamines in combination with a decongestant (as in Dimetapp). These compounds dry secretions, including those in the mouth, and make them harder to expel. Some also contain a cough suppressant (PediaCare). They can have side effects such as varying degrees of sedation, nightmares, and, in what's known as a paradoxical effect, agitation. One study of ninety-six children who received an antihistamine-decongestant, a placebo, or no treatment found no significant differences in cold symptoms among the three groups.

Oral decongestants are usually made of phenylpropanolamine, phenylephrine, or pseu-

doephedrine. In many over-the-counter drugs, these chemicals are combined with an antihistamine. Compared to other decongestants, pseudoephedrine (Sudafed) causes much less stimulation. However, all these drugs can cause jitters, agitation, and insomnia.

Nasal decongestants include phenylephrine (Dristan, Neo-Synephrine, and others), oxymetazoline (Afrin, Dristan Long Lasting, Sinex, and others), and xylometazoline (Neo-Synephrine II). Use of decongestant nose drops or spray for more than three or four days can result in rebound congestion, which causes the person to want to use the drops again and again and again. Most physicians limit use to three days.

Cough suppressants usually contain dextromethorphan, thus the DM in the names of cough medications such as Robitussin DM. This compound is an opium derivative without addiction potential. Cough suppressants can come in handy when a cough is dry and hacking or it interferes with sleep. But when a cough is loose and rattly—indicative that there's a lot of respiratory mucus—a child needs to cough it up and get rid of it, not suppress that reflex. Massive overdose of these drugs can depress respiration.

Expectorants, drugs that help a cold sufferer cough up sputum usually contain guaifenesin. Their efficacy is questionable. A person taking expectorants needs to drink plenty of fluids for them to help; they haven't been found effective for children.

wise, one study found that patient satisfaction did not hinge upon receiving a prescription. Parents of children with colds mostly want to exclude the possibility of more serious illness.

The only over-the-counter treatment Linda has used with some measure of success is nasal decongestant drops. She reserves their use for times when her children complain that nasal stuffiness interferes with sleep. We feel that for the short term, occasional use of these drops is okay, but their overuse can lead to side effects, mainly rebound congestion.

Antibiotics and Colds

What about when the nasal discharge turns green? Aren't antibiotics needed then? Not necessarily. Nasal discharge (your children surely have more appropriately yucky names for it) commonly changes color toward the end of a viral upper respiratory infection. One study compared well children, children with clear nasal discharge, and children with greenish nasal discharge. The two groups of kids with runny noses showed no significant difference in how long they were sick overall or whether they suffered complications.

In another study, researchers cultured the nasal discharge of 142 kids who had the green stuff. They then randomly assigned the children to receive either an antibiotic, an antihistamine/ decongestant, or a placebo. Although much of the bacteria grown in the cultures is often associated with respiratory disease, neither drug treatment significantly affected the children's nasal discharge, overall clinical course, or their rate of complications when compared to the placebo treatment. The decongestant/antihistamine, however, produced significant side effects.

Bottom line: Neither antibiotic nor decongestant/antihistamine treatment improves the outcome of a cold. You'll also find that most over-the-counter medications contain significant amounts of sugar or saccharin, artificial colors, and preservatives.

Home Management of Colds

So if none of that stuff works, how *can* a parent help a child deal with a cold? We prefer to give our children good food, herbs, rest, and love. An uncomplicated cold is an illness you can almost always handle at home. Here are a few of our favorite tricks.

Feed your child "warming" foods such as ginger, garlic, onions, peppers, soups, grains, and herb teas. Throw in a few shiitake mushrooms for their immune-supporting effect (or see Immune-Boosting Soup, page 51). Avoid cold, refined, high-sugar foods such as ice cream, soda, and crackers. If your child is suffering from nausea, there are better, more nourishing strategies than the soda-and-crackers routine; see Chapter 16, Nausea and Vomiting.

Encourage your child to drink lots of fluids such as teas, diluted juices, and soup broths. Staying well-hydrated helps thin respiratory secretions, making them easier to expel. We recommend diluting juices because fruit juice contains large amounts of sugar—even if it is fructose—and sugar can depress immune-cell function. Some health practitioners say that dairy products produce mucus, a theory not tested by scientific studies. But because clear liquids do more to reduce respiratory congestion and are easier to digest, we prefer to offer herb teas, broths, and water instead of dairy products when our children have colds.

Humidify your child's room unless you live in a humid climate. If you use a humidifier, be diligent about keeping it clean; otherwise it will spew not just water droplets but also fungi and bacteria around the room.

Use steam. Your child can inhale steam from a pot of heated water with a few drops of essential oils added. Older kids can take a steamy shower.

If you suspect your child has food sensitivities, by all means avoid those foods during a cold.

Use salt-water nose drops to thin secretions. This loosens congestion and makes it easier to expel the excess mucus. These drops work best after inhaled steam loosens secretions.

Gently remind your child to wash her hands often, especially after blowing or wiping her nose. You can also encourage her not to touch her eyes after touching her nose. Good luck.

Teach your child how to use a tissue (the preferred receptacle for nasal goo, rather than mittens, knuckles, and shirt cuffs). Show her how to clear her nostrils. Tell her to blow gently and avoid pinching her nostrils together so that she doesn't force mucus backward into the sinus or middle ear. This extra pressure could propel infection-laden mucus up into the middle-ear cavity and start an ear infection.

Herbal Remedies for Colds

We don't have a cure for the common cold; nobody does yet. We can, however, offer many home remedies to alleviate your child's symptoms.

Echinacea is the best-researched herb for colds, and one of the best-selling herbs. It enhances immunity by stimulating a type of cell called a macrophage (our resident garbage disposals) to engulf and destroy invading microbes and to produce chemicals such as interferon, which has antiviral activity. Echinacea helps activate our natural killer cells to combat viruses, bacteria, and other threats to our natural immunity.

In a clinical trial, 108 people prone to upper respiratory infections such as colds, sinusitis, sore throats, and bronchitis took either a placebo or 4 milliliters twice a day of the fresh-pressed juice of

> ## SALINE NOSE DROPS
>
> *1/4 teaspoon salt*
> *1 cup warm water*
>
> Mix the salt and water together. Have your child tip back her head or lie on her back while you put in the drops. (If your child is an infant, you can gently draw out the drops and nasal secretions with a suction bulb. Toddlers and preschoolers, however, will probably not allow you to invade their space in this way. Instead, persuade them to blow their noses gently into a tissue.)

E. purpurea for eight weeks. The echinacea group remained healthy more of the time and enjoyed 1.6 times as many infection-free days. When infections did occur, symptoms were less severe and abated more quickly.

Echinacea's best effects are seen when it is taken at the very first sign of a cold, the early scratchy-throat and runny-nose stage. At that point, we give our children three to four cups of tea or the same number of doses of liquid echinacea per day, following label instructions for weight and age to calculate dose amounts. We continue to give that dose for several days, until all symptoms are gone. The nice part about echinacea is that it's nontoxic and safe for children. We find that echinacea glycerites generally have the best flavor, but capsules, tinctures, and tea can be used as well.

Antiviral Herbs

Elderberry has shown potent antiviral activity against influenza and other respiratory viruses. We've used elderberry tea for years for our kids' viral illnesses, and only recently learned of research that backs up its tradition of use. Dried elderber-

Herbal Steams

If your child is four or older, you may want to try using an herbal steam to help moisturize and soothe irritated nasal membranes and loosen coughs.

Heat two quarts of water (purified or filtered water is best) until it barely simmers. Turn off the heat, add a handful of fresh or dried herbs, cover, and let steep five minutes. Herbs to try include eucalyptus, thyme, cedar leaf, pine needles, lemon grass, sage, marjoram, oregano, bay, or rosemary. All contain antiseptic essential oils. Or you can add two to three drops of the essential oil of any one of these plants to the water. (Because the oils evaporate quickly, don't drop them in until your child is poised to breathe the steam.)

Remove the pan from the stove and set it on the table with a folded towel or trivet under it. If your child is small, you can set the pot on a sturdy chair and have him stand beside it or sit on a stool. Test the steam yourself for temperature, and show him how close to put his face to the pan. If the temperature of the steam feels comfortable to him, drape a towel over his head so that it forms a tent around the pot. Then ask him to breathe deeply in and out for a couple of minutes—through his nose if he has a cold or sinus infection, through his mouth if he has a cough. Stay close, especially if your child is young, to guard against burns or scalds. Talking or reading aloud can help pass the time.

Caution: Do NOT apply essential oils directly to the skin or mucous membranes, and don't put more essential oil into the pot than this recipe specifies. If your child has asthma, first try steam alone. If steam inhalation triggers coughing or wheezing, stop. If your child tolerates steam, add one or two drops of essential oil. If this aggravates symptoms, discontinue treatment.

ries and elderberry products are available in health food stores, or you can make your own at home. If you are harvesting the berries yourself, do take care to properly identify *Sambucus nigra* or the other edible species in your area. The berries of some *Sambucus* species are toxic, especially red ones.

Lemon balm, also known as balm or melissa, is an essential cold-remedy ingredient. While most research points to lemon balm's effect against the herpes virus, we use this herb freely when our children have colds. Kids like the taste.

Garlic has broad-spectrum antibiotic and antiviral properties. Try a garlic-honey tea by steeping two or more cloves of fresh, peeled garlic in hot water for five to ten minutes and adding honey to taste. Of course, some kids will prefer capsules. Either way, garlic's aromatic oils are excreted through the lungs, placing its medicinal properties right where you want them.

Licorice root. Licorice contains a diverse group of chemicals, particularly polysaccharides, that have been shown to activate the immune system and destroy viruses, too. Licorice mimics the effects of hydrocortisone, an anti-inflammatory drug. Add a little licorice root to your child's favorite tea blend when she has a cold.

RUNNY NOSE TEA

For ages: 1 and over
Yields: 3 cups

This tea helps open nasal passages, fight viruses, and reduce watery secretions from eyes and nose. All herbs used are dried; if fresh ones are available, double the amount.

2 tablespoons echinacea root, chopped (immune stimulant)

4 cups water

1/2 teaspoon boneset leaf and flowers (immune stimulant)

1 teaspoon lemon grass (antiviral)

1 teaspoon lemon balm leaves (antiviral)

1/2 teaspoon sage leaves (antibacterial)

1/2 teaspoon peppermint leaves (optional) (decongestant)

Honey or maple syrup to taste

Create a decoction of the echinacea root by gently simmering it in the water, partially covered. Keep an eye on the pot and reduce the amount of liquid down to about 3 cups. Remove from heat, add the remaining herbs, and steep for five to ten minutes, but not longer, because the tea will become too bitter for children's tastes. Cool and strain. Lightly sweeten the tea with honey or maple syrup and serve hot in 1/2-cup doses. Label and keep in the refrigerator for two to three days, reheating as needed.

Astringent Herbs

The herbs below are good alternatives to over-the-counter antihistamines. Not all act by blocking histamines, but their astringent action helps slow the flow of secretions.

Eyebright is a good choice to dry up a runny nose or watery eyes. It also avoids the undesirable side effects sometimes seen with commercial antihistamines—drowsiness and dry mouth, for instance. Research is not abundant on this herb, but folklore and Sunny's experience show that kids with runny noses get relief twenty to thirty minutes after taking eyebright. You will find eyebright in children's herbal formulas; otherwise, make a tea at home by infusing 1 teaspoon of the herb in 1 cup of hot water for five to ten minutes.

Sage is an astringent herb that owes its action to its tannin content. Its throat-soothing, antiseptic action is a welcome addition to our households' time-tested tea recipe of sage, honey, and lemon.

Nettles are the same stinging nettles many of us have accidentally run up against in the woods. In their dried form, nettles have an age-old reputation of benefit for hay fever, colds, and coughs. Fresh stinging nettles contain a trace amount of histamine that causes skin irritation, yet, when used dried, or prepared in capsules, extracts, or tea, helps reduce nasal secretions. Kids generally don't mind the taste of nettle tea, but be sure to use only dried nettle leaves.

Headache-Easers

Feverfew isn't just for fevers. It relieves pain and works well on headaches, especially migraines. But it tastes quite bitter, so you'll want to use capsules.

Ginger opens small blood vessels and creates a sensation of warmth. It's wonderful for upset stomachs, but not for use during fevers due to its warming effects. Grate fresh ginger into teas for extra flavor, or take it in extract or capsule form, following packaging directions.

Peppermint adds flavor and relieves mucous-membrane congestion with its mentholated aromatic oils. We rely on peppermint's effects during common colds; it opens clogged nasal passages, provides relief to congested lungs, and just tastes good. Our kids love growing peppermint in the summer and drinking tea from the harvested leaves during the winter. Combining one part peppermint with one part lemon balm makes a great tea blend for colds.

For Aches and Pains

Boneset. Warming to the whole body, boneset is credited with immune-enhancing properties when used in the first stages of a cold or flu infection. It was one of the most favored herbs of early American settlers and was used frequently by the Eclectic physicians of the mid-1800s to early 1900s for the aches associated with respiratory infections and coughs.

Calming Herbs

Chamomile is both calming and antispasmodic, wonderful for infants and toddlers during a common cold. Chamomile makes a delightful tea or glycerite. It's not sedative, but seems to take the edge off when kids are having a hard time settling down.

Skullcap gently calms the nerves. Larger doses act as a sedative. It's bitter, but glycerine masks its taste. It's a good herb to use for tightly wound kids or those who are too ill to sleep.

California poppy is nicely sedating for children. It's also safe and effective for helping stuffed-up kids get to sleep, especially if you help out by raising the head of the bed an inch or two. Sometimes California poppy is all that kids need to help them take a good, long rest and let their own recuperative powers fight a virus. It's not especially tasty, however.

Caution: Children taking MAO-inhibiting antidepressants (Nardil, Parnate, and others), St.-John's-wort, or ephedra should not take California poppy.

Nutritional Supplements for Colds

Two supplements are particularly useful for colds.

Vitamin C. Some, but not all, of the voluminous research on vitamin C has found that supplementation reduces the number of colds per year. Most show that vitamin C results in milder symptoms and reduces the duration of a cold by about a third. Vitamin C works best when taken at the onset of symptoms. Ideally, you and your

GOLDENSEAL AND THE COMMON COLD

Over the last twenty years, Americans have enjoyed a re-emergence of herbal medicine. One of the most popular herbs, goldenseal (*Hydrastis canadensis*), has gained an erroneous reputation for stimulating the immune system and being *the* herb for treating a common cold. While a great deal of research does document its antibacterial chemicals' capabilities, goldenseal is NOT antiviral. It doesn't kill rhinovirus or adenovirus, the two most common infectious agents in the common cold. It can help dry up a drippy nose, however—so if that's the symptom your child is fighting, it may be of help. Purchase only cultivated goldenseal, because it is endangered in the wild.

children can get your vitamin C from food. Good candidates include citrus, strawberries, guava, bell peppers, broccoli, red cabbage, and mangoes.

Zinc gluconate lozenges. Proper immune functioning requires zinc. In a study of adults with colds, people who took one lozenge containing 13.3 mg zinc every two hours while awake got rid of colds more quickly, within 4.4 days for those who took the zinc lozenges, compared to 7.6 days for those who didn't. The zinc group also had less headache, hoarseness, nasal congestion, nasal drainage, and sore throat. Some of them did, however, complain of poor taste and nausea, but no serious side effects.

If you use zinc gluconate lozenges, do so with care. We would restrict their use to children old enough to suck on a lozenge without the risk of choking (age three and up) and a dosage of one lozenge a day for three or four days. Some people dislike the taste and find that zinc upsets the stomach. Taking too much can actually depress immunity and decrease the body's level of

---

RUNNY-NOSE GLYCERITE

For Ages: 1 year and older
Yields: 10 2-ounce bottles

This is the remedy Sunny uses when her kids show the first signs of a cold. Made in advance, this combination will keep well for several years. It's important, however, to use distilled water—it's the simplest way to ensure that water-borne bacteria won't multiply in your glycerite.

*1/4 cup echinacea root
    (immune stimulant, antiviral)*

*1/8 cup eyebright leaf and flowers
    (astringent)*

*1 tablespoon boneset leaf and flowers
    (immune stimulant)*

*1 teaspoon lemon grass
    (antiviral)*

*1 teaspoon lemon balm leaves
    (antiviral)*

*1 teaspoon sage leaves
    (antibacterial)*

1½ cups vegetable glycerine

1 cup distilled water

Directions: With an electric coffee grinder, grind all dried herbs into a coarse powder. Mix well and set aside. In a clean quart jar with a tight-fitting lid, mix water and vegetable glycerine. Add herbs, cover, and shake until all herbs are moistened. Set jar upside down to check that the seal is tight, and put in a cool, dark room. After a day, check the seal on the jar's lid; if no leaks have appeared, store your jar right side up. If the seal is leaking, find a new lid, or line the one you have with waxed paper and check again.

Every day for the next two weeks, shake the jar well. After two weeks, strain the glycerite through several layers of cheesecloth into a clean jar. Gently squeeze the wad of herbs to get the last few drops. Strain again through a clean, finely woven cloth. (Don't, however, moisten the cloth with tap water, as it could cause the glycerite to mold.)

Pour into previously boiled, dry, cooled, one- or two-ounce dropper bottles, available at pharmacies and natural foods stores.

copper. Zinc-containing foods include oysters, lamb, pork, beef, liver, turkey, wheat germ, pumpkin seeds, ginger, pecans, Brazil nuts, sunflower seeds, eggs, and brewer's yeast. Any whole grains, such as wheat, rye, oats, and buckwheat, are good sources of zinc, and wheat germ and wheat bran are especially good. Legumes such as split peas, green peas, lima beans, black beans, peanuts, and lentils are good sources, too. Eating more of these foods has no side effects.

PINKEYE AND STIES

Pinkeye, or conjunctivitis, is a mild inflammation of the conjunctiva—the clear membrane covering the eye (except the cornea) and eyelid. When a child has it, the white of the eye appears pink or red. The eyes water and may burn and exude a yellowish discharge. Newborns less than four weeks old who develop pinkeye should be taken promptly to a doctor. Chances are the redness is caused by eyedrops given soon after birth, but a doctor must evaluate this.

Viruses most commonly cause pinkeye, often along with a cold. Untreated, such cases usually go away within three to seven days. However, herpes viruses also can cause pinkeye and sometimes damage the cornea, so consult your doctor if your child develops *both* cold sores (or fever blisters) and pinkeye.

Bacterial pinkeye turns the white of the eye almost red and produces a heavy greenish-yellow discharge. For significant redness and discharge, physicians may prescribe antibiotic eye drops or ointments.

We like to treat pinkeye early with an eyewash of infection-fighting, soothing herbs including eyebright leaves, yarrow flowers and leaves, Oregon graperoot, or rose petals. Make a tea using about one teaspoon of herbal material per cup just-boiled water as described in the recipe below. Four times a day, apply this tea to the eyes. You can pour it into an eyecup, have your child lower his head until the cup covers his eye, and encourage him to open his eye in the solution for one minute. Wash the eyecup thoroughly with antibacterial soap and repeat on the other side. Or place several drops into each eye and wash the outer eye with a cloth moistened in the tea.

Viral and bacterial pinkeye are very contagious, so encourage your child to wash her hands often, using only her own towels. Have her avoid touching her eyes. Keep her at home until she has completed one full day of antibiotic or herbal treatment, and the discharge has stopped.

Take your child to a doctor if:
pinkeye doesn't improve within twenty-four hours of treatment; —the eyelids are red, swollen, and tender

you suspect a middle ear infection

your child becomes very sick

Sties

A sty is basically a pimple at the base of the eyelash—a bacterial infection that produces a red, tender bump. When the sty bursts, pain stops and the wound heals quickly.

Sties are not dangerous and need no treatment. Discourage your child from touching or squeezing the sty, and hasten healing by applying warm herbal compresses made with the tea described above. Apply for ten minutes, four times a day. To alternate hot and cold compresses, apply four minutes of heat followed by two minutes of cold. Repeat twice, ending with heat. When the sty bursts, rinse the eye thoroughly with warm water.

A sty doesn't require a doctor's attention unless redness, tenderness, and swelling involve both eyelids and your child feels ill. If this occurs, seek immediate medical attention.

HERBAL EYEWASH FOR PINKEYE AND STIES

For ages: 1 year and up
Yields: 2 cups, enough for 3 days

4 teaspoons eyebright herb
    (soothing, astringent, antibacterial)
2 teaspoons yarrow flowers and leaves
    (anti-inflammatory, antibacterial)
1/4 teaspoon Oregon graperoot
    (antibacterial)
A pinch of salt
2 cups distilled water (do not substitute
    tap or well water)

Tools

Eye cup
Tincture bottle, dropper and lid
    disassembled
Clean, tightly woven cloth for straining
Clean strainer
2 paper coffee filters
1 quart non-aluminum pan

Directions: Sterilize eyecup and bottle parts by boiling in tap water for ten minutes. Wring out straining cloth in boiled water; discard water. Dry eyecup and bottle parts on a clean towel. Mix Oregon graperoot and distilled water, cover, and boil for 10 minutes. Off heat, add eyebright, yarrow, and salt. Stir well and cool.

Strain liquid through damp cloth and once through each coffee filter. Assemble dropper and lid; pour eyewash into bottle, add top, and label. Up to five times a day, shake well and apply to the eyes using an eyecup or dropper. Store in refrigerator up to three days.

Caution: Don't use a yarrow eyewash if your child is allergic to flowers in the daisy family (Asteraceae). Never place tinctures or glycerites into the eyes, as they can cause further irritation.

Chapter 10

FLU

Colds and the flu are often discussed in the same breath—the same weakened, congested, exhausted breath. But they're very different. The French word for influenza is *la grippe*—and when your child has the flu, he may feel as though he's definitely in the grip of something—perhaps a taloned, fire-breathing dragon. Generally speaking, the flu is worse than a cold; it makes your child feel bad all over. A group of tricky, rapidly changing viruses causes flu. And because antibiotics kill bacteria, not viruses, they won't help. Worse yet, flu viruses are transmissible by air, making them highly contagious. Fortunately, there are many herbs that not only ease symptoms of the flu, but actually help fight the virus itself.

First questions first: Does your child have a simple cold or influenza? Generally speaking, cold symptoms restrict themselves to the upper respiratory passages. In other words, from the shoulders down, your child feels pretty good, although she may be more tired than usual. The flu, however, comes on quickly and causes total-body malaise. So if your child suddenly loses appetite and feels achy, shivery, feverish, and exhausted, it may be flu.

For a detailed chart of cold vs. flu symptoms, see page 97 in Chapter 9, Colds.

The two most common influenza viruses (as opposed to other viruses that cause flu-like symptoms) are A and B. Type A is the most prevalent, but specific strains vary yearly. Several additional viruses, including parainfluenza and adenovirus, can cause similar symptoms. Flu viruses change constantly in order to outwit their host's immune defenses. For this reason, those who depend on flu shots for protection have to get a new one each fall.

Diagnosing The Flu

Usually, it's easy to tell whether a child has the flu by the symptoms. There are viral cultures or rapid tests for viral antigen that your doctor can perform, but such measures usually aren't necessary. Flu begins with symptoms including fever, chills, and malaise—that all-over weak and sick feeling. Teens and adults may also notice muscle aches, backache, headache, and sensitivity to light. Soon respiratory symptoms set in. Kids primarily have a runny nose, sore throat, and cough. Some of the viruses that produce flu symptoms also give rise to croup and conjunctivitis, or pinkeye—an inflammation of the lining of eyeball and lids. Influenza does not produce gastrointestinal symptoms, so "stomach flu" is a misnomer.

The worst of flu miseries usually subside after two to five days, although weakness and fatigue may linger for a couple weeks. If your child's symptoms have worsened, or have not begun to improve within a week, complications may have set in. Such complications usually involve a secondary bacterial infection such as pneumonia, sinusitis, or middle-ear infection. Each can make a child quite ill and warrants a doctor's exam.

Prevention Tips for the Flu

Flu is catching—and you merely have to share air to get it from someone. For this reason, the more crowded and closed-in your child's environment, the higher her risk of catching flu viruses. That's why outbreaks usually happen in winter, in crowded buildings with shut windows. The virus incubates—in other words, it multiplies inside your child but doesn't produce symptoms—for about two days. Flu sufferers are contagious as long as they have a fever. If one family member has been exposed, prevention becomes more compelling for all family members.

To avoid flu, we recommend maintaining your family's immune strength through sufficient sleep, relaxation, and a natural-foods diet that avoids immune-depressing sugars. Try not to over-schedule your child's day, and allow her ample time to unwind.

Eat in season. Michio Kushi, the father of macrobiotic healing in the United States, opened our eyes to eating seasonally. To macrobiotic diet experts, fruit juices, tropical fruits such as oranges and bananas, and concentrated sugars are not appropriate foods for children in northern climates during the cold and flu season.

We take a moderate path with our own kids: Instead of forcing or eliminating orange juice, for example, we allow six to eight ounces per

SHOULD YOUR CHILD GET A FLU SHOT?

The Public Health Service's Advisory Committee on Immunization Practices recommends flu shots for kids with the following chronic illnesses.

Lung disease (asthma or cystic fibrosis)

Heart disease

HIV infection

Leukemia, cancer, or other immunosuppressive disease

Diseases requiring long-term aspirin therapy (such as juvenile rheumatoid arthritis), metabolic disease (diabetes mellitus)

Kidney disease

That said, some people advocate flu vaccination for children because they often get the flu and frequently share it with other kids, teachers, and family members. However, we don't think the average, generally healthy child needs vaccination. If a member of your household is elderly, has a chronic illness, or has increased exposure to the flu, you may want to discuss vaccinating your children with your doctor.

The following people should NOT receive flu shots.

Pregnant women in their first trimester

Those sensitive or allergic to eggs (the vaccine viruses are grown in chick embryos)

day. During flu season, we often serve warm beverages and acorn squash garnished with plenty of ginger and cinnamon.

Immune-system herbs that can keep your child's natural flu-fighters in top form are easy to add to foods. Garlic and ginger are the two most common; astragalus is another herb that, once you're familiar with it, is simple to incorporate in a soup or tea. They're all discussed below in this chapter's herbal remedies section.

Finally, Grandma was right: Keep your kids warm. Dry wet hair before sending them outside. The same goes for taking off wet mittens and socks promptly. While it's viruses, not the chill itself, that causes colds and flu, letting your child get chilled can tax his immune system and lower resistance.

Conventional Treatment

Because so few antiviral medications exist, doctors seldom prescribe drugs for the flu. Sometimes antiviral drugs such as amantadine, sold under the trade name Symmetrel, and rimantadine, sold as

Flumadine, can help prevent or lessen severity of influenza A if taken within forty-eight hours of symptom onset. About 5 to 10 percent of people who take Symmetrel have nausea, dizziness, and insomnia; a few have had seizures or aggravations of psychiatric illnesses. Flumadine produces similar side effects, but not as often. Antiviral treatment of people at high risk for severe illness makes sense. In the absence of a secondary bacterial infection, antibiotics do not.

Home Care for the Flu

Encourage fluids, because fever accelerates fluid losses. Offer your child water, diluted juice, herbal tea, or soup broth frequently; see Chapter 4 for a recipe for Immune-Boosting Soup. The flu often slows down a normally energetic child enough to help her enjoy a cup of herbal tea. If she is a picky eater, start off with the best-tasting teas: chamomile, lemon balm, organic orange peel, or plain lemon juice in hot water.

You may be surprised how many children like garlic, ginger, and honey tea, all of which have antimicrobial properties. To a cup of just-boiled water, add one chopped garlic clove and a generous pinch of grated fresh ginger. Allow to steep for ten minutes; strain and add honey to taste.

Homemade ginger ale is a snap to make. Add a small amount of freshly grated ginger and honey to room-temperature sparkling soda water or heated water. Ginger can relieve a stomachache and gently warm a chilled body by stimulating circulation. Many commercial ginger ales no longer contain ginger, so if you're buying this beverage bottled, be sure to read the label. Look for real ginger; "natural flavors" may not contain the medicinal constituents you want.

Let your child eat to appetite. Kids with flu often don't feel like eating and should not be

WHEN TO CALL A DOCTOR ABOUT FLU

Call a doctor if your child:
Is under six months old

Acts very sick, with extreme irritability or lethargy or fever greater than 104°F (40°C)

Develops new symptoms: earache, severe cough, or chest pain

Experiences worsening symptoms or symptoms fail to improve significantly after seven days forced to do so. If your child feels chilled and will eat, serve foods spiced to his taste with warming herbs such as garlic, ginger, and hot peppers.

Relieve stuffiness with an herbal steam or bath; for instructions on setting up an herbal steam, see Chapter 9, Colds, page 102. Appropriate essential oils or herbs to add to the steaming water include eucalyptus, bergamot, thyme, rosemary, marjoram, or peppermint. If you're adding herbs, a quarter cup is plenty; for essential oils, start with two to three drops and don't use more than five to a quart of water.

To ease the aches that come with the flu, try massaging your child gently with a soothing oil. We like to use a quarter cup of almond oil containing four to six drops of chamomile or lavender essential oil. Lavender reduces pain, relaxes smooth muscles, and has some antimicrobial properties. Chamomile relaxes the child and may have a slight stimulating effect on the immune system.

To help your child get through that part of the flu when everything hurts, you can use a tea or bath tea with peppermint, elder flowers, yarrow, and boneset. See Achy-Braky Tea on page 95 in Chapter 8, Fevers.

Herbal Remedies

Immune-Supporting Herbs

Echinacea boosts the immune system and stimulates the production of interferon, our body's natural substance that contains numerous antiviral compounds. At least one clinical trial supports echinacea's use for influenza. Researchers randomly assigned 180 flu victims to receive a placebo, 90 drops of echinacea root tincture, or 180 drops of the tincture. Those who took 180 drops reported a significant reduction in flu symptoms, including chills, sweating, weakness, muscle aches, sore throat, and headaches.

However, echinacea is most effective if you start administering it immediately—in fact, as soon as you know your child has been around someone with the flu. Echinacea may take up to a day to reach its full effect.

Dosage depends on the product you're using, but for a 50-pound child, start with one dropper of glycerite or tincture, one capsule, or three-quarters cup of tea three to five times a day. We carry bottles of echinacea glycerite with us in purses, diaper bags, travel bags, and auto first-aid kits so we can start our kids on it at the first sign of illness.

Echinacea has an excellent safety record, but use good judgment. Follow label directions and limit your use to ten days at a time before taking a four- or five-day break. You can use echinacea at the same time as other herbs or antibiotics.

Caution: In very rare cases, if your child is allergic to flowers in the daisy family *(Asteraceae)*, he may also be sensitive to echinacea. If your child has had a severe allergic response to a flower in this family, you probably shouldn't give him echinacea. If you're not sure, start with a tiny dose. If no reactions appear, work your way up.

Astragalus. This herb is known as an adaptogen, an herb or substance that helps our bodies cope with stress, or what Traditional Chinese Medicine calls "pernicious influences"—bacteria, viruses, pollution, and physical or emotional stress. Astragalus boosts immunity and shows activity against some viruses. Whether it's directly active against influenza virus remains to be seen.

Look for astragalus sticks (they look like tongue depressors) in the bulk herb section of health food stores. One astragalus stick decocted in one cup of water makes a sweet tea that kids enjoy. You can also just drop in a stick when making soup or cooked grains.

Schisandra. Like astragalus, this herb is known as an adaptogen. Traditional Chinese Medicine practitioners call it "Five Tastes." Schisandra helps during times of exposure to pathogens and stress, possibly by scavenging free radicals. In fact, its antioxidant power exceeds that of vitamin E. Many herbalists consider it an all-around tonic to support the immune system during cold and flu season. Look for it in immune formulas, or purchase the spicy/sour berries at a reputable Chinese herb store.

Antiviral Herbs

Garlic. Studies show that fresh garlic is clinically effective against influenza and colds. Some active ingredients are released through the lungs, placing them right where you want them to combat infection that can be a complication of flu. You can purchase garlic capsules or make fresh garlic tea with honey. We use lots of garlic in our cooking during the winter. Like echinacea, garlic is a safe herb for nursing mothers to take when their baby has a cold—unless mom is on a garlic- and onion-free diet to reduce the baby's colic.

If your kids hate the taste of garlic, you can make a mild garlic oil to apply topically. Steep three minced cloves in a half-cup of olive oil overnight. Do a patch test of the oil on a small part of your child's foot the first night. If no redness results, rub the oil into both soles before bedtime, and cover with clean socks. Garlic's healing oils will be absorbed through the skin to circulate antiviral compounds throughout your child's bloodstream. Hard to believe? Smell his breath or skin the next day!

Elderberry. For more than twenty years, virologist Madeleine Mumcuoglu, Ph.D., has investigated the impact of one species of elderberry (*Sambucus nigra*) against the influenza virus and has found at least two active ingredients. Apparently, elderberry can inhibit the enzyme that flu viruses use to penetrate our cell membranes.

Mumcuoglu and a team of researchers found that elderberry extract inhibited varieties of both type A and type B influenza viruses in a test-tube. The investigators also gave the extract daily for three days to children and adults in the early stages of flu. Of the flu sufferers who got the extract, 90 percent were cured in two to three days; those who got a placebo took six days. The elderberry extract had no side effects and was inexpensive to boot. The children in the study took a dose of two tablespoons per day of prepared syrup.

Ginger. According to James Duke, Ph.D., one of America's foremost authorities on herbs, ginger contains ten antiviral compounds. It also has anti-inflammatory and analgesic effects, properties that can help ease flu miseries. In traditional herbal medicine, it is believed to reduce pain and fever, suppress coughing, and provide a warming effect when kids are chilled. It's also very helpful for upset stomachs. Feel free to cook liberally with ginger during cold and flu season.

Licorice root soothes irritated mucous membranes such as the throat. Test-tube studies show that the constituent glycyrrhizic acid inactivates and inhibits the growth of a range of viruses. Somewhat like echinacea, the polysaccharide ingredients of licorice can induce the body's production of interferon and can activate various white blood cells. Most kids like the sweet taste of licorice, providing the tea is not steeped more than ten minutes.

Mullein. This herb makes a soothing, antiviral tea for coughs and throat irritations. While mullein flowers do not completely inactivate flu viruses, we recommend their use during colds and flu to relieve coughing and support inflamed respiratory tissue. Warning: the fuzzy hairs on mullein leaves can irritate the throat, so strain this tea through a tightly woven cloth or very fine filter before serving it to kids.

St.-John's-wort. According to test-tube studies, this herb can inhibit influenza A viruses and parainfluenza virus. It also has been shown to act against parainfluenza infection in mice.

Calming and Sedative Herbs

Sometimes fretful sick kids need, more than anything, to relax. A number of herbs can help.

Skullcap. Several studies on the chemical compounds in a closely related plant, *Scutellaria baicalensis,* show activity against several types of influenza viruses. Whether this antiviral ability extends to American skullcap (*S. lateriflora*) remains to be seen. The taste is quite bitter, so look for it in extract or capsule form. You may want to try some of this herb yourself—parents often can use a little herbal unwinder when their children are sick and cranky.

FLU FIGHTER GLYCERITE

For ages: 1 year and up
Yields: 3 cups — enough to share

*1/4 cup echinacea root and/or seed
  (immune stimulating, antiviral)*

*1/4 cup astragalus root, chopped
  (adaptogen, immune stimulating)*

*2 tablespoons schisandra berries
  (immune supporting)*

*1/8 cup thyme leaves
  (antiviral, eases upper respiratory
  symptoms)*

*1/8 cup lemon balm leaves
  (antiviral, calming)*

*1 tablespoon licorice root
  (antiviral, adaptogen)*

*1 tablespoon red clover blossoms
  (liver support)*

*3 cups vegetable glycerine
2 cups distilled water*

Directions: Grind all herbs in a clean coffee grinder. Place in a 2-quart jar with tight-fitting lid. Mix glycerine and distilled water together and pour over the herbs. Shake well; cover tightly. Keep in cool, dark location for two to three weeks, shaking daily. Strain well, pour into 24 one-ounce or 12 two-ounce clean dropper bottles. Store in the refrigerator up to one year.

Dosage: At the first signs of colds or flu, give a 50-pound child 20 drops three or four times per day. Increase or decrease dosage proportionately according to weight—give a 25-pound child 10 drops, or a 100-pound child 40 drops.

Chapter 11

SINUSITIS

Your child has had a cold for a week and a half. Time for it to be over. You go into his room to wake him for school. You put your hand on his head. It feels hot. He opens his eyes and tells you his face hurts and his nose feels stuffy. His breath smells bad. His face looks slightly puffy. He sits up and coughs. What's going on?

He may have a sinus infection. Anything that inflames the nasal passages can set off a sinus infection, but the common cold is the usual culprit. Most kids get three to eight colds a year and up to 5 percent wind up with bacterial sinusitis as a complication. That's a lot of sinusitis, even when other causes of the illness aren't counted.

Here's the million-dollar question: How can you tell the difference between a viral cold and a bacterial sinus infection? With an uncomplicated cold, your child should experience only minimal fever or none at all. Sore throat and sneezing should resolve within three to six days. Nasal discharge will often turn from clear to yellow, then dry up between day ten to fourteen. Coughing may linger into the third week.

When a sinus infection complicates a cold, nasal and sinus congestion hangs on beyond ten to fourteen days or worsens. Yellowish-green discharge persists or increases—unless the duct draining the sinus becomes blocked, in which case discharge is scant to nonexistent. The color of the discharge isn't as important as the persistence of cold symptoms.

Other signs that a cold has progressed to sinusitis include fever, bad breath, unpleasant taste in the mouth from postnasal drip, fatigue, dizziness, and malaise. Older children and teens may complain of headache that worsens when they bend over or lie down, pain or pressure in the sinus area, or pain in the upper teeth. Mouth-breathing during the night may cause morning sore throat, and post-nasal drip may induce daytime coughing.

How Sinusitis Happens

The way the sinuses are built and how they work is key to understanding how sinusitis happens. In a healthy child, the paranasal sinuses are sterile, air-filled spaces above, below, between, and behind the eyes. The sinuses between the eyes, or ethmoid sinuses, are present at birth. The sinuses above and behind the eyes, the frontal and sphenoid sinuses, begin to appear at the age of five or six but don't fully form until adolescence. The sinuses below the eyes, or maxillary sinuses, don't completely develop until the child is between sixteen and twenty-one years old.

The lining cells of the nose and sinuses produce mucus. Ducts connect the sinuses with the nasal passages, allowing air flow and mucus drainage. The opening of these ducts into the nose is about the size of the tip of a ball-point pen, and easily obstructed. Hair cells called cilia sweep this mucus, along with pollen, dust, microbes, and pollutants that it has trapped, into the nasal cavities and to the back of the throat, where it is swallowed.

Chances of sinusitis rise when natural defenses are challenged—during times of stress, exposure to pollution, or after taking antibiotics. The condition usually begins with the common cold, but sinusitis is also associated with cigarette smoke, air pollution, food and respiratory allergies, dry air, infection or trauma to the upper teeth, and anatomical problems such as polyps or a deviated septum. When these irritants or conditions cause swelling, increased mucus production, or damage to the cilia, the sinus ducts can become blocked, creating a sealed breeding ground for microbes.

Diagnosing Sinusitis

Doctors usually diagnose sinusitis based upon symptoms and physical examination. If your child develops chronic sinusitis, an otolaryngologist will look up his nose with a thin, flexible, fiber-optic instrument called an endoscope and use it to withdraw infected mucus from the sinuses for a culture, and perhaps do minor surgical procedures. Sinus X-rays are an unreliable diagnostic test, in part because ordinary conditions like the common cold can produce abnormal results. Of these tests, only a culture of sinus

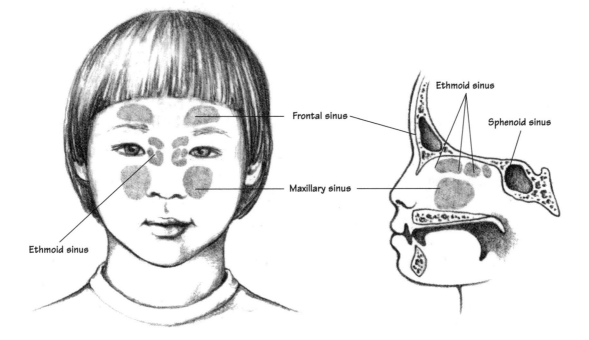

Locations of the paranasal sinuses

mucus can distinguish between viral and bacterial sinus infections.

Conventional Medical Treatment

Conventional medical treatment involves medications for relieving pain and lowering fever, improving sinus drainage, and eliminating the infection. Beware of the many over-the-counter sinus drugs that contain antihistamines. Instead of helping mucus drain from the sinuses, these ingredients thicken it, making it harder to expel. They cause drowsiness, too.

In fact, a study of children with nasal congestion from colds has found that taking a placebo or no treatment is just as effective as taking Dimetapp. Scrutinize drug labels of sinus medications and avoid those that contain antihistamines (diphenhydramine, brompheniramine, chlorpheniramine, phenyltoloxamine).

A pure decongestant can relieve stuffiness. This type of drug works by constricting small blood vessels, which, in turn, reduces the swelling of the mucous membranes. Oral decongestants (e.g., pseudoephedrine, phenylpropanolamine, phenylephrine) can produce side effects: jitteriness, insomnia, and increases in heart rate and blood pressure.

Alternatively, your child can use decongestants as a nasal spray. This way, the drug acts locally, largely avoiding the side effects above. Do take care to avoid rebound congestion by limiting use to only two or three days.

The objective of antibiotic therapy for sinusitis, of course, is to eliminate the infecting bacteria. The usual culprits of acute sinusitis are the same bacteria that cause most middle-ear infections: *Streptococcus pneumoniae, Hemophilus influenzae,* and *Moraxella catarrhalis.* Because doctors don't routinely take sinus cultures, they often select an antibiotic effective against all three. Unfortunately, such antibiotics are usually expensive, and getting therapeutic levels of oral antibiotics into infected sinus cavities isn't easy.

Like acute middle-ear infection, acute sinusitis often disappears without antibiotic treatment. A study of children with acute sinusitis found that antibiotics had little effect on the time to improvement. In fact no studies have yet shown that antibiotics work to help kids with sinusitis.

Is there harm in treating sinusitis with antibiotics? Possibly. In a telephone interview, Erdem Cantekin, Ph.D, Professor of Otolaryngology at the University of Pittsburgh School of Medicine, cites four reasons antibiotics can actually worsen sinusitis.

1. Antibiotics kill bacteria in larger numbers than does the immune system. The toxic debris left behind from bacterial overkill, which can't be cleared fast enough by immune cells, can temporarily damage the mucous membranes and result in further congestion.

2. Antibiotics kill the nasal passage's natural flora, which maintain health by preventing other bacteria from growing.

WHEN TO CALL A DOCTOR ABOUT SINUS PROBLEMS

Your child has failed to improve despite three days of home care, or his symptoms worsen

Your child acts very sick

Your child develops symptoms of middle-ear infection, which often occurs along with acute sinusitis

You suspect your child has stuck a foreign object up his nose

3. Overuse use of antibiotics puts pressure on the infecting bacteria to mutate, leading to the emergence of antibiotic-resistant "super bugs."

4. If the infection is actually viral, antibiotics not only fail to work but actually slow recovery by impairing immune function.

Our take-home message on antibiotics for sinusitis: If your child seems to have a mild to moderate case, follow our guidelines for home care and stay in touch with your health-care practitioner. However, if one of our children became sick with presumed sinusitis, and if natural therapies hadn't helped much, and if our physician recommended antibiotics, we would go ahead and fill that prescription.

Surgical Treatment

If medical treatment fails and the sinusitis becomes chronic, an ear, nose, and throat specialist may recommend surgery to correct structural abnormalities or to enlarge the opening to the maxillary sinus. Our advice: If your doctor recommends surgery for your child, get a second opinion. If no anatomic problem underlies the chronic sinus condition, consult a holistic health practitioner to help you investigate possible allergies, and food intolerances or explore other options.

Home Care for the Sinuses

As always, encourage your child to eat well and drink lots of fluids, especially warm liquids such as tea and broth.

Humidify your indoor air, especially during winter months, and keep the machine clean.

Keep your child away from cigarettes and other sources of smoke. Generally strive for clean

---

IF SINUSITIS BECOMES CHRONIC

Take your child to an otolaryngologist to make sure there's no anatomic abnormality or foreign object lodged in the nasal passages.

Get serious about cleaning up your indoor air. You may want to invest in an efficient air cleaner, such as a high-efficiency particulate-arresting (HEPA) filter or negative-ion generator. The latter is said to eliminate dust, pollens, animal dander, and microbes while adding health-enhancing negative ions to the air.

Identify and treat underlying allergies and food intolerances. Obtain the help of a medical or naturopathic practitioner with training in allergies.

If your child has airborne allergies, regular nasal douching can reduce allergens that adhere to the nasal passages. Freeze-dried stinging nettles taken internally have been successfully used to treat allergic rhinitis and may provide a natural alternative to over-the-counter antihistamines; you can also use steamed or dried nettles.

Consider Chinese Medicine. We believe acupuncture can help correct imbalances that may underlie chronic infection. A well-placed needle can stimulate sinus drainage. See a licensed acupuncturist for assistance.

Acupressure follows the same principles as acupuncture, using finger pressure instead of needles.

indoor air. If you don't need a wood stove for heat, don't use it.

Give your child lots of TLC and rest. For many children, television and movie videos are not restful; instead, try music, or books on tape.

Help your child to safely inhale steam, our favorite home treatment for nose and sinus congestion. Steam helps loosen mucus, soothes dry membranes, decongests, and may relieve sinus headache. By adding antiseptic or decongestant herbs such as eucalyptus, peppermint, thyme, sage, and lemon grass, or two to three drops of their essential oils, you can increase the steam's therapeutic effect.

Let your child wash out her nose. Sounds yucky, but it works. Nasal irrigation decreases congestion, diminishes sinus pain, and washes away pollutants, microbes, and infected mucus (it works best if you first use steam to loosen the mucus). Make a salt-water solution by mixing 1/4 teaspoon of salt in one cup warm water. Pour the salt water into a spray bottle or fill an ear syringe, a small cup, or a container with the solution.

Demonstrate for your child how you irrigate one nostril at a time, closing the other nostril with your finger. Holding your head sideways over the sink with your forehead slightly higher than your chin, gently pour the solution into the uppermost nostril. For very small children, use an eyedropper to put ten to twenty drops of salt solution into each nostril, then gently suction out the fluid with a bulb syringe. Never force water up the nose. You can also add antibacterial herbs such as a cooled, strained decoction of Oregon graperoot to the salt solution. Alternatively, add a few drops of a glycerite. (*Never add alcohol tincture, which irritates the mucous membranes.*)

Warm baths can also help your child feel better, especially if you strain the herbal infusion from your steam inhalation pot into the tub.

A wet, hot-to-tolerance towel placed over your child's face can promote drainage and increase blood flow to the sinuses. Some children prefer to ice the area. A good compromise is to alternate heat and cold.

Teach your child the art of gently blowing her nose into a tissue, then disposing of it properly and washing her hands. Kids tend to sniff, which can suck infected secretions into the sinuses and may create extra pressure on the eustachian tubes, which drain the middle ears.

Herbal Care for Sinusitis

Herbs to Relieve Stuffiness

Although studies have not found that inhaling aromatic herbs measurably improves airflow to the lungs, this technique often helps a sinusitis sufferer feel better.

Lemon balm is soothing to the mucous membranes and calming to sick kids. It also tastes great in a glycerite or served as tea with honey. Lemon balm has documented antiviral and antibacterial activity.

Mint. Peppermint and spearmint decrease sinus stuffiness and pain and are antiseptic. Both taste good, too.

Cayenne. According to Chinese medicine principles, this herb is warming, helps move the blood, and remedies the malaise of colds and flus. Like many spicy foods, it creates the sensation of "opening the sinuses." Taken internally, it helps relieve headaches. If your child can easily swallow tablets, give her a capsule that you've half emptied, then reassembled. Be sure that she can swallow it, though; there is nothing more irritating to the esophagus than a half-swallowed cayenne capsule! Always take cayenne with food.

Horseradish is antimicrobial and also produces that sinus-clearing sensation. When your child complains of sinus congestion, start adding horseradish to the diet. Green Japanese horseradish, or wasabi, is exceptionally powerful and makes a great condiment for rice dishes and sushi. A dash of wasabi the size of a pencil eraser is usually enough to clear the sinuses (and possibly bring tears to the eyes).

Ginger is warming, which can help if your child feels chilled or has a lot of mucus; don't use it, however, if your child is feverish. It is also antimicrobial and anti-inflammatory. Like cayenne and horseradish, it acts as a circulatory stimulant to loosen thick mucus.

Ephedra, also known as *ma huang,* contains the alkaloid ephedrine, from which the over-the-counter medication pseudoephedrine is derived. This herb is a powerful and appropriate decongestant, but must be used carefully. Because it

stimulates the central nervous and cardiovascular systems, it shouldn't be used for long, nor in high doses. We advise you to reserve ephedra for children over seven years old or weighing over 50 pounds. Because dieters and those seeking a legal "high" have abused ephedra, resulting in harmful side effects, children under the age of eighteen cannot purchase the herb in some states.

Nettles have been used successfully in clinical studies in freeze-dried leaf form to reduce the symptoms of allergic rhinitis (hay fever), especially if inhaled allergens have provoked the nasal congestion. Nettles must be steamed or dried to destroy their sting. We've found that liquid extracts and capsules are as effective as freeze-dried nettles. A 50-pound child could take one capsule per day for several days, increasing to three times per day if the herb is well tolerated.

Herbs to Support Natural Immunity

Echinacea boosts natural immunity. Research shows it is antiviral, antibacterial, and anti-inflammatory. We start giving three or four doses a day to our kids the minute we suspect they may have a cold, flu, or sinus infection.

Astragalus supports natural immunity. Like echinacea, it increases the production of interferon, the body's own antiviral compound. It also helps prevent viruses from infecting the respiratory tract.

Licorice root. This herb is anti-inflammatory and soothes irritated mucous membranes; test-tube studies indicate that it interferes with viral replication and the activity of some bacteria. Most kids like the taste of licorice, providing the tea is not brewed for more than ten minutes.

Herbs to Relieve Sinus Headaches

Meadowsweet contains salicin, the pain-relieving precursor to aspirin. Although a bit bitter, it's safe for children; we often add it to pain formulas.

A COMBINATION PRODUCT FOR SINUSITIS

Sinupret is a popular over-the-counter herbal formula in Germany. It contains five powdered herbs: gentian root, cowslip flowers, sour dock or sorrel, elder flowers, and European vervain. The German Commission E has approved it for treatment of acute and chronic sinus inflammation. The herbs seem to work mostly by breaking up mucus so that it is more easily expelled.

Four studies have compared Sinupret favorably to either placebo or conventional treatment. Although Sinupret isn't yet available in the United States, at least one American company has started selling a product using these plants.

Feverfew relieves the pain and inflammation of migraine and other headaches, perhaps because of anti-inflammatory effects similar to those of aspirin. In test-tube studies, parthenolide, a chemical contained in feverfew, inhibits the growth of certain yeasts and bacteria, including *Staphylococcus*. The herb's antihistamine ability also shows great promise, a potential boon for allergy-related sinusitis. Feverfew tastes bitter, so it goes down best in capsules or glycerite.

Willow bark was used by dozens of Native American tribes and American settlers for pain; however, it tastes very bitter.

Antibacterial Herbs

Oregon graperoot helps reduce excess mucus. Although older herb books may recommend goldenseal for sinus inflammations, we suggest you try Oregon graperoot instead; it's safe and effective.

Usnea lichen helps combat many bacteria including strep, the most common cause of bacterial

---

SINUSITIS-FIGHTING GLYCERITE

For ages: 1 year and up
Yields: 1½ cups

1/4 cup Oregon graperoot
    (antibiotic, astringent)

1 fresh garlic clove
    (antibiotic, antiviral)

1 tablespoon echinacea root and seeds
    (antibiotic, immune stimulant)

1 tablespoon eyebright herb
    (anti-inflammatory, astringent)

1 tablespoon thyme leaf
    (antibacterial, expectorant)

1 teaspoon peppermint leaf
    (decongestant, antibacterial)

1 teaspoon licorice root
    (anti-inflammatory, antiviral)

1 teaspoon ginger
    (anti-inflammatory, warming)

1 teaspoon ephedra leaf
    (for children over 7 years only;
      decongestant, stimulant)

2½ cups vegetable glycerine

1⅛ cups distilled water

Directions: Mix glycerine and water. Grind all dried herbs to the consistency of coarse powder in a clean coffee grinder. Chop garlic fine. Pour herbs into a quart canning jar; cover with glycerine and water mixture, and shake until all herbs are moist. Cap tightly and store in a cool, dry area. Shake daily. After two weeks, strain well, once through cheesecloth, then a second time through a fine cloth. Pour into clean, brown-glass dropper bottles and label with formula name, date, and dosage. Refrigerated, the glycerite should be good for a year or more.

Dose: As needed to prevent and relieve symptoms of sinusitis. For a 50-pound child, start at 20 drops once a day, increasing to 20 drops three times a day if tolerated. Use for seven days, then take a two-day break before continuing.

Caution: Ephedra is a very effective nasal decongestant, but its stimulant effects are contraindicated for children under age 7. Some children will have difficulty sleeping if given products containing ephedra after 4 P.M.

sinusitis. It's also anti-inflammatory and boosts immune function. In Europe, a small clinical trial showed that children who took a preparation of usnic acid had greater resistance to colds and flu. Because usnea's helpful ingredients extract poorly into water, we recommend using a tincture.

Garlic is partially excreted via the lungs. When your child exhales through his nose, he gets some of the active ingredients right where you want them. Garlic is a potent antibiotic and antiviral.

Garden sage decreases excess secretions, contains ingredients that are active against staph bacteria, and has antiviral activity. The aromatic oils in sage help create a tasty infusion that's high in minerals; add a little honey for flavor. Sage tea makes an effective gargle for sore throats, too. Just don't mistake sagebrush for garden sage—they're completely different plants. Sagebrush is very bitter and toxic when taken in large doses.

For Further Reading

Ivker, R. *Sinus Survival: The Holistic Medical Treatment for Allergies, Asthma, Bronchitis, Colds, and Sinusitis.* Los Angeles: Jeremy P. Tarcher, 1995.

SINUS-CLEARING HERBAL INHALER

You can make your own inhaler. To do so, you'll need:

A clean, 1-ounce glass jar and tight-fitting lid (a tincture bottle with the glass dropper removed works well)

4 drops essential oil of peppermint, eucalyptus, rosemary, thyme, or a combination.

Cotton ball

Chopstick

Directions: Press the cotton ball into the bottle with the chopstick. Drop the essential oil onto the cotton. Seal.

Voila! You have a simple, inexpensive herbal inhaler. The scent should last at least a week or two; discard after use.

Caution: Allow kids to use the inhaler only with adult supervision. Keep out of reach of small children.

SUNNY'S APPROACH: SINUSITIS ON THE ROAD

On a road trip, my husband and I stopped at a hotel late at night, and Doug developed uncomfortable sinus inflammation. He was coming down with a minor head cold, but the sinus pain came on suddenly after driving over the Rocky Mountains to a lower elevation. Stuck in a hotel room in a strange town, we found an all-night market and bought a piece of ginger. We diced the fresh ginger into tiny pieces with a pocket knife and twisted them into a hot, moist washcloth. Placing this hot, home-made poultice directly over Doug's nose and cheeks brought quick relief.

For the next hour, we put hot washcloths on top of the gingerroot compress every few minutes. Doug awakened in the morning with all pain resolved.

To use this poultice on your child, just be sure that the washcloth isn't too hot; check after the first few minutes for skin reactions.

Chapter 12

EAR INFECTIONS

You might just as well say, "Misery for all concerned, especially the child."
But earaches aren't just painful, they're prevalent—the number-one reason that parents take their kids to the doctor, and the number-one
physician's diagnosis for children under two years old. Two-thirds of kids
suffer one or more episodes of middle-ear infection during the first year of
life, and half have endured three infections by the age of three years.
Most kids stop getting middle-ear infections after age seven, but for
their worried parents, it can seem as if that magical time will never come.

Accurate diagnosis of ear infections isn't easy. Many experts feel the illness is overdiagnosed and overtreated with antibiotics. Even worse, middle-ear inflammation can persist or recur. Plus, ear infections can hurt. They can make a normally placid child whine or wail—for hours. No wonder parents of children with recurring ear infections have a particular, shell-shocked, sleepless look.

Middle-ear infections are just one of three types of ear inflammation that children can get. There are also outer-ear infections and inner-ear infections. In small children, however, middle-ear infections are the most common and bothersome. Here's why.

Structure. The eustachian tube connects the middle-ear cavity to the throat, allowing air to be exchanged and secretions to drain. Compared to adults and older children, an infant's eustachian tubes are shorter, less angled, and have less carti-lage to keep them open. These factors increase the likelihood that microbes will migrate from

the throat up the eustachian tubes. During a cold or allergic reaction, these microorganisms can become trapped in the middle-ear cavity, setting the scene for a classic ear infection.

Lymphoid tissue. This is the stuff of which ton-sils and adenoids are made. Infants have a lot of it in their throats. This tissue, while valuable for immune functioning, can swell and block the eustachian tube, resulting once again in the kind of environment bacteria love—a closed one.

Immune immaturity. The immune system's ability to react to harmful bacteria doesn't begin to form until around the sixth month of life and doesn't mature until the second year. Because of immune-system immaturity, some infants can catch frequent colds, and colds often precede ear infections.

Genetics. If your child has inherited flat eustachian tubes or a congenital anatomic prob-lem such as cleft palate, he may be predisposed to recurrent ear infections.

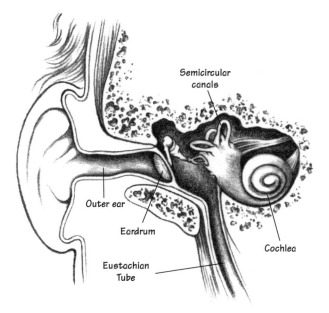

The structure of a child's ear, with its shorter and more horizontal eustachian tube, makes it prone to ear infections.

In other words, the major causes of ear infections are outside your control. Here are a few causes that *can* be controlled.

Day-care attendance can expose your child to increased viral upper respiratory infections; small children in day care run twice the risk of repeated ear infections. Children in day care who are on antibiotics to prevent recurring middle-ear infections may carry, and hence pass along, antibiotic-resistant organisms. Experts blame increased day-care attendance for the corresponding increase in middle-ear infections over the past two decades.

Using pacifiers seems to increase the risk of middle-ear infection.

Siblings at home mean more exposure to respiratory infections, especially colds. This doesn't mean you should send the older kids off to boarding school. We handle this problem by giving each child immune-supporting herbs at the first signs of illness.

Tobacco smoke contributes to 3.4 million doc-

tor's visits for acute middle-ear infection and 110,000 surgeries for persistent middle-ear fluid or persistent middle-ear inflammation. Any smoke, including that from wood-burning stoves, can cause problems.

Baby formulas lack the immunologic goodies provided by breast milk, and infants can develop allergies to the cow's milk and soy proteins upon which formulas are often based. Bottle-propping can cause fluids to flow backward up the eustachian tube, promoting ear infection.

Cold weather brings with it many respiratory tract viruses, and dry indoor air, especially with forced-air heating, can irritate the upper respiratory tract. Being cooped up inside with windows shut increases kids' exposure to germs. Cold weather itself does not cause infections.

Recurrent antibiotic use wipes out the "friendly" bacteria that normally thwart disease-causing bacteria from colonizing the respiratory tract. In addition, antibiotic use increases bacterial resistance, rendering commonly prescribed antibiotics ineffective.

Food intolerances are suspected to play a role in recurring ear infections. See Chapter 7, Allergies.

Symptoms of Middle-Ear Infections

As with colds, most middle-ear infections occur in winter. And a cold usually precedes the ear infection, although allergies and air pollutants can also initiate the process. The first step is inflammation, usually of the throat, tonsils, adenoids, or ears; infection comes later. Coughing, sniffling, and nose-blowing can propel bacteria and viruses from the nose and throat into the middle ear. Swollen respiratory passages and mucus block the eustachian tube, interfering with air pressure regulation and trapping secretions and microbes in the middle ear. (Bacteria cause most—70 to 90 percent—but not all middle-ear infections.)

The child's immune system dispatches white blood cells to the middle ear. These cells kill bacteria, but they also aggravate inflammation. The resulting fluid accumulates and distends the eardrum, often causing piercing pain.

Many middle–ear infections result in the sometimes inconsolable fussing and crying that tries parents' nerves. Other ear infections produce only minimal symptoms. Symptoms of ear infections may include fever, crying, irritability, clinginess, ear pain, or tugging at the ear. The child may also have pinkeye; his appetite declines because it hurts to swallow. Babies with ear infections may cry when they suckle, because this action aggravates pain-producing pressure changes in the ear. The pain can disrupt sleep for the child (and for anyone else in the house).

After the infection subsides, middle-ear fluid can persist for several weeks, but it usually resolves without treatment.

Diagnosing a Middle-Ear Infection

Your health-care practitioner will examine the ear drum with a lighted instrument called an otoscope. The examiner inserts the tapered tip into the ear canal and puffs in air with a hand-held bulb. A diagnosis of acute middle-ear infection requires the following: the eardrum appears red (or yellow when pus collects behind it), thickened, and barely moves with the puff of air. A sure diagnosis requires all three signs.

But accurately diagnosing acute middle-ear infection is challenging, particularly in infants who have tiny ear canals and rarely cooperate with the exam. Also, their eardrums slant away from the horizontal plane and don't move as freely with the air puffs. Throw in a glob of ear wax and, unless the examiner can scoop it out, she can't see a thing. Even trained practitioners, using the best instruments, often can't make a firm diagnosis, so we don't advise spending a lot of money buying your own otoscope.

Conventional Treatment

Physicians typically treat middle-ear infections with pain relievers, decongestants, antihistamines, and antibiotics.

The pain relievers may be taken orally—acetaminophen, for instance—or applied as ear drops that contain benzocaine and antipyrine. A

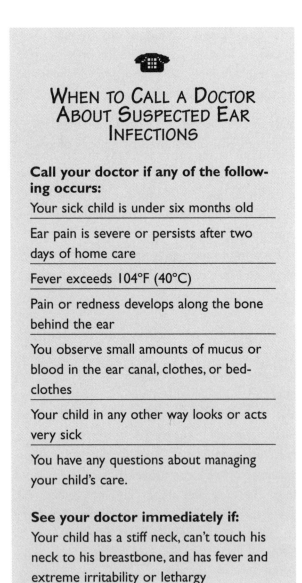

WHEN TO CALL A DOCTOR ABOUT SUSPECTED EAR INFECTIONS

Call your doctor if any of the following occurs:

Your sick child is under six months old

Ear pain is severe or persists after two days of home care

Fever exceeds 104°F (40°C)

Pain or redness develops along the bone behind the ear

You observe small amounts of mucus or blood in the ear canal, clothes, or bedclothes

Your child in any other way looks or acts very sick

You have any questions about managing your child's care.

See your doctor immediately if:
Your child has a stiff neck, can't touch his neck to his breastbone, and has fever and extreme irritability or lethargy

commonly used brand of pain-relieving ear drops is Auralgan Otic.

Decongestants and antihistamines are prescribed in an effort to eliminate the fluid behind the ear drum, despite studies that show such medication is ineffective. In addition, decongestants can make children feel wired and irritable. Antihistamines dry respiratory secretions, making them harder to expel, and this buildup thwarts other efforts toward healing a cold. Antihistamines also can provoke nightmares, sleepiness, and sometimes a paradoxical agitation.

SEVEN WAYS TO REDUCE YOUR CHILD'S RISK OF MIDDLE-EAR INFECTIONS

You can't change the structure of your children's ears—but you can help tip the odds in their favor. Here's how.

Maintain a smoke-free environment.

If possible, breast-feed your babies for six months or more. Mother's milk is not only rich in immunities, but the baby's position and sucking action decrease the risk of fluids entering the middle ear. Compared to formula-fed babies, infants exclusively breast-fed for the first four months have half the number of ear infections during their first six months of life. Furthermore, prolonged nursing (six months or more) decreases the risk of allergic diseases, and diminished allergies decrease the risk of middle-ear infection.

If you bottle-feed your baby—and we realize breastfeeding isn't always feasible—hold your child with her head higher than her chest, and never put her to bed with a bottle.

Delay solid food until six months, unless your physician advises differently, to short-circuit the development of allergies.

Find optimal child care. As we mentioned in earlier chapters, exposure to more kids means exposure to more colds. Look for a situation where your young one will share a room with six or fewer children.

Let kids older than three chew gum. Chewing gum helps exercise the muscles around the eustachian tube. In one two-month study of 306 children in 11 day care nurseries in Finland, kids who chewed two pieces of xylitol gum five times a day after meals and snacks for two months suffered about 30 percent fewer bouts of middle-ear infections than kids who chewed a sucrose gum. Both xylitol and sucrose are sweeteners, but xylitol inhibits *Streptococcus pneumoniae,* a common cause of ear, throat, and sinus infections. In another Finnish study, kids who recieved either xylitol gum or syrup also contracted fewer ear infections. We expect to see more research on xylitol products, because they also help reduce cavities. (Infants and children three or younger shouldn't have gum because they could choke on it.)

Keep your child out of deep water. If your child experiences middle- or outer-ear infections, he probably shouldn't go off the diving board or submerge his head in more than two feet of water until the infection is completely cleared. Water skiing raises the risk of eardrum ruptures.

The most frequent reason for children's antibiotic use in the United States is middle-ear infection. Doctors sometimes prescribe antibiotics when they're not certain of the diagnosis but want to eliminate bacterial infection as a possible cause of discomfort.

Children suffering from mild or moderate middle-ear infection can benefit from watchful waiting—a cautious but attentive approach that begins with relieving pain symptoms, but refrains from giving antibiotics unless the child's condition worsens. However, it does mean that, if symptoms continue, the doctor must see the child two or more times in a short period to evaluate the progress of the infection. Many pediatricians, particularly in Europe, have adopted this restrained approach, reserving drugs for the estimated one out of seven children who can benefit from antibiotics either because they are overwhelmed by infection or because complications seem imminent.

Many American pediatricians have also called for restraint, recommending that antibiotics be reserved for children who have substantial signs and symptoms of infectious illness, not just middle-ear fluid. The consensus is that antibiotics, a godsend when really needed, are just plain overused.

But here's the rub: Early in the course of the illness, it's hard to know which kids will develop more serious disease. For watchful waiting to work, a physician must feel confident that the parent will bring the child back for a follow-up appointment. This approach, then, requires a trusting relationship between the doctor and the parent.

Can Ear Infections Cause Hearing Loss?

The jury's still out on whether the temporary hearing loss that accompanies middle-ear fluid has any long-term effects on language development and hearing. Numerous studies have failed to show a significant correlation between children's ear infections and long-term hearing loss.

According to Donna Whitman, a physician assistant specializing in otolaryngology in Montana, the average ear infection causes about the same temporary decrease in hearing as wearing a pair of inexpensive ear plugs— in other words, mild. But even a small hearing loss could prevent a young child from picking up subtle speech and language clues, possibly delaying development.

Ear Tubes: A Last Resort

When middle-ear infection resists antibiotic treatment, when infection recurs, or when middle-ear fluid persists longer than three months and creates hearing loss in both ears, the doctor may recommend the placement of tympanostomy tubes, or ear tubes. While the child is under general anesthesia, the doctor (usually an otolaryngologist, a specialist in ear, nose and throat concerns) inserts tiny tubes through incisions in the child's eardrum.

The idea is that these tubes facilitate ventilation of the middle ear, allow secretions to drain, and restore hearing ability. Yet middle-ear fluid tends to resolve on its own and recurs frequently in small children, and no proof exists that this surgery prevents hearing loss. Nevertheless, ear-tube insertion is one of the most commonly performed operations on American children, and about 20 percent of kids end up with a second set of tubes when the first ones fall out after a few months and middle-ear fluid accumulates again. Although most experts acknowledge that ear tubes, when truly indicated, help kids by reducing recurring infections, they also agree that this surgery is done too often. Ear-tube surgery does carry potential complications: chronic perforations, scarring, and weakening of the eardrum.

As with most treatments, ear tubes have their place. The toddler years, critical times for speech and language development, require good hearing. If chronic ear fluid interferes with your child's hearing and speech or he suffers from frequent middle-ear infections, he may benefit from tubes. Talk it over with your doctor.

The Other Ear Infections

Outer-ear infections, commonly known as "swimmer's ear," explains the most typical cause.

In young children, foreign bodies such as beans, peas, or small toys lodged in the ear canal also can generate an outer-ear inflammation, marked by pain, ear discharge, and possibly diminished hearing. Treatment involves cleaning the ear canal once or twice a week, eliminating infection with antimicrobial drops, reducing pain, keeping the child out of the water, and, if a foreign body is present, removing it. Unless you can see the foreign body hanging out of the ear canal, don't try to remove it.

MIDDLE-EAR INFECTIONS AND ANTIBIOTICS: THE RESEARCH

Below are the results of some studies of the effectiveness of using antibiotics to treat middle-ear infections.

Researchers in the Netherlands compared antibiotics, myringotomy (a surgical incision on the eardrum to allow drainage of middle-ear fluid), and placebo treatment of middle-ear infection and found no significant difference in how kids healed.

A Scandinavian study found that kids who received penicillin or placebo fared equally well after one week. Penicillin diminished ear pain by the second day of treatment. No complications occurred in either group.

In a large trial, 4,860 Dutch children with middle-ear infections initially received only nose drops and analgesics for symptomatic relief; more than 90 percent recovered within a few days. When antibiotics were used for the sicker children, they responded well and without complications.

In an international study, researchers found that antibiotic use for middle-ear infection varies widely. In Australia, Great Britain, New Zealand and the United States, 98 percent of patients with middle-ear infections receive antibiotics, but only 31 percent of Dutch patients recieve them. Doctors in the United States typically recommend antibiotics for eight to ten days, but European doctors delay antibiotics for two or three days and then give them for five to seven days. Regardless of where and how used, the study found that antibiotics do not improve the rate of recovery.

An analysis of twenty-seven trials involving 6,932 patients shows that three to five days of antibiotics works as effectively as ten days.

A Scandinavian study found that giving antibiotics at the onset of an ear infection increases the chance of recurrent infections nearly threefold. Delaying antibiotics until complications threaten only raises the recurrence rate by a third. Why does prompt use of antibiotics increase disease recurrence? No one knows. One theory is that a child's immune system doesn't have a chance to recognize and mount a response that can lead to later immunity.

You could unintentionally damage the eardrum. Far better to have your health-care provider do this.

Inner-ear infections typically show up as a rare complication of a viral or bacterial infection originating outside the ear. Symptoms include dizziness and often nausea and vomiting. Treatment involves easing nausea and treating the underlying infection. If you suspect your child has an inner-ear problem, take her to your doctor. This isn't a case for home remedies.

Home Care for Middle-Ear Infections

Don't hesitate to call your doctor when your child shows signs of a middle-ear infection. Use these home-care measures as a complement to, but not a substitute for, medical treatment.

Cut down on congestion because congestion can spread to the middle ears. Encourage your child to drink lots of fluids, such as herbal teas and soup broths. Dilute or restrict juice, because its fruit sugars can reduce white-blood-cell activity. If secretions become thick and difficult to clear, you can give your child salt-water nose drops three times a day; mix your own by dissolving 1/4 teaspoon salt in an 8-ounce cup of warm water. Your older child may benefit from inhaling steam; see Chapter 9, Colds, for an herbal steam recipe. Run a humidifier in his room and clean it every couple of days.

Herbs that reduce congestion include eyebright, thyme, licorice, peppermint, and ginger. This blend is particularly appropriate if you suspect that colds, allergies, or food sensitivities contribute to your child's ear infection.

Ease pain. Most pediatricians recommend acetaminophen (Tylenol and other brands). Occasional use of acetaminophen is okay, but taking it regularly or in large doses can damage the liver.

Warm and cold packs can ease ear pain, too. If cold makes your child's ear feel better, use an ice pack or a bag of frozen vegetables—peas work well—covered with a clean cloth. If warmth is better, use a hot-water bottle or warm washcloth. We've filled a clean athletic sock with rice or

HOME TREATMENT FOR SWIMMER'S EAR

Remove water from the ear canal (outer ear) by irrigating the area with rubbing alcohol, the primary ingredient in most over-the-counter swimmer's-ear drops. Rubbing alcohol absorbs water lodged in the outer ear and dries the canal. Do not use for more than three days in a row to avoid further irritation, which could then increase the risk of bacterial infection.

After the ear has thoroughly dried from the alcohol wash, irrigate the ear canal with a solution of diluted vinegar to re-establish the natural acid balance in the ear (this neutralizes the alkalinity of the pool water). The recipe is simple: 1 tablespoon distilled vinegar and 1 tablespoon distilled water. Make fresh daily. Many kids who are in the pool daily use this solution before and after swimming to prevent swimmer's ear.

Avoid using herbal oils for your kid's case of swimmer's ear. While warm ear oils can greatly relieve the pain of a middle-ear inflammation, they can actually make things worse because the ear canal must dry out to heal swimmer's ear.

Call your health care provider if the irritation continues after three days of home care, or if your child develops a fever or yellowish ear discharge.

lentils, knotted it at the top, and microwaved it till warm. Always test the heat level of a warm pack on your own body first.

Elevate your child's head and chest. This may improve middle-ear drainage, and decrease the pressure and resulting pain of the infection. Slide a one- to two-inch stack of books under the head of your child's mattress; adding extra pillows may just give her a sore neck.

Use warm herbal oil. Ear oils relieve the pain of earache, although they don't directly relieve middle-ear infection. Relieving pain is half the battle, however, especially considering that many ear infections resolve without treatment. Health-food stores carry herbal ear-oil blends, but homemade oils are equally effective. St.-John's-wort oil works well; there's a recipe for it on the following page. Other herbs for ear oils include willow bark, meadowsweet, garlic, and mullein flowers. Because it takes two weeks to steep, you'll want to prepare before you need it.

To use ear oil, warm it first by placing the tightly-capped bottle in hot water for five to ten minutes. Remove the bottle, shake, and test the oil on your inner wrist; it should be quite warm, but not hot.

While your child lies on his side, put two or three drops into his ear canal. Push gently on the small flap of skin in front of the ear canal to force the air out of the canal and allow the oil to settle. Loosely plug the ear with cotton. Repeat up to four times a day and during the night as needed.

If you are visiting a doctor in the next few hours, we suggest that you just use a hot water bottle over the ear to relieve pain because the oil can interfere with the ear exam.

But let's say that you used these drops in the middle of the night to relieve your child's ear pain. The next morning, your child remains fussy and feverish. Wisely, you decide to take her to your doctor.

This means you'll need to clear the oil from the ear canals so the doctor can see the eardrum. First, make sure there is no blood or mucus on

HOME TREATMENT FOR IMPACTED EAR WAX

For children over two years old with excessive ear wax, fill a clean, 1-ounce bottle with cooking oil, preferably almond or olive. A clean tincture bottle with a dropper, sterilized by boiling, works well, too. Tighten the lid and place the entire bottle in a pan of hot water for five to ten minutes. Do not microwave.

Remove, shake, and test the oil on your inner wrist. The oil should be warm, but not hot. Place several drops in each of your child's ears before bedtime and cover each ear with clean cotton. In the morning, you will find that your child's ear wax has softened and dripped out.

We do not recommend the use of ear candles to remove wax from children's ears. From doctors and accident reports, we've heard several horror stories of burned ear canals.

CAUTION: Put nothing in the ear canal if your child has ear tubes, will soon be examined by a doctor, or shows signs of a perforated eardrum (drainage of pus or mucus from the ear).

Keep the otolaryngologists' motto ever in mind: "Never put anything smaller than your elbow in your ear." Tell your child that things in the too-small category include cotton swabs, hair pins, buttons, beads, peas, and Lego pieces.

the child's bedclothes or in her ear canal. Then instill several drops of room-temperature hydrogen peroxide into the ear canal. Push gently on the flap and the area just in front of the ear canal. Have your child lie on her side with that ear down so the oil and peroxide can drain out. Repeat on the other side. Do not insert cotton swabs into the ear canal, as injury to the ear drum could occur.

Compensate for antibiotic use. When your child needs antibiotics—and sometimes kids really benefit from them—replace normal intestinal flora with *Bifidobacterium bifidus* (for children under two) or *Lactobacillus acidophilus* (for those two years old and up).

Herbal Remedies

Immune Boosters

Echinacea is tops for fighting infection. It boosts the immune system, fights microbes, and augments the body's natural production of antiviral interferon. Echinacea is nontoxic, but this doesn't mean that if some is good, more is better. Reserve echinacea for times of illness and stay within recommended dosage guidelines. It's not necessary to use it when your child is well.

When our children start to show signs of an ear infection, we give them echinacea tea, glycerite, or capsules right away. The typical 50-pound child can take one capsule, one cup of tea, or one dose of liquid extract three times a day for a maximum of ten days.

EAR INFECTION INFUSED OIL

For ages: All
Yields: 1/3 to 1/4 cup
This oil can be used to relieve the pain of ear infection. The St.-John's-wort and calendula may also be used fresh; double the amounts.

1 to 4 cloves fresh garlic
    (antimicrobial, antifungal, antiviral)

2 tablespoons St.-John's-wort flowering tops
    (antibacterial, anti-inflammatory)

2 tablespoons calendula flowers
    (antifungal, anti-inflammatory)

1/2 cup extra virgin olive oil
    (carrier)

1 500-I.U. vitamin E oil capsule
    (antioxidant, preservative)

Crush or chop the garlic and other herbs. In a small, clean pan, mix the herbs and olive oil. Cover and heat at lowest temperature for 30 minutes. Stir frequently. Do not allow herbs to sizzle or burn, because essential oils will evaporate; crock pots are too hot. Remove from heat and allow to cool. Pour all ingredients into a small jar and cap tightly. Store at room temperature out of sunlight, shaking daily. After two weeks, strain through a tightly woven cloth to remove all herb residue. Puncture the vitamin E capsule and add the oil. Stir, pour into dark-colored, one-ounce dropper bottles and label. Refrigerate; the oil is good for one year.

Caution: Place nothing in the ear canal if your child has ear tubes, drainage from the ear, or will soon be examined by the doctor.

WHEN OUR KIDS HAVE MIDDLE-EAR INFECTIONS

Linda's approach: When my children were infants and toddlers, I took them to the pediatrician if I suspected middle-ear infections. I have an otoscope and can use it, but when they were little, scoping their ears only upset them, and I couldn't summon the tenacity for a good look. Ear exams on infants are tricky, even if the baby cooperates—which almost never happens. Also, babies can get sicker quickly.

If three things coincided—the doctor's exam disclosed a red, bulging eardrum, my child felt miserable, and the doctor believed antibiotics would relieve her suffering—I gave the prescription medicine (fortunately, this didn't happen often). To reduce pain and inflammation, I used warm herbal eardrops after the exam. My husband and I also fed our kids nutritious meals and gave the one who was ill herbal immune boosters and *acidophilus* or *bifidus* supplements.

When my kids were old enough to cooperate with an ear exam, I looked at their ears but still consulted their pediatrician whenever they acted very ill. If the exam and my child's symptoms suggested the early stages of an infection, I soon learned that I could often nip it in the bud with herbal ear-drops, immune boosters, and antimicrobials including Oregon graperoot and lots of garlic.

Sunny's approach: Both of my children have had several ear infections along with colds. Each time, they woke up in the middle of the night with blood-curdling screams from middle-ear pain and pressure. I examined and touched their ears and mastoid bones, looking for signs of infection or perforated eardrum. Finding none, I applied warmed herbal ear oil in both ears. Almost as soon as the warmth touched the ear canal, their crying stopped. The pain relief from the combination of heat and moisture seemed almost instantaneous.

I followed up by giving them good-sized doses of echinacea and Oregon graperoot glycerite, and skullcap or other calming herbs to settle them down. Sometimes we stayed up for a while, rocking, with a warm, moist washcloth on the inflamed ear. Before putting them back to bed, I elevated the head of the bed and turned on the humidifier.

For the next four days, my husband and I gave the kids echinacea, Oregon graperoot, and an antiviral herbal glycerite blend containing lemon balm, lemon thyme, and lemon grass. If the pain recurred, we used the ear oil. We cut dairy and soy from the diet to reduce congestion, and kept the kids home for a day or two. Sometimes we did herbal steams with a few drops of eucalyptus oil in a hot pot of water. We've never had an infection quickly recur.

Would I use this same approach for a child with painful, recurrent ear inflammations? Yes, but I'd also seek professional care from a naturopathic doctor to get down to the serious business of finding the root of the problem.

Oregon graperoot possesses strong antibiotic action against strep bacteria, the most common cause of bacterial middle-ear infections. Give your child fifteen drops of glycerite or one capsule three times per day; discontinue after seven days. (We generally don't blend Oregon graperoot into herbal ear oils because it stains when it drips out.)

Caution: Not for use during pregnancy or nursing.

Grapefruit extract is a commercial product made from the seeds and pulp of grapefruit. Besides acting as a broad-spectrum antibiotic, it's antifungal, too. Dilute it before using to protect your child's tender mucous membranes; read the package directions. Very dilute solutions can be used as an ear wash for swimmer's ear, and capsules or liquid taken internally help against middle-ear infections.

Garlic fights bacterial infections, including strep. Because it also works against fungus infections, use garlic during and after antibiotic therapy to combat the possibility of yeast infection.

Antiviral herbs such as astragalus, echinacea, lemon balm, St.-John's-wort, thuja, and thyme can help combat the common cold. Because upper respiratory congestion can block the eustachian tube, nipping a cold in the bud may drop the risk of a resultant middle-ear infection.

Lymph-Stimulating Herbs

Every day, the lymph nodes scattered throughout the body filter microbes and foreign bodies from the lymph. When infection strikes, lymph glands work extra hard. We use our favorite herbs to support our children's lymph flow.

Red root, a staple healing herb of the Choctaws, Eastern Shoshones, Lakotas and Ojibwa, was traditionally used to treat diarrhea, colds, and lung and stomach problems. Herbalist Michael Moore likes it for "kick-starting" congested lymphatic tissue. Red root must be used in alcohol-tincture form; its oils just won't extract into glycerine. We usually avoid alcohol tinctures for children, but a seven-day course of red root is considered safe. A 50-pound child can take 10 drops, three times a day. To prevent the tincture from irritating your child's throat, you can put the drops directly onto a small piece of bread or dilute them in a cup of water, tea, or juice.

Cleavers are usually used for urinary tract inflammations, but this herb is also effective as a lymphatic cleanser. If your child suffers from chronic ear inflammation, make a tea of this safe and gentle herb and give it three times a day for a week; you may notice a slight diuretic action. The fresh herb is much preferred to the dried.

Sedative Herbs

Don't forget the herbs that calm the nerves of kids (and their parents) during trying or painful times, including ear infections. Some of our favorites include chamomile, lemon balm, wild oats, skullcap, passionflower, and California poppy. Flower essences, particularly Rescue Remedy, also can help calm a fretful child; they're handy for those middle-of-the-night crying jags.

Other Complementary Therapies

Homeopathy. Many people swear by homeopathy, and there is some scientific evidence that homeopathic remedies can help ease the symptoms of ear infections. If you want to learn how to use homeopathic remedies for acute infections, you can take a class or consult one of the many books on homeopathy, such as *Homeopathic Medicine for Children and Infants* by Dana Ullman (Jeremy P. Tarcher, 1992). For best results, work with a professional homeopathic practitioner to find the correct remedy.

Traditional Chinese Medicine. We have both spoken with practitioners of this ancient system of medicine who believe that Chinese herbs and acupuncture can help heal ear infections. Both of us would turn to such a practitioner for additional support if a child had chronic ear infections.

Nutritional Support

Vitamins and minerals can supply necessary healing agents to a child's body. If your child has a poor diet or is just a picky eater, be sure to provide him with a multivitamin and multimineral supplement each day. Make sure he gets ample vitamin C and carotenes.

Essential fatty acids can provide tremendous anti-inflammatory dietary support for a child with recurrent ear infections. Several manufacturers now make flavored flaxseed oil and fish oil liquids and capsules that are palatable.

If Ear Infections Recur

If your child has chronic middle-ear fluid, allergies may be to blame. Most studies show that 85 to 93 percent of kids with chronic ear infections have allergies to inhalants, foods, or both. In this case, using antibiotics to kill bacterial infection in the ear doesn't get to the source of the problem: the congestion that builds up from the allergies.

A recent study of the impact of food allergens on chronic middle-ear fluid has found that eliminating common food allergens from children's diets improves their ear problems significantly. If you have an older child with recurrent middle-ear infection, consider working with an allergy specialist or naturopathic doctor. Also see Chapter 7, Allergies.

Recommended Reading

Schmidt, Michael A. *Healing Childhood Ear Infections: Prevention, Home Care, and Alternative Treatment.* Berkeley: North Atlantic Books, 1996.

WHEN AN EARDRUM RUPTURES

Sometimes the eardrum ruptures naturally. Most children with an eardrum tear will have a cold, pain, crying, and difficulty swallowing or nursing. Then again, some won't.

Suspect a ruptured eardrum when your child's severe ear pain suddenly vanishes; this perforation releases the pressure from infected mucus, and relieves the pain. You may notice a very small amount of blood-tinged pus or mucus on your child's clothes, bedclothes, or inside her ear canal.

To treat a ruptured eardrum, see your doctor as soon as possible for a diagnosis and antibiotic treatment. Put nothing into the ear—no herbal oils, no cotton swabs—because doing so could introduce infectious agents into the middle ear.

Ruptured eardrums generally heal all by themselves. Your child will need antibiotics to protect against infection and beneficial replacement bacteria such as acidophilus for digestion, but other treatment is rarely required. Very few children sustain significant, permanent hearing loss from a single rupture.

Chapter 13

SORE THROATS

Scratchy, hoarse, burning, throbbing: The discomfort of sore throat varies, depending upon the cause and the nature of the child. Rooting for your team at a swim meet can make you hoarse. Hay fever can give you a scratchy throat. Mouth-breathing during sleep can dry your throat, especially in arid climates. But the usual source of significant sore throat in kids is infection, most commonly viral infection. When bacteria are to blame, however, the culprit is usually strep, a microbe that parents should take seriously.

Sore throat ranks right up there with earache as a common reason for parents to take their child to the doctor. Parents make the trip for two main reasons: to seek a way to ease their child's pain and to find out if the cause is strep. If the sore throat has come with the other symptoms of a cold or the flu, the discomfort typically lasts three or four days, goes away without any medical treatment, and antibiotics won't do a lick of good. But if strep (or one of the rarer bacteria) has caused the illness, antibiotics can help. Sore throats of both kinds are quite contagious. The incubation period (the time between exposure and onset of symptoms) takes two to five days, so apparently healthy kids can spread the infection.

Types of Sore Throats
Viral Causes

Viral sore throats are often part of the package of a viral respiratory infection. With a cold, a child sniffles, sneezes, coughs, and may complain of a scratchy throat. Hoarseness or laryngitis develops when the voice box, or larynx, becomes inflamed. The sore throat your child may suffer when he has the flu goes along with other hallmarks of that syndrome: muscle aches, cough, headache, fever, and chills. Adenovirus causes flu-like symptoms with sore throat and pinkeye. Infectious mononucleosis—the "mono" that mainly afflicts teens and young adults—causes sore throats with fever, extreme malaise, fatigue, poor appetite, and enlarged lymph nodes.

So how do you tell—or at least hazard a guess—whether the cause of a sore throat is viral or bacterial? Runny nose and cough along with a sore throat usually indicate a viral respiratory tract infection. These rarely accompany strep.

Bacterial Causes

Strep (infection with the *Streptococcus pyogenes* bacteria) accounts for about 15 percent of all sore throats. During some times of the year, however, up to half of kids' sore throats may be due to strep. Prime symptoms are marked throat pain that worsens with chewing or swallowing and a fever above 101.3°F (38.5C). Kids may also complain of headache and stomachache, sometimes with vomiting. Their throats look fiery red, and often—but not always—have a whitish crud resembling cottage cheese on the tonsils and back of the throat. The lymph nodes in the sides of their necks become enlarged and tender.

Some strep bacteria occasionally produce toxins that cause other diseases. For instance, scarlet fever or scarlatina can develop after a day or two of fever and sore throat. The tongue at first looks white and furry, then very red, and tiny red dots appear in the throat, usually on the soft part above the uvula (the waggly thing that hangs down).

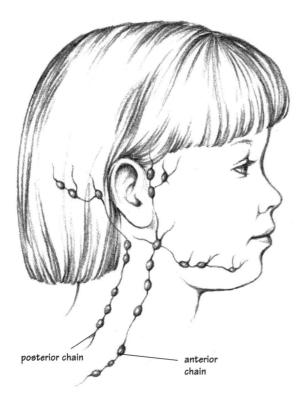

The cervical lymph nodes. In strep throat, the lymph nodes that run down the front of the neck—the anterior chain—become enlarged and tender.

Small bumps that feel like sandpaper appear on the base of the neck, face, and upper trunk, then spread. Most noticeable in the skin folds, the rash rarely affects the palms of the hands and soles of the feet. Later, the skin peels. This illness usually afflicts children between four and eight years old; by the age of ten, most kids have developed lifelong antibodies against this strep toxin, but not future strep infections.

Rare Bacterial Throat Infections

Deadly **diphtheria** epidemics once swept the United States, but this bug is now rare except among unvaccinated children. (The "D" in the DTP vaccine stands for diphtheria.) The illness, with symptoms that include sore throat, fever, diminished appetite, and enlarged lymph nodes, is distinguished by the formation of a grayish membrane around the tonsils that can span the throat. Diphtheria requires prompt treatment with antitoxin and antibiotics; don't try to manage this disease at home.

Epiglottitis is a potentially life-threatening bacterial infection of the flap of tissue that covers the upper airway during swallowing. The resultant swelling can impede or even stop airflow. Fortunately, vaccination against *Hemophilus influenzae*, called Hib vaccine, has greatly reduced incidences of epiglottitis and meningitis.

Distinguishing epiglottitis from croup may be tricky. Epiglottitis tends to strike rapidly and dramatically, with neither a recent cold nor a barky cough. Unlike croup, it often results in muffled voice, high fever, such difficulty swallowing that the child drools, and extending the neck forward to breathe. Croup tends to affect kids six months to three years old; epiglottitis affects kids from three to seven years old.

This serious illness requires immediate medical treatment with antibiotics and perhaps insertion of a tube into the airway. If you suspect your child has epiglottitis, call 911 for emergency transport to the hospital. Your child's epiglottis is behind the tongue; the adenoids are behind the nose.

Noninfectious Causes of Sore Throat

Hay fever can cause a mild throat irritation, and frequent clearing of the throat from the postnasal drip can aggravate it. Air pollutants or direct trauma, as from swallowing a very hot drink, can make the throat sore. People who breathe through open mouths at night may awaken with sore throats, especially if they live in dry climates. Kids with food or environmental sensitivities can have chronic hoarse voice. So can those with vocal nodules, which can be formed by chronic overuse or misuse of the voice.

Diagnosing Strep Throat

The main objective behind going to the doctor is to find out whether your child's sore throat has a viral or streptococcal origin. Distinguishing between the two can be tricky. The main strep symptoms—lack of cough, fever greater than 101.3°F (38.5°C), white crud on the tonsils, and tender lymph nodes in the neck—predict a positive throat culture only 50 percent of the time. Definitive diagnosis requires a positive result on one of two tests: a rapid strep test (based on recognition of strep antigens, substances that stimulate an immune response) or a throat culture. The rapid test gives results within fifteen to thirty minutes. Although you can trust a positive result, occasionally the result is falsely negative. This is why health practitioners usually follow this test with cultures that give results within one to two days. While these tests may add a few dollars to your bill, they're important for determining appropriate treatment.

Treating Sore Throat

If viral infection has caused the sore throat, antibiotics only wipe out the beneficial bacteria normally present in the body, thus eradicating a natural defense against infection. But if lab tests reveal strep, antibiotics can improve symptoms, usually within twenty-four to forty-eight hours. Doctors usually prescribe a ten-day course of penicillin, a relatively inexpensive antibiotic, for strep infections, but some newer drugs work just as effectively within five days. In addition to helping your child feel better sooner, the antibiotics can prevent complications such as scarlet or rheumatic fever. After twenty-four hours on antibiotics, your child is no longer contagious and can return to school if he feels up to it and you feel it's wise.

When antibiotic treatment for strep fails, it's often because the patient didn't take the antibiotic as prescribed. Because antibiotics—and antibacterial herbs—reduce symptoms within a day or two, it's easy to forget about taking the rest of the medication or to think it's no longer needed. Not completing the course, however, may contribute to developing antibiotic-resistant bacteria in the throat and perhaps a rebound infection with similar or worse symptoms. Be sure to give your child all the antibiotic prescribed. The same guideline holds for antimicrobial herbs such as echinacea, Oregon graperoot, thyme, and others: Keep taking them for several days after symptoms disappear.

Strep complications. Kids with strep need antibiotics because the infection can spread from the throat to the tissues behind the throat, middle ears, sinuses, lymph nodes, and lungs. Other complications—rheumatic fever or glomerulonephritis—can occur one to three weeks after infection.

Rheumatic fever manifests in a variety of symptoms, including some combination of fever, painful and swollen joints, a jerking movement known as chorea, heart inflammation, and skin rash. Sometimes it permanently damages the heart valves. Antibiotic treatment within a week of the onset of strep throat prevents it. Rheumatic fever is sneaky, though—sometimes it can appear after full treatment of strep, and in one-third of cases, after very mild infections.

WHEN TO CALL A DOCTOR ABOUT SORE THROATS

Call your pediatrician if:

Your sick child is under six months old

She complains of severe throat pain

He has a fever, sore throat, swollen lymph nodes in the neck, and no runny nose or cough

Her very sore throat is accompanied by voice changes and difficulty opening her mouth (signs of an abscess in the tissues behind the throat)

He makes a harsh sound when breathing in and has a barky cough (signs of croup)

One to three weeks after a sore throat, your child develops a red rash, fever with painful or swollen joints, involuntary jerking movements, rust-colored urine, or swelling of the eyelids, scrotum, feet, or legs (signs of complications of strep infection).

Dial 911 for emergency transportation to a hospital if:

Your sick child looks ashen, has such trouble swallowing he begins drooling, and speaks in a muffled voice (signs of epiglottitis)

Glomerulonephritis is an inflammation of the kidneys that follows infection of the throat or skin by certain strains of strep bacteria. Signs include elevated blood pressure, blood and protein in the urine (rust-colored pee), and swollen eyelids, scrotum, feet, and legs. Antibiotic treatment of the initial strep infection has only a small preventive effect, but antibiotics play an important role in treating it. Most children who develop this complication recover fully.

Our Antibiotic Compromise

If your child develops strep throat, she needs antibiotics. You can, however, support your child's health using natural strategies.

Know the typical symptoms of strep and those that point to a viral illness. If you suspect your child has a strep throat, go to your health practitioner for a rapid strep test and/or culture. If your child's rapid strep test is negative, you may safely choose to avoid antibiotics until results from the throat culture become available—usually two days.

Most pediatricians recommend that a child with a positive throat culture receive antibiotics to avoid complications of strep. Always finish the antibiotic prescription. If the label says to continue taking the pills for ten days, do so even if symptoms disappear.

Support your child's immune system with herbs at the very first signs of a cold or sore throat. (See a discussion of immune-boosting herbs in Chapter 9, Colds.) Use the herbs consistently: Give four to five child-sized doses during the first days of illness, and continue at least three times a day throughout the course of the sore throat and for several days afterwards.

During antibiotic therapy and for ten days afterwards, replenish your child's beneficial digestive-tract bacteria with a high-quality acidophilus/bifidus blend for children. Check the refrigerator section of your natural foods store for a brand with a high active-organism count and follow label directions. Keep acidophilus refrigerated at all times.

Home Remedies for Sore Throats

To relieve pain, we recommend tried-and-true home remedies. First, make sure your child drinks plenty of warm liquids such as herbal teas and vegetable broth.

Keep your child's neck warm. You can make a neck warmer by partially filling a long, clean sock with a grain such as rice, lentils, or split peas, knotting it at one end, and microwaving it for a minute or less until comfortably warm to the touch. Wrap the warmer around the neck, holding it in place with a bandanna.

If you'd like, first apply to the neck a mild aromatic salve containing thyme, eucalyptus, or other aromatic herbs, or two to three drops of these essential oils in a teaspoon of olive oil or almond oil. (Test a tougher area of skin, such as the arm, before using vapor balms or essential oils on young children's sensitive chest and neck skin.) Occasionally, a child with a warm constitution will ask for a cool washcloth instead of warmth.

Herbal Therapies for Sore Throats

For immune-enhancing herbs with a special affinity for sore throats, we often turn to echinacea, thyme, Oregon graperoot and astragalus. See the recipe on the following page for a general immune supporting glycerite.

Antimicrobial Herbs

Most studies of the infection-fighting power of herbs are test-tube studies—researchers drop some of the herb or some of its constituents on the bugs and see if they die. Positive results tell us nothing about whether the herb gets from the stomach to the site of infection in sufficient concentrations to kill microbes there, or in an effective form.

Such studies do suggest that applying particular herbal preparations to the infection may do some good. With strep throat, you can do this by spraying the preparation onto the back of the throat or by gargling with infusions or decoctions.

Garlic and **onions** both show lots of antiviral

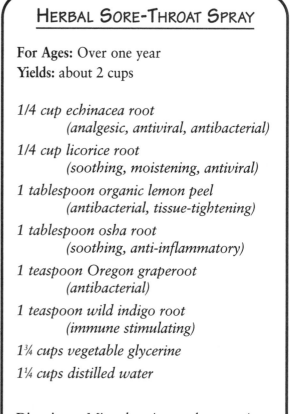

HERBAL SORE-THROAT SPRAY

For Ages: Over one year
Yields: about 2 cups

1/4 cup echinacea root
   (analgesic, antiviral, antibacterial)
1/4 cup licorice root
   (soothing, moistening, antiviral)
1 tablespoon organic lemon peel
   (antibacterial, tissue-tightening)
1 tablespoon osha root
   (soothing, anti-inflammatory)
1 teaspoon Oregon graperoot
   (antibacterial)
1 teaspoon wild indigo root
   (immune stimulating)
1¾ cups vegetable glycerine
1¼ cups distilled water

Directions: Mix glycerine and water in a clean canning jar. Grind herbs in a clean coffee grinder. Add to jar and seal tightly. Shake the jar daily for two weeks. Strain the herbs out of the glycerite and discard. Pour glycerite into one-ounce spray bottles available from your pharmacist or natural foods store. When needed, shake well and spray on irritated throat up to four times daily to relieve irritation and fight infection.

Caution: Not for use during pregnancy.

and antibacterial activity, including action against strep bacteria. Raw garlic is best for medicinal effect, but let's get real: all but the most hardy kids will want their garlic cooked.

Elecampane is antibacterial, relieves coughs, and soothes the inflammation of laryngitis; it also destroys herpes simplex II virus, and herbalists suspect it acts against other viruses as well. It's used as an expectorant for dry, irritable coughs and asthma.

Elecampane is generally sold in root form, so you can decoct it by boiling and disguise its bitter taste with honey, unless your kids prefer capsules.

Caution: Unless medically supervised, avoid elecampane during pregnancy or with diabetes.

Oregon graperoot contains a main constituent, berberine, that specifically destroys many types of bacteria, including strep. Its taste is bitter, so try it in glycerite form or capsules.

Lemon balm acts against a broad spectrum of disease-causing microbes. In test-tube studies, its volatile oils destroy bacteria—including strep—and a variety of viruses, including some that cause flu symptoms. Add this sweet-tasting herb to any healing tea or glycerite.

Usnea lichen is the green-gray "old man's beard" that hangs from tree branches. Besides making great costumes, this strange-looking lichen works against strep throat and other upper respiratory infections. Usnea also serves as a broad-spectrum antibiotic, reduces inflammation, and stimulates the immune system.

The strongest usnea products use alcohol to

IMMUNITY GLYCERITE FOR STREP THROAT

For ages: Over one year
Yields: About 24 one-ounce tincture bottles

1/4 cup echinacea root
       (antibacterial, immune support)

1/8 cup astragalus root
       (immune enhancing, lung support)

2 tablespoons thyme or lemon-thyme leaves
       (antibacterial, antiviral)

1 teaspoon Oregon graperoot
       (antibacterial)

1 teaspoon chamomile flower
       (antibacterial, anti-inflammatory,
          calming)

1 teaspoon plantain leaves
       (antibacterial, demulcent)

1 teaspoon hollyhock root or marshmallow
    root
       (antibacterial, immune supporting,
          demulcent)

2¾ cups vegetable glycerine

1¾ cups distilled water

3,000 mg vitamin C powder or ground
       tablets

In a blender or coffee grinder, grind all herbs to a coarse powder and set aside. Mix vegetable glycerine and distilled water in a 2-quart canning jar. Stir in herbs until all are moist. Cover tightly and shake well daily for two weeks. Strain once through loosely woven cheesecloth to remove herbs, and a second time through a tightly woven cloth or coffee filter to catch the fine particles. Add vitamin C powder to preserve. Bottle and label; shake well before each use. You'll have plenty, so share with your friends who have children. Store in refrigerator for up to one year.

Dosage: For a 50-pound child, give 20 drops, 3 to 4 times a day.

extract the herb's constituents into a tincture, although traditionally it was decocted into a tea. One herbalist in the Pacific Northwest, Cascade Anderson Geller, has made usnea spaghetti. The lichen must be boiled three times, in three different batches of water. In other words, bring the lichen, covered with water, to a boil and pour off the water. Again cover the usnea with water, boil, and decant the water. The third time, simmer the lichen for twenty minutes or so.

Geller warns that the lichen will still be chewy. "Eaten without this parboiling," she says, "it could make you sick and will definitely irritate your mouth. As for palatability, without a flavorful sauce, that is debatable."

Caution: Studies indicate that usnea is probably safe during pregnancy and nursing, although large doses in children or adults can cause vomiting.

Shiitake mushrooms can cost over ten dollars a pound—but we don't care. We love to cook with this powerful and tasty medicinal food. Luckily, just a small amount is effective; one to three lightly sauteed mushrooms per person is an adequate dose. Shiitakes have enjoyed a tremendous resurgence since research has confirmed their antiviral and immunostimulating effects. Unless your kids hate mushrooms, shiitakes are an excellent addition to vegetable soups and stir-fry meals during sore-throat season.

LINDA'S APPROACH: A MOM COPES WITH STREP

Both my children have had strep throat. My son, Alex, the older of the two, had a bad case when he was about three. I had been treating his sore throat with herbs, although I didn't know then to give them every two hours. After Alex had been sick a couple of days, he became suddenly more feverish and miserable, with flushed cheeks, strawberry tongue, and the beginnings of a scarlet-fever rash. Alex began taking antibiotics right away and recovered fully and quickly.

Last year, I got strep throat. For four days, I had a sore throat so wicked that I could barely swallow my own saliva, along with headache, malaise, fatigue, muscle aches, and poor appetite. My strep test was positive.

My birthday was the next day. Friends were flying in to help me celebrate, and we planned to go skiing. I intended to have fun, but I didn't want to expose everyone to strep—I filled the prescription. By evening, I felt much better.

At dinner in the mountains, however, Darcy,

our daughter, looked pale and complained of a stomachache. By morning, she had fever and chills, nausea and vomiting, but denied sore throat. Her lymph nodes and tonsils seemed huge. She vomited everything, including the herbs I hoped she would take. I took her to the clinic for a strep test. Positive, with low blood oxygen—possibly from mild altitude sickness or combined upper respiratory inflammation plus dehydration. We got Darcy an oxygen tank and antibiotics, and by the next morning she felt well enough to build a snow fort.

My advice: If your child has a severe sore throat, high fever, and swollen lymph nodes—especially in the absence of cold symptoms such as runny nose and cough—take her to the doctor. If the strep test is positive, give her antibiotics. After that, you can make her strong again by replenishing her normal digestive bacteria with acidophilus and bolstering her immune system with herbs.

Chapter 14

COUGHS

"Love, and a cough, cannot be hid," said seventeenth-century poet George Herbert. Coughing still turns heads, especially when it erupts from a small child. When it's your own child coughing, it can feel as if the world is watching, sitting in judgment of whether you're a good parent and wondering whether your child should be out in public at all. And is your child contagious to their children?

But there are coughs, and there are coughs. There are the lingering, harmless coughs that follow ordinary colds, and there are coughs that can signal serious illness or complications of minor illness. The key to parental peace of mind is knowing how to manage the harmless coughs, and how to identify the ones that signal a need for medical attention.

What causes this staccato sound, anyway? A cough is the body's reflexive response to irritation of the respiratory tract lining, from the throat on down into the lungs. Picture the respiratory tract as an upside-down tree. The trachea, or windpipe, is the trunk, the bronchial tubes the larger branches, and the bronchioles the twigs. The alveoli, or air sacs, bud off from the bronchioles, like leaf buds on the twigs. These delicate structures, with linings only a single cell thick, are ideally designed for the exchange of carbon dioxide and oxygen with the blood.

When infection or another form of irritation strikes your child's airways, however, the mucous membranes lining them swell and secrete more mucus. The hairlike cilia that usually propel mucus toward the mouth are temporarily para-lyzed or destroyed. The extra mucus is an irritant, and the cough is your child's body attempting to get rid of the extra mucus and any microbes, allergens, or other particles.

Causes of coughs include inhalation of allergens, pollutants (especially cigarette smoke), or other foreign matter; upper or lower respiratory allergies and infections; reactive airway disease such as asthma; and heart and lung disease. In kids, infections most commonly set off acute coughs, and viruses cause the vast majority of infections.

With viral infections such as colds and flus, runny nose, sneezing, or sore throat are first to appear, but usually subside after three or four days. A cough often begins after a day or two but can linger for two to three weeks. When flu viruses are to blame, a cough can hang on for up to eight to twelve weeks. Usually the cough is dry the first couple of days, then becomes productive. The sputum, initially clear, turns yellow after a few days as dead respiratory-lining cells and white blood cells accumulate and are coughed up.

A common cough associated with a cold can be managed at home if your child is normally healthy. For serious illness with cough or chronic lung disease, your child needs professional care.

Coughs Unrelated to Colds

One of the problems parents face in deciphering what their child's cough means is the medical vocabulary. Some coughs are by-products of mere colds; others are the most prominent symptoms of specific infections. Some terms, such as bronchitis, refer to the location of the infection.

Croup

This fairly common infection, which can be caused by several viruses, affects the larynx, trachea, and bronchi and tends to hit small children between three months and three years of age. Some children get croup only once; others have recurrent attacks.

Transmission occurs by direct contact with someone infected with the virus. Symptoms typically begin two to six days later, usually heralded by a runny nose. As the virus inflames the larynx and trachea, the airway narrows, making breathing more difficult and causing hoarseness. A seal-like barky cough and what doctors refer to as "stridor on inhalation"—a sound like dragging

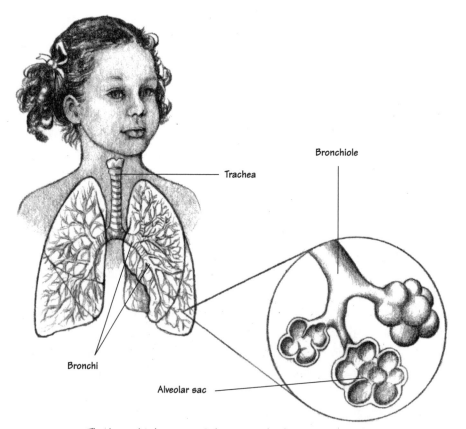

The bronchial system: where coughs happen

your foot through gravel—are typical of croup, as is fever. Your child's breathing rate may rise to 35 to 45 breaths per minute as compared to a normal rate of 20 to 30 per minute for kids under age three. Symptoms fluctuate over the course of the day, often growing worse at night. The illness usually resolves within four days, although the cough may persist longer.

Home management of croup is often based on keeping the air humid, although some studies show no significant benefits. Still, many parents

WHEN TO CALL A DOCTOR ABOUT COUGHS

Call during your practitioner's office hours if:

Your one-to-three-month-old infant's cough persists beyond three days

Your child's mild to moderate cough lasts longer than three to four weeks

Coughing interferes with sleep or causes chest pains

You suspect your child may have whooping cough

Your child has a barky cough and noisy inhalation

See a doctor right away if your coughing child:

Is under one month of age

Has difficulty breathing—shows rapid or labored breathing, sucking in of the skin between the ribs or above breastbone, develops bluish lips or fingernails

Develops high fever, chills, rapid and shallow breathing, and/or chest pain (signs of pneumonia)

Passes out or gets blue lips with coughing spasms

Dial 911 if:

You suspect your child has inhaled a foreign object. This usually results in sudden choking, trouble speaking, coughing, and sometimes a high-pitched noise with each breath.

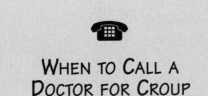

WHEN TO CALL A DOCTOR FOR CROUP

Call a doctor right away if your child:

Is under 12 months old

Has poor skin color or blue-tinged lips

Has severe stridor—harsh, noisy breathing

Shows retraction—sucking in of the skin —between the ribs when he inhales

Demonstrates extreme restlessness or lethargy

Shows dehydration: Your child won't drink much, hasn't peed within the last eight hours, cries without tears, has dry lips and, in infants, a sunken soft spot (fontanel)

Call 911 if your child has:

High fever, very sore throat, muffled voice, drooling due to difficulty swallowing, and difficulty breathing. These are signs of epiglottitis, a serious infection of the epiglottis, or little flap at the back of the throat.

A WORD ON BREATHING RATE

In the animal kingdom, the general rule is that the smaller the critter, the faster it breathes. Babies breathe faster than children, who breathe faster than adults. A number of factors, such as exercise, anxiety, or fever, can increase a person's respiratory rate, but prolonged rapid rate usually signifies lower respiratory tract disease.

Here are some guidelines for normal respiratory rate. Note that the range for infants is wide. You should check your child's breathing rate when she's healthy and at rest to get an idea of her normal rate. Because babies and little kids are abdominal breathers, it's easy to count breaths by watching tummy movements.

Newborn: 20 to 100 breaths per minute, with an average of 30 to 40

Infants and toddlers: 20 to 40 breaths per minute

Older children: 15 to 25 breaths per minute

About age 15 to adult: 16 to 20 breaths per minute

attest to having broken croup attacks by cranking on a hot shower, closing the bathroom door, and letting the child breathe the steamy air. Sometimes taking the child outside into the chill night air gives relief; you'll have to see what works best for your child.

Croup can be frightening for both child and parent. Keep your child calm because agitation usually aggravates the condition. Rescue Remedy and the antiviral herbs listed on page 147 can help. But kids who have stridor even at rest need to see a doctor. Children with severe croup are usually admitted to the hospital.

Bronchitis

Bronchitis refers simply to infection or irritation of the bronchial tubes, or bronchi. It begins as a dry, hacking cough that becomes loose and productive as the illness comes to an end. Fever may or may not be present. It usually resolves without treatment.

Viruses are the most common cause of bronchitis, but many doctors treat it with antibiotics. When bacteria and bacteria-like organisms produce bronchitis, antibiotic treatment is appropriate.

Whooping Cough

This disease, also known as pertussis (the "P" in the DPT vaccine), is bronchitis caused by *Bordetella pertussis* bacteria.

Pertussis rates have actually risen since the early 1980s, apparently in part because teens and adults can get it. Another reason may be parents who cannot or will not immunize their children.

Whooping cough is highly contagious and potentially fatal to babies—a good reason to keep your newborn away from crowds. Young children under five years of age, and especially infants under six months who have not had all three DPT vaccinations, are most susceptible. Among immunized children, whooping cough is rare but not impossible; vaccination provides immunity for a maximum of twelve years.

The bacteria that cause whooping cough spread through airborne droplets unleashed by a cough or through contact with contaminated objects. Symptoms begin in about seven days—sneezing, runny nose, watery eyes, and low fever. A persistent, dry, hacking cough worsens to recurrent fits of spasmodic coughing—a burst of five to ten short, rapid coughs upon a single exhalation. While coughing, the child's face may turn red or bluish while his eyes bulge and his tongue protrudes. The sudden inward breath that follows makes the high-pitched, whooping sound. Afterward, the child may vomit.

Coughing fits can number five to forty a day and continue for four to six weeks. In extreme cases, exhaustion sets in. Treatments with pertussis antibodies and antibiotics are not highly effective, but help most if begun promptly. This illness can be serious, so call your doctor if you suspect your child has it.

Bronchiolitis

Infection or inflammation of the bronchioles, the tiny airway tubes that open into the alveoli, or air sacs, is called bronchiolitis. Viruses cause up to 75 percent of cases, especially respiratory syncytial virus (RSV).

Highly contagious, the RSV virus spreads by hand-to-nose and hand-to-eye contact and from touching contaminated objects. Epidemics of RSV occur annually in the United States, usually from December to April, and lead to 100,000 hospitalizations per year. Infants eighteen months and younger are particularly susceptible.

Bronchiolitis often begins like an ordinary cold—with a runny nose, congestion, cough, and perhaps low fever. Wheezing with increased respiratory rate follows. Lethargy, irritability, and poor feeding occur as well. In three to seven days the infection eases, but some infants experience diminishing episodes of bronchospasm (marked narrowing of the airways) for the next two years. Complications include dehydration, periods of temporarily suspended breathing, and, rarely, respiratory failure.

See your pediatrician if your infant under three months has a severe cough or if you suspect your older child has bronchiolitis. Treatment depends upon the severity of the disease. For home care, your doctor may recommend breathing humidified air to correct dehydration. Children under three months of age and those with respiratory distress or significant dehydration are usually admitted to the hospital for treatment. Antibiotics don't help this illness unless it is complicated by bacterial pneumonia.

Pneumonia

The alveoli are the end of the line for respiratory tract infection. When infection—pneumonia—occurs here, the microorganism has outwitted or overcome all the body's natural defenses protecting the lungs. Cases of viral pneumonia outnumber those that are bacterial; rarely, the cause may be fungi or breathing in toxic fumes or stomach contents. Mild viral pneumonia may produce few or no symptoms, but bacterial pneumonia or any such infection in an infant or toddler causes obvious illness.

Clues that your child has pneumonia include cough, fever, chills, chest pain, and signs of respiratory distress—rapid respiratory rate, retraction of the skin around the ribs and collarbone, flaring of the nostrils, and a bluish tinge, especially to the lips, nail beds, and around the mouth. With your ear to your child's chest, you may hear moist rattling or crackling sounds that don't clear with a good cough.

Call your doctor right away if you suspect your child has pneumonia. The doctor will carefully examine your child's chest and perhaps check her blood oxygen. Sometimes chest X-rays are necessary.

Pneumonia treatment includes close observation, lots of fluids, excellent nutrition, and plenty of rest. Bacterial pneumonia warrants antibiotic treatment but viral infection does not, although doctors sometimes prescribe it to prevent bacterial infection. Hospitalization is reserved for very sick children, particularly sick infants.

Managing Coughs At Home

If you live with a smoker, for health's sake, ask him or her to smoke outside. Cigarette smoke irritates the respiratory tract and impairs the clearing of mucus.

Make sure your child drinks lots of water. When your child drinks plenty of liquids, the respiratory secretions will become thinner and easier to cough up.

Expectorants may aid in expelling mucus. For severe coughing that prevents sleep, your physician may recommend a cough suppressant. Otherwise, most health practitioners don't interfere with the cough reflex, particularly when it is producing sputum; coughing defends against pneumonia.

Humidify, humidify. Steam inhalation can calm a dry cough and thin secretions so they're easier to expel. An easy method is to boil a pot of water, remove it from the burner, and set it on a sturdy table. See Chapter 9, Colds, for instructions on doing an herbal stream.

Humidify the child's room with a clean, fine-mist humidifier. Be diligent about cleaning the humidifier every couple of days.

Along with steam treatments, try chest rubs. Tiger Balm salve—for kids, the white type—contains circulatory stimulants. Chest rubs with menthol-containing herb balms seem to help relax the airways and increase local blood flow, creating a warming effect. The best part, however, may be the curing power of a loving touch.

A modified slant board relieves congestion in an old-fashioned but effective way. First, if the child is old enough, have him take a hot-to-tolerance shower, then dress warmly; otherwise, let him inhale steam from a pot or commercial steamer. Next, elevate the foot of his bed two to three inches with books or bricks. Have your child get into bed and lie on his stomach with his head and upper body lower than his mid-section. After two to four minutes, have him roll onto his back for another few minutes. At this point, he may want to take a break and slowly sit up—he may feel dizzy. Then ask him to lie on one side, then the other.

To increase mucus drainage, gently tap your child's chest with the pinky side of your palms. If this repeatedly triggers coughing, stop.

Try a mustard plaster. Sunny has used this time-tested remedy on her kids to stimulate circulation to the lungs and expectoration during stubborn coughs. Many people born in the 1940s or earlier remember this simple home treatment. To use one, see the recipe on the following page.

Dietary Support

Some health practitioners recommend that parents withhold dairy and soy products from their kids' diets during colds and flus. Practitioners of Traditional Chinese Medicine consider milk and soy milk to be "mucus-forming."

These practitioners also identify fruit juice as "mucus-forming," and it's packed with fruit sugars. Sunny avoids giving cold fruit juices to her kids during respiratory illnesses. Linda reduces her kids' consumption of cold juices or blends them with herb teas and serves them warm.

Teach your child to use a tissue when coughing, and to spit politely into it when the cough is productive. Our society is a little squeamish about spitting, but swallowing lots of mucus can cause stomach upset. Gently remind kids to wash their hands frequently during cold and flu season to prevent transmission of viruses.

Healthy Treatments

Many herbs help with respiratory infections in more than one way. Thyme, for instance, relieves cough spasms while fighting bacteria. Many of the other herbs listed below are powerful allies when children are suffering from coughs.

Demulcents

Mucilaginous herbal teas made with marshmallow root, plantain leaf, and mullein leaves and flowers can coat the throat with a temporary "mucous membrane" when coughing dries the throat. Research has confirmed marshmallow root's immunostimulating and cough-suppressant effects. Licorice root adds a sweet flavor—if your kids like the taste—and it fights microbes while inducing the body to produce its own antiviral chemical, interferon.

Immune Stimulators

Echinacea. At the first cough, begin using echinacea root to support the immune system.

Osha is another good choice because it particularly helps soothe both dry and productive coughs. It also supports the immune system, fights viruses, and acts as an expectorant. Don't harvest osha yourself—it has been overharvested in many areas, and besides, it looks a lot like poison hemlock!

Antiviral and Antibacterial Herbs

Elderberry is one of the few medicines, herbal or otherwise, that has been shown to be effective against influenza viruses and RSV. Elder flowers have also been used for centuries for children's fevers, and the berries make a great herbal syrup.

Garlic is an excellent herb for respiratory infections, especially bacterial ones. Its aromatic oils

are excreted through the lungs, where they act directly to kill infection and expectorate mucus.

Mucus–Clearing Herbs

Mullein leaves and flowers contain saponins, chemicals that gently nudge the lungs to expecto-

---

MUSTARD PLASTER

For ages: Over 3
Yields: One treatment

1 teaspoon dried mustard powder (counterirritant, stimulates circulation)

1 teaspoon wheat flour (adds mucilage, dilutes oils of mustard)

About 1 teaspoon very warm water

About 1 teaspoon carrier oil (almond, olive, etc.) (protects skin)

Directions: Mix mustard powder and flour. Gradually add hot-to-tolerance water to make a moist paste. To protect your child's skin and make it easier to remove the plaster, first cover the child's chest with the carrier oil. Spread the paste over the affected area, cover with a plastic bag or plastic wrap to protect bed clothes, then cover with a warm, moist cloth. Stay with your child and read her a story. Do your best to keep her quiet while the plaster remains on. Remove the plaster in five minutes with the spatula, then clean her skin with soap and water. **Do not lose track of time,** because the volatile oils in mustard can easily blister a child's sensitive skin.

SCIENCE EXPERIMENT FOR KIDS AT HOME WITH COUGHS

2 large organic onions
1/2 cup sugar
1/2 cup honey
2 wide-mouth quart jars

After an adult slices the onions into 1/2-inch thick rings, kids can put 1 set of onion rings on the bottom of each jar. Cover the onions in one jar with about 1 tablespoon of sugar. Cover the onions in the other jar with 1 or 2 tablespoons of honey. Place another layer of onion rings in each jar, and repeat the process until you've used up all the onion slices, honey, and sugar.

Take a good look at each jar, cover them with a lid, and leave them alone for 3 hours. Now take a look at the jars. How did the liquid get into the jars? Is the honey in your onion jar thicker or thinner than when you started?

The jar with the sugar may have a thin, watery syrup. The honey in the other jar will be thinner than when you began. Typically, the sugar pulls more liquid out of the onions than the honey.

Congratulations, kids! You've just made your very own cough syrup! Onions attack the germs that bring on the cough, so this syrup will help you get over it. Take one teaspoon of the syrup four times every day until your cough is gone. Hope you feel better!

rate. Make a simple tea by steeping one teaspoon of dried leaves per cup of water for five to ten minutes. Strain it through a clean, finely woven cloth to remove the irritating little hairs from the leaves, and then add a bit of sweetener. We generally use this herb with others in a tea blend (see recipe on the following page).

Elecampane root fights bacterial infection while provoking expectoration with its essential oil, helenin. We choose elecampane when our kids have lots of respiratory mucus and need a bit of herbal help to make their coughs productive.

Several other aromatic plants contain antiseptic volatile oils that, because they're excreted through the lungs, act as expectorants. Some good choices are peppermint, hyssop, and eucalyptus. With eucalyptus, a little goes a long way; a pinch of leaves in a cup of tea is good, but too much makes it bitter. Two or three drops of essential oil of eucalyptus enhance steams and can be used, diluted in almond oil, to make a chest rub, but *never* use essential oils internally.

Cough Relievers

Thyme and **lemon thyme** help reduce spasmodic coughing. Thyme also provides an antimicrobial oil, thymol; many commercial antibacterial cleansers made today include a synthetic form of thymol. The German Commission E lists thyme as safe for children and useful for symptoms of bronchitis, whooping cough, and upper respiratory mucus. Thyme thrives in warm climates or indoors, so it's easy to grow. Most kids like the taste of thyme tea or glycerite. Pour one cup of boiling water over one teaspoon of thyme leaves, steep five minutes, and strain for a powerful, cough-relieving tea.

Lobelia leaf has a history of traditional use for relaxing spasmodic coughs such as croup. The herb both sedates spasmodic coughs and encourages expectoration.

It's safe for kids only when used cautiously, because the tea, in large amounts, can cause vomiting; its other well-earned name is puke-wort. Use it only for kids over five with deep, productive coughs, but start by infusing no more than 1/4 teaspoon dried herb per cup of hot water. A 50-pound child can drink as much as one cup of this dilute tea three times daily. Expect the child to cough up plenty of mucus; then you may see a relaxant effect. Don't exceed this recommended dose, and discontinue if your child doesn't tolerate the tea.

Cough Suppressants

Use herbal cough suppressants only when the cough is dry or it interferes with the child's sleep.

Cherry bark inhibits the cough reflex. Sacajawea benefited from cherry bark tea in 1805 on the Lewis and Clark expedition; her ailment remains unknown, but she was so ill that Merriwether Lewis despaired that she would die. By drinking cherry bark tea and water from a naturally antibacterial sulfur spring, she recovered completely.

With its strong antispasmodic effects on the lungs, cherry bark is tremendously helpful for reducing the hacking cough that keeps kids (and their parents) awake at night; we count on it when nothing else works.

Look for a cherry bark glycerite or cough formula, or make tea with two cups of water and two teaspoons of dried bark, simmered for ten minutes or less and sweetened to taste. Adding equal parts of honey and water creates a simple cough syrup. Limit use to three half-cups tea per day for a child of 50 pounds for up to one week.

Caution: Cherry bark contains a glycoside similar to cyanide; don't harvest the bark in the fall, when the glycoside is highest. Avoid it during pregnancy.

TEA FOR LOOSE, GURGLING COUGHS

For ages: Over two
Yields: 3 cups tea

1 teaspoon dried horehound leaves (expectorant)

1 teaspoon dried mullein leaves (soothing expectorant)

1 teaspoon dried boneset herb (immune support)

1/4 teaspoon dried peppermint leaves (decongestant; stomach soother)

1/4 teaspoon dried skullcap herb (sedative)

A pinch grated fresh ginger (warming)

1–5 drops propolis tincture (optional) (antimicrobial, anti-inflammatory)

Honey to taste

3 cups just-boiled water

Combine all herbs in a non-aluminum teapot or pan; add water. Cover and steep for 5 to 7 minutes. Strain and add honey to taste. Serve warm in 1/4- to 1/2-cup doses throughout the day and evening, up to five times a day.

Optional: After brewing, add the propolis tincture to taste. Propolis is a bee product, so don't use it if your child is allergic to bee stings.

Licorice calms coughs and acts as a demulcent. Fringe benefits include antiviral, anti-inflammatory, and immune-boosting properties.

Anise seed has a pleasant licorice-like taste that most kids like; in Germany, physicians use it regularly to calm children's coughs. Decoct one teaspoon of the seed in one cup of water. Strain and serve several times a day. Anise seed is antibacterial, expectorant, relieves stomachaches, and can help stop coughing. Some sources advise against using medicinal quantities of this herb during pregnancy.

Sedative Herbs

Sleep is a powerful healer. Sedative herbs not only grease the sleep wheels, but relax muscles, including those of the respiratory tract.

California poppy, a classic, gentle children's relaxant, tends to calm irritable coughs.

Passionflower leaves do the trick for relaxing overtired kids who just can't stop coughing. Glycerites and teas of this herb help bring on sleep and are usually readily available.

Skullcap and **valerian** are the herbal "big guns" on the sedative scale for kids. Taken as a tea or the tastier glycerite form, skullcap and valerian make excellent ingredients for a nighttime cough tea or formula. If your child can swallow capsules, he can avoid these tastes entirely.

Recommended Reading

Gagnon, D. and A. Morningstar. *Breathe Free: Nutritional and Herbal Care for Your Respiratory System.* Wilmot, WI: Lotus Press, 1990.

EXPECTORANT SYRUP FOR STUBBORN, DRY COUGHS

For ages: Over 1 year
Yields: About 4 cups syrup

*4 teaspoons dried cherry bark
   (relaxes coughs)*

*2 teaspoons echinacea root
   (immune stimulating, antibacterial)*

*1 teaspoon licorice root
   (soothing, antiviral)*

*1 teaspoon marshmallow root
   (moistening, immune stimulating)*

*1 teaspoon pleurisy root
   (moistening to mucous membranes)*

8 cups water

1½ to 2 cups honey

*1–5 drops cinnamon or orange natural
   flavoring (optional)*

Combine herbs and water in non-aluminum pot. Simmer for 10 to 15 minutes partially covered so that steam can escape; do not allow to boil. Continue simmering until liquid is reduced by half. Remove from heat and strain. Return to low heat, slowly stirring in honey until a consistency of watery syrup is reached. Remove from heat. The syrup will thicken as it cools. When cool, add cinnamon or orange flavoring.

Dosage: Use up to 4 servings per day to reduce spasmodic coughing.

Under 20 pounds	1/2 teaspoon
20–40 pounds	1 teaspoon
40–75 pounds	1 to 1½ teaspoons
over 75 pounds	2 teaspoons

Chapter 15

HAY FEVER

Ah, spring. It either makes you want to run amok in the greenery, or don a surgical mask and stay indoors. Hay fever has become surprisingly common in children. By the age of two to three years, 20 percent of children have symptoms of upper respiratory allergies. By age six, 42 percent have them. As with asthma, cases of childhood hay fever have increased recently; a survey of Swedish schoolchildren showed that both maladies doubled between 1979 and 1991.

What causes these allergies? The mechanism is still somewhat of a mystery. Basically, the immune system over-reacts to particular molecules present in the environment. It treats these allergens as though they threatened the body's health, as though they were, say, cold viruses. This response liberates chemicals such as histamine, leading to inflammation of the nose, eyes, and throat. No one knows why some people are more susceptible than others.

Hay fever, a.k.a. seasonal allergic rhinitis, generally refers to airborne allergens in the form of pollens from trees, grasses, and flowering plants. The worst offenders are ragweed and other plants in the compositae family, including sagebrush (*Artemesia*) species.

In perennial allergic rhinitis, symptoms persist year round. Common allergens include house-dust mites, molds, feathers, animal dander, and food allergies and intolerances. Many allergy sufferers react to more than one type of allergen. A study of fifty kids with allergic rhinitis found that 50 percent tested positive for inhaled allergens, 20 percent had identifiable food allergies, and 30 percent had both. Their common food allergies included shellfish, tomatoes, rice, and peanuts.

The symptoms that plague sufferers range from annoying to nearly incapacitating. Nasal congestion tops the list. You may notice that your child breathes through her mouth, snores at night, speaks with a nasal tone, sneezes, sniffles, and scratches her nose and eyes. If the allergic rhinitis has become chronic, you may see the following classic signs in your child: a crease across the top of the nose from constant rubbing and "allergic shiners," a darkening of the skin under the eyes. Postnasal drip can cause coughing. Occasionally, seasonal allergens can trigger asthma. Your child may also have trouble sleeping and may generally feel and look puny. At school, she may have trouble concentrating.

Risk factors for hay fever include early introduction of foods or formula, heavy parental cigarette smoking, especially in the child's first year of life, and parents who have allergic disorders. Air pollutants play a role, too. One study found that kids who live on heavily trafficked streets have twice the chance of developing asthma and hay fever than those who live on streets with low traffic.

Complications and associated diseases can develop when hay fever lingers: recurrent nosebleeds and middle-ear infections, pinkeye, chronic cough, asthma, sinusitis, and lack of energy or interest in life. If the mention of middle-ear infections piqued your interest, here's what happens in a nutshell: When a young child's upper respiratory tract becomes congested from allergies or viral infections such as the common cold, the tube that allows drainage

from the middle ear to the throat can become blocked. If bacteria begin to grow in the secretions trapped in the middle ear, a middle-ear infection occurs. Some 40 to 50 percent of kids over the age of three with chronic middle-ear infections also have hay fever. You may want to read Chapter 12, Ear Infections, for tips on how to manage these symptoms with herbs and other complementary therapies.

Medical Treatment

Conventional treatment involves, first and foremost, avoiding exposure to the allergen. If your child is allergic to many things, this might seem a formidable, even impossible, task, but you can try. You may need to keep your house super clean, switch to dust-free decor (no carpets or drapes), and limit exposure to pets, or

Is It a Cold or an Allergy?

Here are some tips to help you distinguish between the two.

Symptoms	Common Cold	Allergy
Respiratory	Runny nose; sometimes watery eyes and scratchy throat; moderate sneezing; nasal secretions that go from clear to yellowish	Runny, itchy nose and weepy eyes; itchy throat and nose that trigger sneezing; nasal secretions that stay clear
Fever	Mild to none	None
Seasonal variation	More common in fall/winter	Most often seen in spring and summer or year-around
Family history	No relationship	Other family members have allergies, including eczema or asthma
Physical exam	Inside of nose looks red and swollen	Inside of nose looks grayish-blue and boggy
Allergy skin tests	Negative (unless underlying allergies exist)	May be positive

bathe them frequently and keep them out of your child's bedroom. You can encase pillows and mattresses in special allergen-impermeable covers, and buy pillows and comforters stuffed with cotton, wool, or synthetics instead of down or feathers. Wash stuffed animals regularly, and keep them out of your child's bed at night. If your child has seasonal allergies, you can close her bedroom windows and use a high-efficiency particulate accumulator (HEPA) air filter when pollen counts are high.

Antihistamines typically act quickly to control symptoms such as runny nose, sneezing, watery eyes, and itchy nose, eyes, and throat. Older antihistamines caused sleepiness, but the newer medications do not, and they can be given less frequently. But some have other side effects, including dry mouth, blurred vision, stomach upset, and irritability. Be sure your health-care provider has filled you in on the cautions if you use these drugs. Herbal alternatives to antihistamines are available; you may wish to try them first.

Decongestants relieve stuffiness—but not other allergy symptoms—by constricting the small blood vessels in the respiratory mucous membranes. They can be taken orally or as nasal sprays. Oral decongestants can cause nervousness, irritability, insomnia, heart palpitations, and rapid heart rate. Overusing nasal sprays can cause rebound congestion—your child stops using them, and suddenly he's even stuffier.

Cromolyn sodium acts by stabilizing specialized cells called mast cells, which release the chemicals that instigate allergic symptoms. Like many other medications, cromolyn was originally derived from an herb, *Amni visnaga,* an ancient Egyptian medication that is still used by herbalists today in managing asthma. Cromolyn relieves nasal symptoms except congestion. To work effectively, however, it should be taken before symptoms appear. Its effects are short-lived, necessitating doses four to six times a day. Cromolyn is safe but relatively expensive. If your doctor recommends cromolyn for your child, you can take comfort in knowing that side effects are rare.

Intranasal corticosteroids, such as Beconase, Rhinocort, Nasacort, and others, supress the inflammatory response, thereby preventing symptoms. To date, these powerful drugs are approved for children six and older. Compared to antihistamines and decongestants, corticosteroids take longer to kick in—from twenty-four hours to two weeks—but they usually produce great relief. To date, nasal steroids appear free of the serious side effects that come with long-term use of oral steroids. Infrequent side effects include headache, sore throat, nasal drying, and nosebleeds.

Immunotherapy, or allergy shots, involves repeated injections of allergens into the skin. Such treatment is usually reserved for kids whose symptoms don't respond adequately to avoidance and drug therapy. Allergy shots are not a cure, but rather a means to reduce immune reaction; effectiveness varies among individuals. Because of the slight risk of a serious allergic reaction, a doctor should be in attendance when the shots are given.

Home Management of Hay Fever Symptoms

Keep your child's nose clean. And we mean literally. Using nasal salt drops or nasal irrigation helps wash away allergens. Doing steam inhalation first will cut down on congestion and loosen the mucus so that it's easier to expel. See the chapters on colds and sinusitis for recipes and detailed instructions.

Experiment with changing your child's diet. A hidden food sensitivity may be the straw that breaks this camel's back during pollen season. Eliminating food allergies and intolerances helps resolve a variety of inflammatory illnesses. Keep in mind that standard allergy tests may not detect food intolerances. See Chapter 7, Allergies and Intolerances, for more information.

Try carrot juice. It's full of antioxidant and immune-boosting carotenes. Sunny's kids love to make it. Her two-year-old daughter likes to mix carrot juice with a pinch of fresh onions, garlic, and a miniscule amount of horseradish, a great blend for fighting bacteria, opening the sinuses, decreasing inflammation, and providing lots of vitamins. All of these qualities help kids' bodies cope with hay fever.

Some foods can cause histamine release. Susceptible people can experience hives after eating some foods, and, less frequently, stomach upset, diarrhea, or headaches. Common culprits include cheese, tomatoes, bananas, strawberries, shrimp, lobster, salmon, pineapple, and chocolate. If you find your child is sensitive to any of these foods, you may wish to avoid them, especially during hay fever season.

Review the stress in your child's life. Stress contributes to dozens of health problems; high stress often equals low immunity, and thus illness.

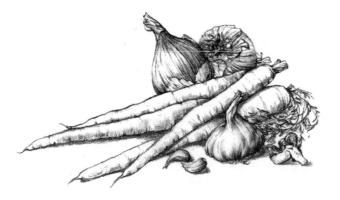

Sunny's kids like carrot juice zinged up with onions and garlic.

Herbal Remedies for Hay Fever

Along with herbs mentioned for individual symptoms in the chapters on allergies, coughs, and asthma, be sure to consider the following botanicals.

Stinging nettle has been shown in one study to relieve allergic rhinitis better than placebo treatment; well over half the adults who took the herb reported it effective. Ironically, this plant's stinging hairs contain histamine, but it nearly disappears when the leaves are air-dried or cooked. Apparently the tiny residual amount of histamine contained in a dose of stinging nettle has a desensitizing effect, and can actually prevent the body's own histamine release from immune cells. Nettle is also rich in several vitamins and minerals, including those with natural antihistamine effects such as vitamin C and magnesium.

Licorice root acts against inflammation and allergies. Other benefits include antibacterial and antiviral effects. Deglycyrrhizinated products—called DGL licorice—don't contain the components needed to help hay fever. Instead, use whole licorice root.

Caution: Do restrict licorice-root dosages. A 50-pound child can take one 500-mg capsule three times a day, or follow package directions. Never use licorice root for more than six weeks at a time, because long-term use has caused increased blood pressure and sodium retention. Pregnant women or anyone with hypertension or taking heart or kidney medications should not use it at all.

Sage is full of the antibacterial essential oil thujone, so sage tea makes a great gargle for throats irritated by post-nasal drip and excess mucus. Just steep 1 teaspoon dried leaves and flowers per cup of water or 2 teaspoons fresh herb, add honey to taste, cool, and serve. Don't confuse garden sage of the mint family with sagebrush (*Artemesia* species) of the daisy family, because sagebrush pollen can cause hay fever.

Caution: Pregnant or nursing mothers should avoid sage; it has slight uterine-stimulant effects.

Eyebright works like a charm for drying runny secretions from the nose and eyes. Follow the label instructions, using Clark's rule if children's dosages are not given.

Fenugreek is a simple cooking herb that also has medicinal activity. It's mildly anti-inflammatory and very soothing to irritated throat membranes. This tiny seed makes a pleasant tea that tastes like a combination of maple syrup and licorice. Combine equal parts of fenugreek, rose hips, and a pinch of gingerroot for a good hay fever tea. Simmer 2 teaspoons of the herbal mix, covered, in two cups of water for five minutes, cool, and enjoy. Sprouted fenugreek seeds can be added to salads.

Caution: Due to a slight estrogenic action, fenugreek should be avoided by pregnant women.

Nutritional Supplements

Vitamin C acts as a natural antihistamine, both by preventing secretion from white blood cells and by increasing detoxification activity.

Onion, garlic, cayenne pepper, and other hot foods contain the natural antihistamine quercetin, which inhibits the body's formation and release of histamine. Quercetin can be taken as a nutritional supplement; the recommended adult dosage of supplemental quercetin ranges from 200 to 500 mg, taken two to three times daily before meals. Check with a dietitian or other health practitioner to determine a safe dose for your child. Laboratory studies have found quercetin to be safe, even at high doses for long periods of time.

Omega-3 fatty acids, abundant in flaxseed oils and cold-water fish such as salmon, herring, and mackerel, can influence the pathways in the body that make chemicals called leukotrienes and prostaglandins that have an effect on the inflammatory process. These fatty acids can actually

---

HAY FEVER TEA

This tea has a sweet and sour taste with drying, decongestant effects.

For ages: *5 and up*
Yields: *7 cups of tea*

*2 teaspoons eyebright herb
(decreases secretions of nose and eyes)*
*2 teaspoons stinging nettles
(decreases histamine response)*
*2 teaspoons schisandra berries
(nourishes adrenal glands)*
*2 teaspoons rose hips
(provides vitamin C, bioflavonoids)*
*1 teaspoon elder flowers
(reduces excess mucus)*
*1/4 teaspoon fresh grated ginger
(stimulates circulation, anti-inflammatory)*
Organic frozen fruit-juice concentrate to taste
7 cups water

Bring water to a boil. Remove from heat. Add herbs; steep 5 to 10 minutes. Strain and sweeten to taste.

Dosage: Start with 1/4 cup, twice a day, for a 5-year-old, 1/2 cup three times a day for older kids. Stores well in refrigerator for up to four days.

tip the process in favor of prostaglandins with anti-inflammatory actions. In this way, they may help reduce allergic reactions. Gamma-linoleic acid, contained in evening primrose, borage, and black currant oils, also fosters production of favorable prostaglandins.

Our families take flaxseed oil daily in capsules or by adding the oil or ground seeds to foods. Note that you can't cook with flaxseed oil because it goes rancid at cooking temperatures. Store flaxseed oil in the refrigerator. Flaxseed oil works well in salad dressing or on top of rice or pasta.

Magnesium has natural antihistamine effects. Some experts recommend that children take 6 milligrams of magnesium per pound of body weight daily in the form of magnesium chloride or magnesium citrate, a dosage higher than the FDA's recommended daily allowance.

If your child eats few dairy products, consider giving her calcium and magnesium together, with two parts calcium to one part magnesium. Start with a low dose and gradually increase, because magnesium can act as a laxative. Food sources of magnesium include nuts, blackstrap molasses, soy products, meat, fish, oatmeal, cornmeal, whole wheat, string beans, spinach, coriander, and dairy products.

Recommended Reading

Rapp, D. *Is This Your Child?* New York: William Morrow and Co., 1991.

Chapter 16

ASTHMA

Few things are more terrifying than seeing your child labor to breathe. You watch, wringing your hands. Your child inhales, the skin drawing inward above his collarbone. He exhales, and you can hear the wheezing from several feet away. His eyes look frightened. You tell him everything will be okay and try not to show your own fear as you usher him into the car for the drive to the doctor's office.

Fortunately, there are many treatments available for asthma, from mild to severe cases. For the mildest cases, a doctor's evaluation and some training in home management are all that is needed. Lifestyle changes can lessen the chance of repeat asthma attacks. Best of all, early intervention techniques can reduce your child's risk of getting asthma and its severity if it does occur.

But first, the bad news: More and more kids, and consequently their parents, are having to cope with this unnerving and sometimes disabling disease. The Asthma and Allergy Foundation of America estimates that twelve to fifteen million Americans have asthma, twice the number afflicted in the early 1980s. A recent study of children living in Bronx County, New York, found that 14.3 percent—one child in seven—has asthma. Although the reasons for this increase aren't clear, experts suspect that diet and environmental pollution play a role.

Doctors view asthma as an inflammatory process, an over-reaction of the airways to various environmental insults. Here's what happens when the lungs of an asthmatic encounter an irritant. The smooth muscle of the bronchi constricts, diminishing the diameter of these airways. A cascade of inflammation reactions causes the membranes that line the airways to swell and produce excessive mucus, further narrowing the air passages. The net result is a temporary and correctable obstruction to the flow of air.

An asthma attack can come on gradually or suddenly. Classic signs and symptoms include increased breathing rate, cough, a sensation of chest tightness, difficulty breathing, especially exhaling, and wheezing. In some children, however, the only clue that they have asthma is a persistent cough and a tendency for colds to go straight to the chest.

What Causes Asthma?

Genetics can play a role in producing asthma; along with hay fever and other allergies, it can run in families. Children born prematurely sometimes have lung damage that predisposes them to asthma.

Many of the things that induce asthma attacks are irritants for most people, but to a lesser degree.

WHEN TO CALL A DOCTOR ABOUT ASTHMA

Any time your child has trouble breathing, get medical help. With asthma, prompt treatment is critical. If a health practitioner has already evaluated your child, there are home treatments that can nip mild attacks in the bud. If you have any doubt about what to do, call your practitioner.

If your child demonstrates any of the following symptoms, call your doctor's office to find out whether you should go there or to the emergency room. While you await help, try to keep your child and yourself calm.

Symptoms of respiratory distress:

Use of the muscles of the neck and shoulders to help force out breath

Flaring of the nostrils

Sucking in of the skin between the ribs on inhalation

Grunting on exhalation

Skin that goes pale, then bluish, especially around the lips

Speech limited to one-word answers.

Upper respiratory tract infections, viral bronchitis, cigarette smoke, air pollution, exercise, emotional distress, food allergies and intolerances, inhaled allergens, accidental inhalation of food, and medications such as aspirin or ibuprofen are a few. While doctors once thought asthma had psychological origins, medical researchers now acknowledge that stress and emotions can play a role, but are usually accompanied by other precipitating factors.

Infection with respiratory syncytial virus (RSV) can cause an infection of the small airways, or bronchiolitis, and pneumonia. This infection produces symptoms similar to asthma—cough, wheezing, and shortness of breath. Once cured, exposure to the virus can also predispose its victims to asthma.

Food allergies also can play a role in asthma. One study found that, in 5.7 percent of asthmatic children, symptoms were brought on by consuming offending foods, most commonly milk, eggs, and peanuts. The children also typically had other symptoms—eczema, bloating, and diarrhea, for example—associated with food allergies. Another study found that food allergies were responsible for 6 percent of asthma cases. Eggs and milk topped the list for allergenic foods, followed by wheat, fish, potatos, and pork. While neither of these small studies proves that food allergies cause asthma in a majority of patients, some practitioners believe that diet, allergies, and food intolerances should be investigated whenever a child has asthma.

13 Ways to Help Your Child with Asthma

1. If your child has a specific allergy, avoid or eliminate his exposure to it. Keeping a journal of your child's asthma attacks may help you pinpoint precipitating foods, drinks, activities, and

emotional stressors. Toss aerosol cleaners, deodorants, and hair sprays and replace them with natural alternatives that don't create synthetic mists. You can also switch to an unscented, biodegradable detergent. Many of the synthetic fragrances in laundry products are known allergens.

2. Keep your house clean. This will help reduce airborne allergens such as dust, mites, molds, pollen, and animal dander. Get rid of allergen-collecting furnishings such as carpets, rugs, curtains, and upholstery. Encase bedding in allergen-impermeable covers, and launder bedclothes weekly in hot water.

3. Keep your child away from cigarette smoke and, when possible, other forms of air pollution. You may want to invest in an air purifier for your home. If you live in a dry climate, you may also want to use a fine-mist humidifier.

4. Encourage your child to drink lots of fluids, especially during an attack. This will help thin respiratory secretions, making them easier to expel.

5. Some spicy foods such as garlic, onion, cayenne, and ginger provide warming circulation to the lung area. Herbalists often use them to increase expectoration and decrease inflammation. Also, garlic's antimicrobial activity can help ward off respiratory infections, which typically aggravate asthma.

6. Use immune-supporting herbs such as echinacea at the first exposure to or sign of a cold. Although asthma involves a hyper-vigilant immune response, keeping your child's immune system in top working order may help her avoid a viral respiratory infection, which, in turn, may set off asthma.

7. Go easy on meat and processed foods made with hydrogenated oils. Large amounts of animal products in the diet tend to tip the balance of prostaglandins, a class of chemicals that influence inflammatory response, in favor of inflammation. Omega-3 fatty acids tend to reduce inflammation. High intake of omega-3 fatty acids correlates with a low incidence of inflammatory diseases, including asthma. Flaxseed oil and cold-water fish such as salmon, mackerel, and herring are good sources of different kinds of essential fatty acids. Some research on supplementing the diets of asthmatic children with fish oil has been positive. Consult your health practitioner and/or a nutritionist about the subject when adding such supplements to your asthmatic child's regime, especially if he or she is under age seven.

8. Avoid food additives. Sulphites, tartrazine, and benzoates can trigger asthma attacks in susceptible people. Become a label reader and stick to food without synthetic preservatives and/or flavorings.

9. Ask your doctor if your child could have a metabolic problem. Here's an example. Some kids with asthma don't properly metabolize the amino acid tryptophan. As a result, the chemical by-product serotonin accumulates and causes airway constriction. If your doctor thinks it warranted, she can test your child's metabolic status.

10. Boost your child's intake of antioxidants. Low intake of vitamin C, the major antioxidant present in the surface liquid of the airways, seems to correlate with asthma. One study found that vitamin C blood levels were significantly lower in children with asthma than those without it. A review of clinical trials on vitamin C supplementation in asthmatics found that, although some studies did not find benefits, others did. As an alternative to giving your child a lot of vitamin C pills, boost her intake of vitamin C-rich foods, such as citrus fruits, rose hips, cantaloupe, papaya, strawberries, broccoli, tomatoes, and most sprouts.

Asthma and Peak Flow Meters

When a child has asthma, both she and her parents can benefit from learning subtle warning signs that may herald an attack. These can include signals such as changes in breathing rate and depth, sneezing, headache, mood shifts, runny nose, cough, fatigue, dark semicircles under the eyes, trouble sleeping, diminished exercise tolerance, and itching of the chin or throat. To monitor changes in breathing, your child can use a peak flow meter. This small, easy-to-use gadget measures the flow of air in a forced exhalation. Anywhere from hours to a day or two before an asthma attack occurs, peak flow rate declines. Asthmatic kids can use the meter at home each day to record how well their lungs are working. Your doctor can help determine optimum peak flow values for your child and give you guidelines for what to do when peak flow drops. To find out more about peak flow meters, ask your doctor or call National Jewish Center for Immunology and Respiratory Medicine's LUNG LINE at 1-800-222-LUNG. Located in Denver, National Jewish is one of the top international centers for studying and treating asthma, chronic allergies, and food sensitivities.

Adapted from *Your Child and Asthma*, 1992, the National Jewish Center for Immunology and Respiratory Medicine, Denver, Colorado

11. Ask your doctor about ruling out immune-depressing infections such as parasitic infestation with *Giardia lamblia* or fungal overgrowth from *Candida albicans*. According to Jacqueline Krohn, M.D., parasites and other chronic gastrointestinal infections can play a role in immune-system suppression.

12. Take your child's emotional pulse. In Traditional Chinese Medicine, the lungs often correlate with the emotion of grief. A skilled childhood counselor may be invaluable for helping release any emotional traumas associated with your child's asthma.

13. Consider helping your child learn a relaxation technique such as yoga, meditation, or guided imagery. Such practices not only improve overall well-being, but can also reduce anxiety, an asthma trigger for some people.

Conventional Treatment

First of all, health practitioners usually recommend avoiding allergic triggers. Various tests can help identify inhaled and food allergies (see Chapter 7, Allergies, for more details).

The asthma medications your doctor recommends will depend upon the severity and frequency of your child's asthma attacks. A wide variety of medications are available, many of which have adverse side effects, either immediately or with long-term use. Be sure that your doctor discusses these side effects with you in detail. Despite these side effects, *conventional treatment of asthma has saved lives.*

There are four basic types of asthma medications:

- bronchodilators, which help open the airways and are chiefly administered by inhalers or nebulizers and less often in tablets;

- anti-inflammatories, which include cromolyn, an inhaled medication used preventively to inhibit the release of inflammation-causing chemicals, and corticosteriods (cortisone-like drugs) taken by inhalation or as tablets when bronchodilators alone can't control asthma;
- anticholinergics, which block the nerves that constrict airways; and
- leukotriene receptor antagonists, a new class of drugs that inhibit the formation or action of inflammatory chemicals.

If your child has asthma, you'll want to do whatever it takes to keep his illness under control. This commitment means researching possible causes, but also taking prescription medications as directed. Please don't take your child off her asthma drugs "cold-turkey"; this could pose serious risks to her health.

Complementary Therapies

Notice we're using the word complementary here. Severe asthma attacks can be life-threatening; parents *must* get a doctor's help in managing this disease. You may also wish to consult an allergy specialist, a naturopathic physician, an herbalist, nutritionist, or acupuncturist. A recent review of sixteen asthma studies showed that, in most of them, acupuncture led to improvement of asthma and other chronic lung conditions. Patients also were able to reduce medication doses. Although we don't know of studies involving acupressure

BREATHING LESSONS

A simple breathing technique, called Eucapnic Breathing or the Buteyko Method, can ameliorate asthma. It corrects asthmatics' tendency to breathe faster than other people, whether they are at rest or under stress. Humans exhale carbon dioxide. Although they need to get rid of some carbon dioxide, hyperventilation causes the body's carbon dioxide levels to fall so low that the bronchi spasm; as a result, less oxygen moves from red blood cells to the tissues. In other words, breathing too quickly and deeply paradoxically decreases the amount of available oxygen. K. P. Buteyko, a Russian doctor, developed a technique to break this vicious cycle. Patients learn to take small, gentle breaths through the nose (which filters, warms, and humidifies the air) and to breathe from the abdomen rather than the upper chest. They also learn that short periods of breath-holding (just long enough for accumulating carbon dioxide to open the bronchi) can interrupt attacks of hyperventilation. Swimming may help asthmatics because of the need to hold the breath between strokes. Buteyko found that 83 percent of asthmatic kids who used his method improved considerably; the other 17 percent showed some benefit. In a 1995 clinical trial, the Buteyko method reduced the need for bronchodilating drugs by 90 percent and reduced asthma symptoms by 50 percent. For more information, check out the Internet site, www.buteykovideo.com. To obtain instructional videotapes, write:

Buteyko Asthma Video Sales, PO Box 41, Annerley, Qld 4130, Australia; phone 61-7-3847-9750; fax 61-7-3397-3832; or e-mail pathein@gil.com.au.

(stimulation of acupuncture points with blunt objects such as the finger tips), we wonder whether learning relevant pressure points might help with the home care of your child.

A number of studies have found that yoga training promotes greater relaxation, increases exercise tolerance, and lessens the need for asthma drugs. In one, teens with a history of childhood asthma found that yoga training improved their scores on pulmonary functions and their exercise capacity. Two years later, the teens' symptoms were still reduced. In another study on adults, asthma sufferers who underwent hypnosis reduced symptoms, improved their scores on pulmonary function tests, and were able to reduce their use of bronchodilating drugs.

If you feel that food sensitivities may play a role in your child's asthma, you may wish to consider an elimination diet. See Chapter 7, Allergies and Intolerances, for more information.

Herbal Therapies

Plant medicines can help maintain your child's respiratory health, reduce his need for prescription medications, or even stave off mild asthma. But don't alter your child's dose of a prescription medication without your doctor's guidance. Because asthma is so serious, we also suggest enlisting a trained herbalist or naturopathic doctor to help you choose among herbal remedies. Go slowly and monitor your child's response.

Mullein is a safe and effective antispasmodic herb, with anti-inflammatory action and a special ability to direct moisture to bronchial tissue. Mullein thins thick mucus in the lungs and makes it easier for asthmatics to breathe. A 50-pound child with chronic asthma can take one to two cups of mullein tea a day for six weeks. Before serving, strain the tea through several layers of fine cloth to remove the tiny leaf hairs.

Want to make a mullein tea taste better? Add antiviral lemon grass and lemon balm, and vitamin-C-rich rose hips and organic orange peels. You can also add dried nettle leaf for its antihistaminic effect.

Ephedra (*Ephedra sinica*), known to Traditional Chinese Medicine practitioners as *ma huang,* has a 5,000-year history of use for the treatment of asthma. It contains ephedrine, similar in structure to the epinephrine our bodies manufacture. Although less potent than epinephrine, ephedrine has similar effects on the body, and it lasts longer. Ephedrine relaxes smooth muscle, creating a larger airway; decreases congestion; and reduces coughing. Although in the same genus, American ephedra (*Ephedra vulgaris, Ephedra viridis*) is not nearly as effective.

Caution: Like epinephrine, however, ephedrine also elevates heart rate and blood pressure and stimulates the central nervous system, and in large doses can produce undesirable effects such as restlessness, anxiety, tremor, insomnia, and headaches. Caffeine-containing products magnify such symptoms. Children with high blood pressure, heart disease, thyroid disease, glaucoma, prostate disease, or diabetes should not use it, nor should pregnant women. Ephedra should not be mixed with other prescriptions for asthma, or with certain types of antidepressants.

Ephedra is a potent remedy for acute situations (like a mild asthma attack), and is not for everyday use by small children. If one of our children over age five were having such an attack, we'd feel comfortable giving him a half-cup of ephedra tea. For other uses of ephedra for asthma, we'd seek the advice of a qualified herbal practitioner.

Marshmallow has had a centuries-long reputation for helping children heal irritated mucous membranes during dry coughs. In the last few years, revered herbal author Michael Moore has hypothesized that marshmallow appears to stimulate the immune system. Now the German Commission E, a branch of the German government that is roughly analogous to our own Food and Drug Administration, agrees. While this makes marshmallow root sound perfect for children's asthma, do take care to sweeten the decocted tea before expecting kids to like the taste. Marshmallow root tea is a bit gooey and is best used for dry, irritable coughs.

Ginkgo has long been used by the Chinese to treat asthma. Its leaves contain ginkgolides, which inhibit a body chemical called platelet activating factor. This substance mediates or slows blood clotting and inflammation and, in high amounts, causes bronchi to constrict. Clinical studies of oral ginkgolides show a reduction in airway over-reactions to inhaled allergens or exercise. Ginkgo leaves also contain the flavonoid quercetin, a natural anti-inflammatory compound. While ginkgo is not a traditional

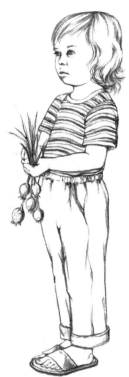

Foods from the onion family contain quercetin, a bioflavonoid that's helpful for asthmatics.

herbal remedy for asthma, its safety record and solid research suggest that it may be worth a try. The recommended dosage for children six to twelve years old is 80 mg of ginkgo biloba standardized extract a day, divided into two to three doses. For children under six, the dosage is 40 mg a day in two to three doses.

Coffee and **tea** both contain caffeine. Caffeine is similar to the asthma drug theophylline; in fact, the body can break down caffeine to theophylline. One study found that people who drank coffee had a 29 percent reduction in asthma symptoms relative to coffee abstainers. The minimum effective dose seems to be about 7 mg of caffeine per 2.2 pounds body weight. Coffee has about 135–150 mg of caffeine per eight-ounce cup, tea about 60 mg. So the dose for a 50-pound child would be about one cup of strong coffee.

We're not suggesting that you start making your child espressos for breakfast. But in an emergency, a cup of coffee may provide relief while you wait for medical help, provided that your child is calm enough to sip it.

Caution: Do not combine coffee or tea with ephedra. Both act on the central nervous and cardiovascular systems, meaning your child could get a double-whammy effect.

Onion extracts have been shown in lab tests to inhibit asthmatic responses. We know that onions, like ginkgo, are rich in quercetin. Onions' benefits for asthmatics, however, may be due to chemicals called isothiocyanates (mustard oils) and thiosulfinates. Either way, eating lots of onions and garlic (and other related foods such as shallots, scallions, and leeks) should become a way of life for kids with asthma. During cold and flu season, a garlic supplement is a good idea. Commercial preparations with parsley can help your child avoid garlic breath.

Elecampane is often used in herb-friendly European countries in pill form. One of

Herbal Steams for Children's Asthma

Inhalation of a steam made with essential oils gives herbal constituents a chance to act directly on the airways, where they're needed. But breathing steam or air laced with essential oil can provoke airway spasm in asthmatic children. You can reduce the chances of this happening by using very dilute concentrations. Start with two drops, if tolerated, and gradually increase to a maximum of five drops in a quart pot of water. You can also begin with your child's face relatively far from the steam/inhaler, then move him closer. Have him take just a couple of breaths; if he coughs, have him move back farther still or discontinue use of this essential oil.

Perhaps a safer use of essential oils during an acute incident of asthma is to make a dilute chest rub of antispasmodic oils. Simply mix two or three drops of essential oil in one-quarter cup of carrier oil such as almond, apricot, or canola oil. Good essential oils to use include lavender, rosemary, peppermint, or German chamomile. Massage this oil gently on your child's back and chest at a time when symptoms are *not* present. If the oil causes no irritation or worsening of asthma, keep the blend handy for use during mild chest constriction.

Stinky Chest Rub That Really Works

Sunny uses this liniment during mild asthma attacks to calm her kids and decrease spastic coughing.

For ages: 1 and older
Yields: 1–2 uses

40 drops valerian tincture or glycerite

1 tablespoon vegetable oil (preferably almond oil), at room temperature

1 or 2 drops chamomile, rosemary, lavender, peppermint, thyme, or lemon thyme essential oil

In a small bowl, mix valerian glycerite or tincture into the vegetable oil. Add the two drops of essential oil. You may want to warn your child that she'll probably notice a funny smell. To engage her imagination and help her relax, create a new name for this stinky but helpful oil. Rub the oil mix between your palms to warm it, then massage generously into your child's chest and back, including the area between the ribs. Wrap your child in an old shirt (the oil may stain) and keep her warm. Within five minutes, she should begin to feel a warm and relaxing sensation in her lungs that allows the airway spasms to subside.

Caution: Never use essential oils internally.

herbalism's most respected and experienced practitioners, the late Rudolf Weiss, M.D., noted that although research hasn't documented exactly why elecampane works, patients with asthmatic bronchitis should expect some help from this expectorant herb if it is used over a period of time. Sunny has used elecampane for spasmodic deep coughs, and has seen it provide benefits quickly. You'll find elecampane in many commercial herb formulas for asthma and respiratory complaints.

Licorice acts as an expectorant and an anti-inflammatory agent. Both effects would suggest that licorice can help asthma sufferers, but clinical trials are needed to test this theory. What *is* known about licorice is that it soothes sore throats and supports the adrenal glands. That's why herbalists often use it in stress formulas. Because licorice occasionally causes retention of sodium and water and loss of potassium, long-term use should be monitored by a qualified health practitioner, especially if your child has high blood pressure.

Horehound also merits inclusion in an asthma formula. Old herbals often credit horehound as a lung strengthener. For asthma we regard it as an effective expectorant, especially for people with a lot of loose, moist mucus in the lungs who need help to get it coughed out.

Horehound has been used traditionally in sugar-sweetened cough drops. To avoid the sugar, you can make horehound into a tea and disguise the bitter taste with natural sweeteners such as honey or maple syrup, or with pleasant tasting

VEGETABLE CHEST POULTICE

For ages: 1 year and older
Yields: one application

For minor lung inflammations, a warm vegetable poultice can have profound healing powers. The heat brings healing blood supply to the area to help the lungs clear out excess mucus and congestion. Sunny prefers carrots for kids with sensitive skin. For others, she chooses onions. Both vegetables have a surprisingly strong ability to dissipate excess mucus and reduce congestion.

2 medium onions, sliced
OR 2 whole carrots, grated
1 old cloth about 12 inches square

Steam your chosen vegetable in a small amount of water over medium heat until slightly softened. Check the temperature of the vegetable against your inner wrist. If it is warm to the skin, but not hot enough to burn, wrap the vegetable into a thin cloth, such as a bandanna or old T-shirt, moistened with hot water. Have the child help you cover the poultice with a warm, moist washcloth or hot-water bottle. Without their interest and cooperation, the job becomes tricky!

For the first application, leave the poultice on your child's skin only five minutes. If no skin irritation develops, replace the poultice for another five minutes, rewarming it if necessary. Repeat for up to ten minutes every three hours. Stop immediately if asthma or coughing increases.

herbs such as peppermint, rose hips, lemon balm or lemon grass. All these flavor-enhancing herbs have medicinal value for asthma.

Valerian is an herbal sedative. Small doses, such as 15 to 20 drops of valerian glycerite for a 50-pound child, can be gently relaxing during a mild asthma attack. In one double-blind study of valerian, patients reported a feeling of stress reduction. In many other studies, valerian has been shown to be an effective sedative.

Red clover is another traditional herb for use in children's asthma. It's a milder expectorant than horehound, but tastes better. Even though red clover's use as an expectorant has not been confirmed by clinical studies, Sunny uses soothing red clover tea as a general tonic to help children recover from any bout with respiratory illness.

Caution: Because of its naturally occurring blood-thinning compound, coumarin, red clover should not be used by children or adults with blood-clotting disorders.

Struggling for a Breath of Fresh Air

In a symbolic sense, the breath of fresh air your child labors for may represent a yearning for change. Healing asthma almost always involves significant changes in your family's lifestyle—not an easy path. Recovery is not an overnight project; sometimes it can be a long, tedious job for both adult and child. If you are the parent or caretaker of a child with asthma, give yourself credit for the wise choices in medical care you have already made. Resolve to continue your education as you unravel this illness. In the meantime, congratulate your child for his bravery and dedication to helping himself feel better.

For Further Reading

Krohn, J., et al. *The Whole Way to Allergy Relief and Prevention.* Point Roberts, WA: Hartley and Marks, Inc. 1991.

Rapp, D. J. *Is This Your Child?: Discovering and Treating Unrecognized Allergies.* New York: William Morrow Co., 1991.

LUNG TONIC TEA

For ages: 1 and over
Yields: 3½ cups

This tea is meant for use during the "asthma season" in your home. Its herbs will tone and support your child's overworked lungs.

*2 tablespoons chopped astragalus root
(adaptogenic, immune stimulating)*

*1 teaspoon horehound leaves
(expectorant)*

*1 teaspoon sage leaves
(antibacterial, expectorant)*

*2 teaspoons mullein leaves
(antiviral, expectorant)*

*Peel of 1/8 organic orange, dried
(circulatory, stimulant)*

4 cups water

honey to taste

Simmer astragalus root in water in a covered pot for 10 minutes. Remove from heat. Add remaining herbs; steep for five minutes (no longer, as the tea will become bitter). Strain and sweeten to taste. Serve warm in small cupfuls throughout the day. Store unused portion in refrigerator for up to three days.

Chapter 17

NAUSEA AND VOMITING

Childhood tummy upsets are the stuff of family legends: the night Sarah threw up on three consecutive sets of clean sheets and blankets, the time that a forty-five-minute jaunt took over two hours because Brady was carsick at every curve in the road, and the afternoon that Kelly's unexplained "stomach flu" turned out to be caused by her secret consumption of a whole bag of marshmallows. Years later, everyone groans and laughs. When it's happening, however, a kid's vomiting isn't even remotely laughable. It can occur suddenly and without apparent cause—Sunny's son once gave her exactly fifteen seconds of warning before throwing up. And although nausea and vomiting are not usually worrisome, certain kinds can signal serious illness.

First, we'd like to distinguish between a baby's spitting up and true vomiting. Spitting up is common among infants and involves the effortless expulsion of one or two mouthfuls of stomach contents, usually soon after a feeding. Most importantly, infants who spit up do not appear ill in any other way. In comparison, vomiting has more force behind it and therefore a more impressive trajectory.

Causes of Nausea and Vomiting

Nausea can be triggered by many things—motion sickness, food poisoning, overeating (especially of high-fat or junk food), food allergies, or infections (most commonly viruses). Migraine headaches or strep throat can make kids vomit. Given sufficient nausea, vomiting usually follows; sometimes your child gets the package deal that includes diarrhea.

With acute viral infection, your child may also have belly pain, fever, and headache. Infectious nausea and vomiting should resolve within one to three days, and are quite contagious.

Swallowing a lot of nasal secretions during a cold can also cause nausea and vomiting. It's not uncommon for kids to vomit after an episode of violent coughing. This occurs in whooping cough.

In rare cases, a congenital abnormality of the gastrointestinal tract can cause vomiting, as can other causes of obstruction of the stomach or intestines. In extremely rare cases, a brain tumor may be the cause. Such cases require medical evaluation and treatment.

Managing Nausea and Vomiting

Vomiting is one of the body's ways of purging itself. For this reason, you don't want to stop it, particularly if the cause is microbes or toxins. Suspect infectious origins if your child acts ill with accompanying symptoms such as stomachache, fever, and diarrhea, has been in contact with someone else who has had a "stomach bug," or has eaten food that is possibly contaminated. The following strategies can help children's bodies recover.

Breast-feeding infants with mild to moderate vomiting can usually continue to nurse. Because small volumes of milk are more likely to stay down, you might want to nurse for only five to ten minutes at a time, or only on one breast at a time. Some mothers may find it useful to first empty their breasts a bit with a breast pump so the child gets only a small amount of milk.

If your infant drinks formula, your health professional may recommend switching to an oral rehydration fluid such as Pedialyte or KAO Lectrolyte for eight hours.

Stop solid foods for kids old enough to eat them for at least eight hours and eliminate milk and other dairy products for a day or two. Prevent dehydration, which can aggravate vomiting, by encouraging clear fluids while the vomiting persists. For the first eight hours, give only tepid, clear liquids in small sips at frequent intervals, even if you must spoon-feed your child. Large volumes of fluid may induce more vomiting.

Fluids to give include diluted juices, teas, soup broths, and sports drinks such as Recharge or Gatorade. This type of beverage contains a

balance of sugar and salts that help make up for mineral loss. Your health practitioner may recommend a children's rehydration fluid. If your older child feels like sucking on ice chips or

WHEN TO CALL A DOCTOR ABOUT NAUSEA AND VOMITING

Vomiting persists for twelve hours if your child is under six months old; or one day if she is between six to twelve months old; more than two days for older children

Your child refuses to drink

Your child seems dehydrated. She has dry skin and lips, cries without tears, urinates less often than every eight hours, and her soft spot is sunken

Your newborn routinely vomits with force (projectile vomiting) after meals

Your child vomits blood

Your child complains of severe abdominal pain

You suspect accidental ingestion of poison

Your child has periodic vomiting that seems unrelated to infectious illness, suggesting possible food intolerance or an emotional component

Your child acts very ill, especially with extreme irritability or lethargy

Your child had chicken pox or flu in the previous two weeks

Your child routinely vomits in the morning and complains of headache frozen pops made from juice or herb tea, that's fine.

After eight hours on clear liquids, reintroduce bland foods such as oatmeal, crackers, white bread, white rice, pureed barley, mashed potatoes, cooked carrots, applesauce, bananas, and brothy soups. Babies already taking solid foods can ease back into rice cereals, pureed carrots, mashed bananas, and applesauce. Go slowly. Small, frequent meals are best.

Use herbal antispasmodics such as gingerroot or peppermint to relieve stomach and intestinal cramps.

On the second day after vomiting stops, try serving your child good-quality, live-culture milk or soy yogurt, which helps replenish beneficial gut bacteria.

Use common sense when it comes to hygiene. Make sure your child washes his hands after he vomits. Wash your own hands frequently when caring for him, handling his laundry, and preparing his meals.

Herbal Remedies for Nausea and Vomiting

Ginger is the herb *par excellence* for controlling nausea. In a study of people susceptible to motion sickness, ginger was superior to Dramamine in reducing gastrointestinal distress.

Your child can take ginger in whatever form he can tolerate—fresh, crystallized, dried, or powdered. Some kids like to chew crystallized ginger, although it's generally coated with sugar. We make ginger tea by grating one teaspoon of the fresh root, covering with boiling water, and simmering five to ten minutes. Once the tea is strained, we add honey or lemon to taste.

Sometimes we give our kids room-temperature ginger ale for nausea. Read the label to make sure the ginger ale contains real ginger; many brands contain only ginger flavoring. You can leave the bottle or can open a while or add a teaspoon of warm water to cut the carbonation.

Studies have generally used a daily adult dose of one to two grams of dried, powdered ginger, which is the equivalent of 1/3 ounce of fresh ginger or one 1/4-inch slice. A 50-pound child can take approximately one-third of the adult dose, and a 25-pound child can take one-sixth of the adult dose.

Peppermint leaf seems like a simple tea herb, but its powerful antispasmodic effects can relieve stomachaches and gas pains. Sunny carries peppermint throat lozenges in her briefcase and car for exactly this reason. In a pinch, you can purchase peppermint lozenges at any convenience store; most contain menthol, the active ingredient in peppermint leaf. Most people like the taste of

---

CHAMOMILE TUMMYACHE COMPRESS

1/2 cup dried or 1/4 cup fresh chamomile flowers

One quart pure water

Soft cloth, approximately 12 inches square (pieces of an old T-shirt will do)

Make a strong tea by steeping the chamomile for 10 to 15 minutes in hot water. Strain. While the tea remains warm but not too hot, soak the cloth in it, wring, and apply to your child's stomach and intestinal areas. Stay with your child and soothe her with lullabies or a story as you reapply the compress every five minutes or so. Keep the compress warm by applying a hot-water bottle over the affected area. Don't allow the cloth to chill, as this may increase her cramps.

peppermint. Or as one child put it: "At least it doesn't taste so bad if you end up throwing up anyway."

Catnip is a time-tested herbal remedy for colic and children's stomachaches. Unlike cats, humans usually experience calming effects from catnip. Healers worldwide use it as a mild sedative and to relax intestinal cramping. Be sure to purchase certified organic catnip, not the pet-store packages; that catnip tends to have been raised with pesticides.

Caution: Do not use while pregnant.

Chamomile. No discussion of children's tummy aches would be complete without Peter Rabbit's favorite, chamomile tea. Many restaurants around the world serve it. We think these tiny flowers smell and taste best when fresh. This is not a wimpy herb: the German Commission E and ample research confirm its antispasmodic, antiseptic, and anti-inflammatory value for relieving digestive distress (including ulcers), mild anxiety, and a variety of skin complaints. One of chamomile's greatest assets is its ability to relieve minor stomach cramps when taken as a tea or glycerite.

Wild yam acts to calm sharp, spasmodic twinges of smooth muscle and consequently helps ease stomachache and intestinal cramping. You can keep a jar of capsules handy and break them open to brew a mild tea; a 50-pound child can drink half a cup, twice daily, for several days.

Caution: The American Herbal Products Association rates wild yam as safe when consumed appropriately, although its safety during pregnancy is not known.

Chapter 18

DIARRHEA AND CONSTIPATION

Few parents need a definition for diarrhea, but here it is: an abrupt and dramatic increase in bowel movements with loose stools. It's common for breast-fed infants to have mushy, even green stools. But when a child shows a radical change in bowel habits, it's usually a symptom of some kind of digestive trouble. Kids can come into contact with a wide variety of microorganisms these days; if diarrhea doesn't clear up in a few days, consult a doctor. Constipation, the opposite bowel problem, can often be cleared up with dietary changes or gentle herbs.

Like vomiting, acute diarrhea is one of the body's ways of ridding itself of a noxious substance. The cause usually is an infectious agent or something ingested. While vomiting usually ceases in twenty-four hours, diarrhea can continue for several days.

The cause of diarrhea can be as simple as drinking too much juice, a common problem among toddlers. Sometimes food can disagree with your child or—more frightening—be tainted with bacteria or the toxins bacteria produce. Viruses can cause diarrhea; rotavirus is one of the more common ones. Bacterial infections are more serious, but much less common, especially in the United States. Parasites can also cause diarrhea. Giardia, one such parasite, is increasingly common in U.S. day-care centers. In general, kids in large day-care centers have an increased risk of getting infectious diarrhea; kids in small home-based child care don't.

Non-Infectious Causes

Toddlers love juice. But excessive juice consumption also loosens stools. Apple juice, which is high in the difficult-to-absorb sugars fructose and sorbitol, is often at the root of chronic diarrhea in small children. If this could be causing your youngster's diarrhea, stop giving her juice and substitute a weak, honey-sweetened herb tea, broth, or other clear liquids. Vitamins taken in high doses, especially vitamin C, can also cause diarrhea; if this is a possibility, take a one-day break and see what happens.

Many antibiotics irritate the intestines, so diarrhea is a fairly common side effect. Check with your doctor about ways to counteract the diarrhea that won't interfere with the medicine your child needs. Often adding supplements of acidophilus/bifidus bacteria can help offset diarrhea caused by antibiotics.

Food allergies can cause recurrent diarrhea, usually accompanied by belly pain, sometimes by vomiting. The most common offender is milk. Studies estimate that 0.3 to 7.5 percent of kids have allergies to milk protein. For infants on milk-based formula, symptoms usually begin around thirteen weeks of age and include vomiting, diarrhea, poor growth, flatulence, excessive

crying, eczema, coughing, and wheezing. About 30 to 40 percent of infants sensitive to milk protein are also sensitive to soy protein. You'll want to check with your doctor about formula alternatives if you are unable to breastfeed and your baby seems intolerant of standard formulas. Older children may also manifest diarrhea from food allergies.

Nursing moms who take laxative herbs should know that any substance they eat or drink can be

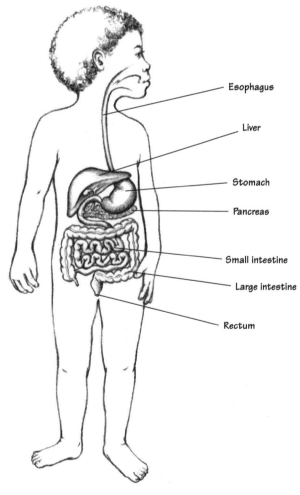

Inside the digestive system

Esophagus

Liver

Stomach

Pancreas

Small intestine

Large intestine

Rectum

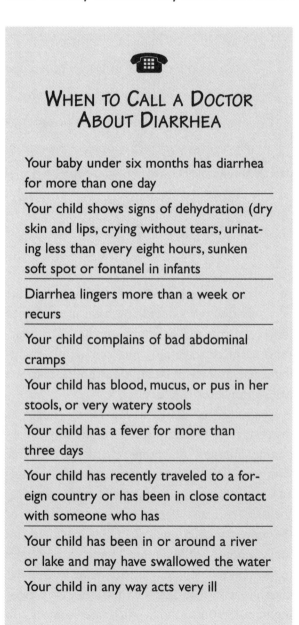

WHEN TO CALL A DOCTOR ABOUT DIARRHEA

Your baby under six months has diarrhea for more than one day

Your child shows signs of dehydration (dry skin and lips, crying without tears, urinating less than every eight hours, sunken soft spot or fontanel in infants

Diarrhea lingers more than a week or recurs

Your child complains of bad abdominal cramps

Your child has blood, mucus, or pus in her stools, or very watery stools

Your child has a fever for more than three days

Your child has recently traveled to a foreign country or has been in close contact with someone who has

Your child has been in or around a river or lake and may have swallowed the water

Your child in any way acts very ill

transferred to their babies. We recommend that nursing moms avoid laxative use, and rely on additional fluids and fiber-rich foods to relieve their own constipation.

Infections in or irritations to other organs, notably bladder infections, can cause loose stools. Some people believe ear infections and teething can be a cause as well.

Infectious Causes

So you're certain it wasn't something your child ate—or at least, not anything that was big enough to see. Unfortunately, a multitude of "bugs" can cause diarrhea—viruses, bacteria, and parasites. These microorganisms can contaminate food products, or be passed person-to-person through poor hygiene. Pets can also transmit them; turtles can have salmonella and dogs, giardia.

Viral Diarrhea

Viruses are the most frequent cause of kids' diarrhea. The two most common types are rotavirus and Norwalk virus. Rotavirus is the most common cause of infectious diarrhea in developed countries such as the United States. Kids under the age of two seem to be particularly susceptible; the virus is very contagious, because it is often difficult to kill. It can become epidemic in day-care centers. Rates of infection hit their peak in winter.

After an incubation period of one to three days, rotavirus symptoms appear, including diarrhea that is watery but without blood, vomiting, and low-grade fever. Symptoms usually go away within five to eight days. Conventional treatment focuses on keeping your child hydrated. A new vaccine called Rotashield™ can be given to infants by mouth in three doses. Three clinical trials have shown it to be effective in reducing the number of infections (particularly those that

APPENDICITIS SYMPTOMS EVERY PARENT SHOULD KNOW

The appendix is a small tube projecting from the large intestine near the point where it joins the small intestine. If a blockage in the appendix causes an infection, it swells and becomes inflamed, resulting in appendicitis. An infected appendix can rupture, spilling its infectious contents into the abdominal cavity—naturally, an occasion every parent would like to avoid. *If you suspect appendicitis, call your doctor immediately. He or she will advise you about how to proceed.*

The main symptom of appendicitis is abdominal pain that begins as cramps in the middle of the belly, then becomes constant and settles in the lower right corner (unless your child is one of those rare people whose organs are switched right to left). Coughing, deep breathing, jumping, or any sudden movement worsens the pain. Pushing on the right lower belly, then quickly letting go, causes a sharp pain.

The following symptoms usually occur with the sharp abdominal pain—but not always. When they occur without the abdominal pain, the symptoms below aren't cause for alarm. The abdominal pain alone or combined with these symptoms signals an emergency.

Loss of appetite, nausea, and vomiting

The urge to pass stool or gas

Fever

Elevated heart rate

cause severe diarrhea), the duration of illness, dehydration, and the need for hospitalization. If your small child attends day care, or is otherwise at risk, you may want to talk to your doctor about this vaccine.

Norwalk virus can affect older kids and adults; incidence peaks in winter. The source is usually contaminated food or water. After an incubation of twelve hours to four days, symptoms begin with nausea, vomiting, and diarrhea; some people also have muscle aches. Vomiting is particularly frequent. Again, conventional treatment's goal is to make sure your child gets sufficient fluids and wait for the virus to run its course—and, of course, to try to prevent transmission to the rest of the family.

Bacterial Diarrhea

Campylobacter particularly affects those at either end of their childhood—infants under the age of twelve months and young adults. Peak infection time is summer and fall. The source is usually contaminated food—frequently raw milk or poultry—or an infected person. Symptoms begin two to four days after exposure. They can include abdominal pain, nausea, frequent diarrhea, headache, muscle aches, and low-grade fever. In severe cases, the diarrhea may contain blood. Usually, campylobacter infections clear up without treatment within a week. Severe or prolonged illness may require a round of an antibiotic such as erythromycin. Sometimes antibiotics are recommended in less than severe cases to prevent the spread of the disease, especially if the child is in day care.

Salmonella has begun to occur more frequently, possibly because of the use of antibiotics in livestock and a resultant rise in antibiotic-resistant organisms. The source of infection is usually infected food—meat, poultry, eggs, or raw dairy. The organism also can be passed from one person

to another by poor hygiene after bathroom use or changing a diaper. Pet turtles and iguanas are another source.

If the source of infection is contaminated food, symptoms begin a few hours to three days after eating. They include severe abdominal cramps, nausea, vomiting, diarrhea, weakness, fever, and chills. The numerous watery stools may contain mucus, pus, or blood. The illness usually resolves within one to seven days. Cases in infants often require antibiotics, sometimes intravenously administered.

Escherichia coli, often referred to as *E. coli,* occurs most often in infants under eighteen months. Most cases occur from late summer to early fall. This organism is a common cause of traveler's diarrhea. Sources usually are contaminated food or drink or other infected people with lax handwashing habits. The disease comes on abruptly, with frequent, foul-smelling stools the color and consistency of pea soup. Kids who encounter *E. coli* also usually have abdominal cramps, vomiting, and possibly fever. Mild to moderate cases resolve on their own after five to ten days, but they can be very rough days. Infants are at particularly high risk of becoming dehydrated and should be medically monitored.

Shigella is more common in developing countries than in the United States. Kids under the age of five are most susceptible to this bacteria, but adults are in no way immune. Sunny was once rafting with a group of people in the Grand Canyon who all suffered from shigella dysentery during the trip. The sources are primarily other people and unclean drinking water. The disease begins suddenly with high fever and weakness. The large-volume, watery stools may contain mucus. The dysenteric form of shigella causes worsening diarrhea over two to three days, severe abdominal pain and tenderness, painful bowel movements, and small-volume stools that contain blood and mucus. Infants and children diagnosed with shigella are generally treated with antibiotics. On the river trip, Sunny and friends drank copious amounts of an oral rehydration mix until they could get to a medical facility.

Parasitic Infections

Giardia is the most common parasitic infection. A Wisconsin study has noted that, between 1981 and 1988, giardia cases increased twentyfold, with most cases and the greatest increase in cases occurring in children between ages one and four. A third of the cases in this age group occurred in kids who attended day care.

Sources of giardia include contaminated municipal water, many lakes and mountain streams, other people, and sometimes pets. Its symptoms may not appear until one to three weeks after exposure, and include abdominal cramps, nausea, flatulence, and watery diarrhea. The stools may smell bad, appear greasy, and float. Symptoms can last between five days and months. Conventional treatment involves antiparasitic drugs.

Amebiasis is caused by an amoeba. Although uncommon in the United States, it occurs worldwide. The source is usually an infected person who contaminates food and water. Gradually appearing symptoms usually include slight fever, abdominal discomfort, and diarrhea; they can be mild to severe. The stools don't smell all that bad (compared to when bacteria are to blame); they can contain clear mucus. But amebiasis is nothing to mess with; these bad bugs can deeply invade the bowel wall and infect other organs, notably the liver. Conventional medical treatment usually involves antiparasitic drugs.

Pinworms don't generally cause vomiting or diarrhea. They can, however, cause abdominal pain, sometimes mimicking appendicitis. They induce irritability, restlessness, and intense anal itching, especially at night when the female pinworms leave the anus to lay eggs. The itching and abdominal pain can interfere with sleep. Some kids lose their appetites.

A simple diagnostic technique for pinworms is to press adhesive cellulose tape right over the anus, ideally first thing in the morning before your child wipes her bottom. Your doctor may instruct you to fold this tape, sticky sides together, place it in a clean jar and bring it in for microscopic examination.

Conventional medical treatment consists of an antiworm medication such as mebendazole, which goes by the trade name Vermox. Holistic medical doctors often agree that Vermox is a relatively safe and easy way to help your child get rid of pinworms and get on with her life.

Home Care for Diarrhea

Most parents can perform basic care for a case of the "runs" at home. But if you suspect your child's recurrent digestive problems are due to a bacterial or parasitic infestation, we urge you to promptly consult a doctor for a diagnosis. Some of these infections, left untreated, can progress to serious conditions. You may also want to explore the treatment options offered by naturopathic physicians.

As with vomiting, diarrhea is the body's way of eliminating microbes and toxins, so you don't necessarily want it to stop. If something noninfectious, such as a food allergy or too much juice, is to blame, removing the offending substance will usually end the diarrhea.

Maintaining Fluid Intake

Perhaps the most important aspect of home care during this uncomfortable time is maintaining fluids. Diarrhea can rapidly dehydrate a child, particularly an infant. Encourage lots of clear liquids. You'll know your child is adequately hydrated if he pees often (every three to four hours) or, if he's an infant or toddler, wets eight diapers a day (granted, in the presence of frequent diarrhea, this isn't easy to determine). Children should drink lots of clear liquids in the form of water, weak herbal teas, sports drinks, and diluted vegetable and fruit juice. Basil tea can help relieve cramping. If your child craves cold beverages, you can try frozen treats made of juice, herbal tea, or a combination of the two. Go cautiously with fruit juices, because they can aggravate diarrhea. One way to give fluids and soothe your child's irritated intestinal tract is to have him sip barley water. Cook three tablespoons dried barley in one and one-quarter cup water until the barley is soft, then strain.

MILK AND DIARRHEA

Although earlier studies showed that milk aggravated diarrhea in kids, a more recent study found that modest intakes of milk were well tolerated. On the other hand, milk allergy and lactose intolerance is a common cause of chronic or recurrent diarrhea. You'll have to see how milk affects your child and act accordingly.

If you suspect milk allergy has caused the diarrhea to begin with, eliminate dairy from your child's diet. You may want to discuss this first with your health practitioner. If your baby takes a formula based on cow's milk or soy (another potential allergen), let your doctor help you find another formula. Antiallergenic formulas are fairly expensive, so reimbursement from insurers or a tax deduction is worth looking into.

What—and When—to Feed

For the twelve to twenty-four hours of moderate to severe diarrhea, your child over one year should take only clear liquids and no solid foods. If the diarrhea is mild, just avoid whole-grain cereals and raw fruits and vegetables. For all degrees of severity, many physicians recommend that kids forego milk products except yogurt for about a week. Continuing a clear liquid diet for more than two days can perpetuate diarrhea, however. Also, your child will lose weight. If removing suspect foods and solids doesn't begin to firm things up in two days, it could be time to call the doctor about a possible viral, bacterial, or parasitic cause for the diarrhea.

If your child with diarrhea is under one year, continue nursing if you breast-feed. In general, breast-feeding reduces the risk of intestinal infections and, compared to formula-feeding, shortens the course of the illness. Breast milk seems to favorably alter an infant's bowel bacteria. It also contains antibodies and compounds such as mucin that protect against intestinal infections, including those caused by rotavirus. And breast milk, although relatively high in lactose, doesn't seem to trouble infants recovering from diarrhea. In more serious cases, a doctor may recommend adding oral rehydration liquids (Pedialyte and others) to your infant's diet to prevent dehydration. And if your baby drinks a soy or milk-based formula and has very frequent stools, your doctor may have you either switch to oral rehydration liquids for about a day or dilute the formula. Under no circumstances, however, should you dilute formulas without a doctor's supervision.

Once the acute diarrhea wanes, you can support your child's return to health with a good diet. She probably won't feel much like eating, but yogurt with live cultures is an easily digested food that tastes good. Yogurt contains beneficial bacteria that have already digested the milk sugar so often troublesome in the post-diarrheal phase. Avoid high-sugar versions, as parasites tend to thrive in high-sugar environments.

After your child's stools become less watery and less frequent, you can reintroduce easy-to-digest foods such as bananas, applesauce, cooked carrots, toast, crackers, clear soups, rice, and rice cereals. Recovering kids often tolerate slightly burnt toast, because the burnt, carbonized portions tend to relieve intestinal spasms. Start with small, frequent meals. Delay whole-grain cold cereals and raw fruits until your child shows she can handle bland foods.

When digestive powers are recovering, concentrated high-protein foods are often difficult to digest, but steamed vegetables and cooked whole grains are great. Cooked oatmeal and barley are excellent recovery foods. Avoid serving your child fried foods and most raw fruits or vegetables. Foods that have been used traditionally to combat intestinal parasites include squash seeds, onions, and walnuts, especially the tincture of the green hulls. If you live in a tropical area, you should know that the stinky durian fruit is a reliable folk remedy for treating malaria and gastrointestinal parasites. And of course, fresh, ripe pineapple, with its naturally occurring digestive enzyme, bromelain, should be a big help if your child's intestinal tract can tolerate it. If not, you may want to try a bromelain supplement.

The Squeaky-Clean Strategy

The organisms that cause infectious diarrhea are highly contagious. You can prevent the spread of infection with good hygiene. Cut everyone's fingernails short and be vigilant about hand-washing with soap, especially after using the bathroom. If your child isn't toilet trained, remind those caring for her to wash hands after diaper changes. Keeping the house and bedclothes exceptionally clean can also help. Wash sheets, pajamas, and underwear daily in hot water with a bit of antibacterial bleach or bleach substitute. Sanitize toilet seats with a mixture of five drops thyme essential oil per two cups water. Keep following a heightened hygiene schedule for two to three days after the diarrhea has resolved.

Herbal Remedies for Diarrhea

If your child's diarrhea has an infectious basis, you generally don't want to use herbs or anything else to stop the elimination of infectious agents, unless he's becoming dehydrated. Check first with your health practitioner.

Carob powder. Carob is a great natural remedy for diarrhea and is generally safe for infants. Plus, they love the taste. Simply mix one teaspoon of carob powder into applesauce or yogurt, cover

MORE WAYS TO COPE WITH FLUID LOSS

If your child isn't taking fluids well, you can increase absorption of water and herbal constituents via herb baths, herbal tea foot soaks, herbal massage oils, and warm compresses applied to the stomach. Make sure the bath temperature is warm, but not hot — don't dehydrate your child further by "sweating" her.

For an herbal bath or soak, simply make a large pot of strong tea, strain, and pour it into the bathtub. Bath or foot-soak herbs to decrease intestinal spasms may include catnip, chamomile, a small amount of peppermint, thyme, lemon balm, fennel, motherwort, or lavender.

all stainable surfaces (including the kids), and let them enjoy their medicine. By the way, carob's flavor resembles chocolate, but carob has no caffeine.

Bentonite clay. Bentonite makes a great "cork" for slowing mild diarrhea. You can purchase bentonite clay powder in bulk form at natural products stores. If your child is over age two, you can stir one teaspoon of powder into a cup of water. Start with one teaspoon of this mix every four hours for kid ages two to four, or a tablespoon every four hours for kids over age four. Serve quickly before it settles, and use cautiously; too much bentonite has a binding effect and can constipate a child when his body still needs to eliminate.

Blackberry or **raspberry leaf** and **root.** Sunny has a friend who swears that after three days of severe diarrhea, he could actually feel his first dose of blackberry root tea puckering up his behind and curing his temporary intestinal problem. It's a gentle way to control diarrhea, without

stopping the elimination of toxins. On the other hand, it's hard to find these roots unless you're willing to dig them up out of your own garden. To make a tea of the roots, chop them and simmer for ten minutes.

The leaves of the two plants are astringent, but not as strong as the roots. Read the labels when buying these teas; you're looking for the actual herb leaves, not raspberry or blackberry flavoring. Serve kids sips of either tea throughout the day, as they are able to take it. Berry leaf teas makes great popsicles, too.

Apple peels contain naturally occurring pectin, a universal remedy for fighting diarrhea. Purified pectin is used to thicken foods such as jams, jellies, and ice cream. Most herbalists suggest making cooked applesauce with the whole apple peel. Use organic apples to avoid pesticides and waxes laden with chemicals. If you mix your homemade applesauce with carob powder, you've got a great-tasting potential cure for mild diarrhea. Very rarely, a child will be allergic to apple peels; discontinue use if the diarrhea seems to get worse. And yes, this fruit works both ways: cooked apples are a time-honored remedy for diarrhea, while raw apples and apple juice can help loosen constipation.

Cooked carrots are antibacterial and rehydrating. Researchers have found that carrot soup actually blocked bacteria, including *E. coli,* from sticking to the small intestines of patients with severe diarrhea. All you need to do is to steam sliced carrots and puree in the blender. Some parents may want to add garlic for its antimicrobial effects, or ginger to ward off chills or nausea, but that depends on your child's food preferences. You may see an orange poop or two, but don't worry; this is natural during times of quick intestinal transit.

Acidophilus and **bifidus** are strains of *Lactobacillus,* a bacteria normally found in the

---

DIAPERS AND DIARRHEA

Diarrhea can be especially miserable for a child who's still in diapers. Protect his bottom with an ointment or herbal salve. Make or purchase one containing comfrey to encourage speedy skin-cell regeneration.

If your diapered child ends up with painful blisters from diarrhea, avoid salves or lotions and try to expose her skin to fresh air several times a day. You can also coat your child's inflamed bottom with a bit of barley water (see page 175, Maintaining Fluid Intake). For more information on diaper rash, see Chapter 18, Skin Disorders.

intestines. The latter predominates in infants and young children. Supplements of these organisms, called probiotics, help prevent and improve recovery from diarrhea. They work in several ways: out-competing undesirable bacteria, preventing "bad" bacteria from clinging to the intestinal lining, strengthening local immune response in the gut, and stimulating white blood cells. (The acidophilus milk you can buy at the grocer usually dosen't have enough organisms to help.)

Herbal Strategies for Bacterial and Parasitic Infections

Kids with some bacterial infections, serious viral infections, and any parasitic infection need to be seen by a doctor. After that, you may want to help any conventional medications do their job with the following herbs.

Garlic is a traditional treatment for several types of parasites. Research has shown that garlic kills several parasites, including roundworm, pinworm, tapeworm, and hookworm. While science hasn't yet proven (or disproven) garlic's use against other parasites, it is always included in traditional herbal parasite formulas, and we wouldn't hesitate to use it on our own children while they were receiving other medical care for parasites. Eating several raw cloves of garlic a day is most effective. You can also give your 50-pound child half of a garlic-oil capsule several times a day with food. (Poke the capsule with a pin to release half of the oil; increase dose to a full capsule if your child tolerates the garlic oil well).

Charcoal. Activated charcoal is very effective for relieving intestinal gas. Sunny knows several people who took several capsules daily during herbal treatment for the recurrent sulphur-smelling gas of giardia. They all proclaim great relief from this simple remedy.

Caution: Charcoal's absorptive abilities are known to affect bloodstream minerals as well. Follow package instructions and do not give your child charcoal for more than one week without a one-day break. Discontinue use if gastric irritation occurs.

Oregon graperoot is a good candidate for treating giardia. It contains the alkaloid berberine, an antimicrobial compound. In one study, children with giardia, ages five months to fourteen years, were given berberine. After ten days, 90 percent of the children were cured, comparable to the percentage cured with drugs. Another study found berberine to be as effective as antibiotics in treating 65 kids with diarrhea caused by *E. coli*, shigella, salmonella, and cholera bacteria.

If one of our children had giardia or other bacterial diarrhea, we would be comfortable giving her a dose equivalent to 500 mg of Oregon graperoot for a 50-pound child, three times a day for ten days. We would also supplement her diet with acidophilus during and for several days after the treatment.

Caution: Herbs containing berberine are not for use during pregnancy.

Raw pumpkin seeds. These are available at natural products stores, often in the refrigerator section. Whether pumpkin's antiparasitic action is due to its essential fatty acid content, high zinc levels, or another factor isn't clear. One herbal researcher suggests that pumpkin seeds can discourage cellular reproduction of the parasite.

The great thing about pumpkin seeds is that they're delicious when fresh. They get bitter if stale or rancid, so we keep our seeds in the refrigerator. Kids love their nutty taste. Due to the high reoccurence rates of several types of parasites, we suggest serving raw pumpkin seeds for snacks several times per week, year round, if your kids have been exposed.

Peppermint. We've found peppermint's antispasmodic action on the smooth muscles of the intestines to be tremendously helpful during giardia. Keep peppermint lozenges or glycerite on hand for quick relief.

Citrus seed extract can be helpful in fighting both bacterial and parasitic infestations. Made from the seed, pulp, and inner rind of grapefruit, this extremely bitter substance is best taken in capsules. Test-tube studies show that grapefruit seed and pulp extract has activity against a broad range of "bugs."

Because of its potency, we recommend this nutritional supplement only for children over seven years old. Start with a low dose: half a capsule for three days. If that is tolerated, give your child half a capsule twice a day, with the final dose being three half-capsules three times a day for a 50-pound child. Use for a maximum of fourteen days.

Linda gave this supplement to her kids as a preventive when they were as young as five. She brings it when traveling to places where the water is questionable, and adds drops to her family's morning juice or gives everyone a tablet. Stir the juice well, she advises. This stuff is really bitter! Linda and her family don't do a lot of foreign travel, but so far, no one has gotten traveler's diarrhea.

Quassia bark *(Picrasma excelsa).* This bark has a strong reputation for treating giardia. Many herbalists and their clients swear by its action—and swear at its taste. Like many digestive herbs with strong effects, quassia is very bitter. For this reason, reserve its use for children over seven years who can swallow a capsule or a vile-tasting tincture.

Several adults whom Sunny knows have taken thirty drops of the tincture three times daily for three weeks to eradicate giardia symptoms. There is no specific research on its safety for children, but the American Herbal Products Association, the main self-regulating body for producers, rates quassia as safe. Follow the package directions and Clark's rule to find a dosage for your child.

Caution: Do not use during pregnancy.

Elecampane contains a potent worm and parasite killer called alantolactone. A beautiful, tall plant, elecampane is generally thought of as an expectorant, but we would certainly try giving small sips of this bitter tea several times a day if our children were diagnosed with intestinal parasites.

Caution: Not for use during pregnancy and nursing.

Echinacea is a useful herb for any inflammatory state, including the digestive upset that accompanies parasites. Give your child echinacea glycerite or tea to help support the immune system during this challenging time.

Papaya contains proteolytic enzymes, making it a natural digestive aid. Make a tea of the leaves or purchase chewable papaya enzymes at a natural foods store. Sunny uses papaya regularly after meals and has also recommended it to help relieve digestive spasms in people with giardia. The greatest quantity of antiparasitical components are in the unripe fruit. Children can chew one teaspoon of papaya seeds per day to treat parasites or pinworms, or the seeds can be crushed and mixed with a lot of water.

Other Complementary Practices

A study involving Nicaraguan children with diarrhea found that, compared to treatment with a placebo, individually prescribed homeopathic medicines significantly reduced the number of stools per day and the duration of diarrhea. If you want to investigate homeopathic medicines for your child's diarrhea, seek out a trained practitioner to help you select the right remedy.

Constipation

Doctors define constipation as infrequent and painful passage of stools. If the stools are soft and don't cause discomfort, then your child may just have a more leisurely rhythm. Some infants and kids habitually go two or three days without a bowel movement. Most pediatricians consider longer intervals as constipation.

Usual causes of constipation include inadequate intake of fluids and fiber and reluctance or anxiety about using the toilet. If your child passes a hard stool that cuts or tears his anus, he may really resist going to the bathroom the next time and create a vicious cycle. Food allergies, particularly allergies to milk, can also cause constipation.

Home Care for Constipation

First, encourage your child to drink more fluids, especially water. If your child is an infant over four months and drinks from a cup or bottle, you can add a little diluted juice. Older children should drink lots of water; add juice in moderate amounts. We say "moderate" because juice contains a lot of fruit sugar without the fiber found in whole fruit. Prune juice remains the all-time favorite laxative juice. Try quarter-cup servings, three to four times a day, rather than one large dose.

Make meals fiber-rich. If your baby is over four to six months old and taking some food, you can enrich her diet with pureed fruits and vegetables. For older children, serve whole-grain breads and brown rice to increase fiber intake. Try to add whole grains, legumes, fresh fruits, and vegetables. Foods good at loosening stools include figs, prunes, blackberries, bran, almonds, and apples.

Go easy on potentially constipating foods: dairy products, especially milk, cheese, and ice cream, and foods made from low-fiber, highly processed grains, such as many supermarket cereals, crackers, and pastries.

Help your child stay active. Exercise encourages good bowel function. We don't mean that your child should get up each morning and work out to an aerobics video. Just encourage him to go out and play with friends, join an athletic team, dance around the house with you, or whatever seems age-appropriate.

If your child develops a tear in his anus from passing a hard stool, try a sitz bath. Add a quarter cup of salt per warm bathtub of water. Or try a comfrey bath. Boil two quarts of water; add a quarter to a half-cup of comfrey leaves and steep for 15 minutes, then strain and add to bath water. After the soak, apply an herbal salve.

Some dietary supplements are constipating, including iron and calcium. Try taking your child off these for a week to see if they are the cause.

WHEN TO CALL A DOCTOR ABOUT CONSTIPATION

Your child has had infrequent bowel movements since birth

Constipation becomes the rule rather than the exception

Your child holds his stools for days, then soils himself (also known as encopresis)

Your child complains of significant belly pain

You seem to have a toilet-training battle on your hands. (Usually the solution is to let your child take charge of his own toileting. A health practitioner trained in behavioral strategies can offer additional help.)

Your child has blood in his stool, or there is often blood on the toilet tissue.

Occasionally, children develop constipation as a reaction to irritating foods. If your child has food allergies or sensitivities, or you suspect he may, see Chapter 7, Allergies and Intolerances.

Natural Remedies for Constipation

The following supplements loosen stools by adding bulk to naturally improve bowel function, *provided enough fluids are consumed with them.* If your child doesn't drink enough, then bulking agents can further harden stools.

Bran. You can add bran to foods such as cereals or applesauce at the rate of about one teaspoon to one tablespoon a day. As always, start with the lower amount and work your way up as needed. The only kids who won't benefit from this are those with wheat allergies.

Psyllium seed comes from a species of plantain (*Plantago psyllium*) and is a great source of fiber. You can buy decent-tasting commercial products, such as Metamucil, that contain psyllium. Or you can just pick up some powdered psyllium seed husks at health food stores and forego the added sweeteners, dyes, etc. (We recommend using only the seed husks, and not the seeds themselves, because the seeds are believed to be able to lodge in intestinal pockets and cause irritation.) Dissolve them in juice or add them to cereal or applesauce. Then have your child drink or eat quickly before the moisture-loving husks create an inedible sludge. Our suggested dose for children over two years is one scant teaspoon dissolved in water or juice, chased with another glass of water. Increase dose to up to one tablespoon for kids over 100 pounds.

Flaxseed is another great bulking agent. Flaxseed also provides a significant source of essential fatty acids. Keep those acids fresh by storing flaxseed in the freezer and grinding small amounts at a time. Better health-food stores carry flaxseed in the refrigerator section.

Kids enjoy drinking or eating these little seeds once they're ground. Mix one teaspoon ground flaxseed per cup of water or juice and have your child drink this slightly thickened mix. You can also sprinkle the seeds directly on foods. If you have a picky eater on your hands, blend ground flaxseed into a smoothie with yogurt and fruit.

Magnesium citrate can have a laxative effect. Try giving your child one to two teaspoons of liquid per day, to equal 200 to 500 mg, for one week. Nuts, blackstrap molasses, whole grains, soy, and seafood are good food sources of magnesium. For everyday use, most nutritionists believe magnesium supplementation should be balanced with two times as much calcium.

A WARNING ABOUT LAXATIVES

Please don't give your child harsh laxatives, either over-the-counter products or herbal ones. Herbal irritant laxatives include senna (*Cassia senna*) and cascara sagrada (*Rhamnus purshiana*). These medications work by irritating the bowel, sometimes causing cramping and diarrhea. Also, bowel function can become dependent upon their use. Daily laxative use, including herbal laxatives, can dehydrate your child thoroughly enough to cause serious medical problems.

Chapter 19

COLIC

How many times have people—even people you don't know—admonished you to cherish your child's early months because they pass so quickly? The phrase "The days are long, but the years are short" takes on new meaning when you have a newborn. If you're the parent of a colicky baby, the first months may seem to stretch into eternity. You have our sympathy. Nothing makes a parent feel more helpless and exhausted than being unable to console a crying infant. But don't despair—you can try a number of coping strategies and herbal remedies, and one or more will probably work.

Colic is defined as persistent, unexplained crying in an infant. Symptoms typically begin during the first three weeks of life and resolve by the fourth month. The baby's piercing shrieks can go on for hours, and she certainly seems to be in pain. During an episode, she may tense her belly muscles, flex her legs, lift her head, and pass gas. Between crying jags, however, she appears content and healthy.

Colic afflicts about 10 to 30 percent of infants worldwide and does not discriminate between breast-fed or bottle-fed babies. A colicky baby may fuss off and on all day, with a peak in screaming in the late afternoon or evening—right about the time her bedraggled parent is struggling to get dinner on the table. Colicky babies also tend to be finicky feeders and poor sleepers.

No one knows what causes colic. Theories include immaturity of the gastrointestinal tract, excessive gas, milk allergy, intolerance to other foods, insufficient friendly gut bacteria, and reflux (backwash) of stomach contents into the esophagus. Other possibilities include nervous–system immaturity, over-feeding, under-feeding, premature introduction of solids, inadequate burping, incorrect positioning of the baby with resultant air swallowing, parental anxiety or depression, and transfer of the caregiver's tension to the baby. Studies have failed to prove that any one of these factors causes colic.

You'd think that if a baby cries that much and that passionately, his very life is at risk. But it's not true; colicky babies grow and thrive as well as more content babies. And your baby's colic is in no way connected to your abilities as a parent.

Treating Colic

Researchers and parents alike have sought a cure for colic in vain. All agree, however, that in cases of colic at least two people need help: you and your baby. Probably everyone else who spends significant time in your household does, too. We believe in starting with simple measures first, trying dietary changes, gentle massage, then herbs, and saving treatment with pharmaceuticals for a last resort.

Get emotional support. You and others who care for your baby need reminders that the colic will pass, probably by the end of the baby's third month of life. You may find help in the form of friends (particularly other parents who have survived a colicky baby), parenting books, and health-care workers, including those with training in mental health. Without such reassurances, colic can interfere with parent-child bonding and wreak havoc on a marriage. If you leave your infant with a babysitter, check to see how the sitter is handling the stress of the baby's colic. Share what you learn with the sitter, or seek one who already knows about colic.

Reduce stress. Don't expect too much of yourself. Some parents feel they've really accomplished something if, in the course of caring for their colicky baby, they manage to squeeze in a shower. So keep your "to do" list short. On the other hand, if you feel frustrated by the many demands of caring for the child, find a sitter so that you can take some time for yourself, and return home relaxed and happy.

Keep your home environment reasonably mellow, full of soft music, quiet conversation, and soft lighting. Easy to say; hard to do if you have other children in the house.

Hold your baby. Some studies have found that infants with colic cry less if they are carried often. Most experts agree that you should respond quickly to your baby's cries and that you can't spoil a newborn by doing so.

Carrying your infant with a front carrier, sling, or backpack (provided he has sufficient head and neck control) leaves your hands free for other activities. Some babies seem to enjoy feeling encased in the carrier, but others dislike the constraint.

The position in which you hold your baby can matter, too. Some babies are more comfortable in a fairly vertical position; others derive comfort from positions that create pressure against their bellies, such as being laid over your lap or shoulders. Still others calm with gentle movement: rocking, swinging, car rides, stroller rides. Notice we specify gentle movement—jostling your crying baby may prevent him from getting to sleep, which could be what he needs most.

Swaddling. Some parents find that wrapping their colicky baby snugly in a light blanket helps to calm the child. The theory is that children with

WHEN TO CALL A DOCTOR ABOUT COLIC

If your baby screams more than you think he ought to, especially if he seems to be in a lot of pain, call your doctor. A physical exam of your baby will determine if he has a treatable problem such as infection, trauma, or improper GI-tract function—or colic.

If you feel that you're reaching the end of your rope with the baby's inconsolable crying, reach for the phone. When you're exhausted, you can't give the baby the care he needs, and part of a health professional's job is to support your parenting efforts. So don't wait until your rope runs out—call for help.

immature digestive systems often have underdeveloped sensory patterns as well. Without swaddling, some babies apparently see their hands swinging wildly in space without knowing that they're actually attached, a situation that possibly creates a cycle of fear and sensory overload. Whatever the case, this technique has worked for numerous babies.

Continue nursing. Don't let grandparents, friends, or acquaintances lead you to believe there's something wrong with your breast milk. In fact, weaning can worsen colic. Frequent feedings seem to yield less distress in babies, so nurse as much as your baby desires.

What you eat, however, may affect your baby's symptoms. One study found that babies' colic improved when their nursing mothers stopped drinking cow's milk. Another study found a 39-percent reduction in colic distress when bottle-fed babies drank a special predigested formula or when nursing mothers avoided common food allergens such as milk, eggs, wheat, and nuts along with artificial food additives.

Other foods you may want to avoid include peanuts, caffeinated beverages, chocolate, cucumbers, hot peppers, and citrus fruits and juices. Some nursing mothers find that avoiding foods that give them gas—typically cauliflower, broccoli, brussels sprouts, cucumbers, peppers, garlic, onions, and beans and other legumes—eases colic. In other words, if mom is sensitive to a particular food, baby may be, too. Eliminate such items from your diet one by one, and watch your baby's digestion for forty-eight hours. You may confirm your own suspicions about these foods.

If your baby drinks formula, talk to your physician about switching to another type. About 1 to 3 percent of bottle-fed babies are allergic to the protein in cow's milk. Clues to milk intolerance include persistent diarrhea and stools that test positive for microscopic traces of blood.

Switching to a soy-based formula may or may not help, because about a third of these infants are also allergic to soy.

Your physician may suggest a formula that contains partially digested protein (Nutramigen, Pregestimil). Because these formulas are expensive, they're usually discontinued if a week's trial does not improve symptoms.

Feeding techniques. During feedings, hold your infant so his head is higher than his belly. This position will prevent backwash of stomach contents into the esophagus and aid expulsion of swallowed air. After nursing or bottle feeding for five or ten minutes, burp your baby. Again, his head should be above the rest of his body.

Try a warm bath. Some babies feel better with warmth—just be careful to check the temperature. Linda found that her son quieted if she nursed him in a warm bathtub, and it relaxed her, too. Of course, there's only so much time you can spend in the tub, but regular soaks may bring a

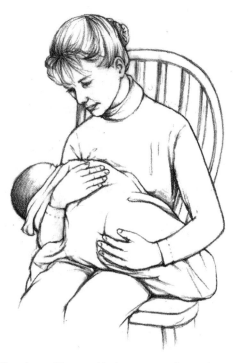

Gentle rocking and being wrapped snugly sometimes soothe a colicky baby.

much-needed respite from the crying, or even lull your baby to sleep.

Try gentle massage. You can massage your baby's whole body to calm him or you can concentrate on his stomach. Use light pressure. Some people advocate moving in circles around the abdomen in the direction that the large bowel empties. Start in the lower right corner of your child's belly (lower left from your perspective), move up, then across under his ribs, and down his left side. Some parents find that cycling their baby's legs (in the motion of riding a bike) helps too. See what your baby seems to like. Of course, his reaction may change from moment to moment.

Herbal Rescue for Colic

One study compared giving infants with colic a liquid placebo or several ounces daily of an herb tea made from chamomile, vervain, licorice, fennel, and lemon balm. With each colic episode, parents offered their baby the tea or placebo drink—up to 5 ounces at a time, not more than three times a day. The tea eliminated colic in 57 percent of infants, whereas placebo treatment helped only 26 percent. Chamomile, fennel, and lemon balm all relax the intestines. Licorice has anti-inflammatory compounds, and vervain is a traditional calmative for crying babies.

The other classic herbs for colic are catnip, dill seed, anise seed, and caraway seed. These herbs contain volatile oils with relaxing, antispasmodic properties. They are safe, tasty, and well-tolerated by babies. Most babies can take an ounce or so of mild herb teas at the breast from an eyedropper slipped next to your nipple. In addition, if you are nursing, you can drink a cup of herbal tea or take glycerites yourself several times a day; try the herbs individually before making a blend.

The essential oils of the herbs should enter your milk rapidly and show peak effect in approximately two to six hours.

Conventional Treatment

The drugs prescribed for colic make a very short list. Simethicone (Mylicon), which helps break up intestinal gas bubbles, could decrease intestinal pressure, and hence the pain of colicky babies. A study comparing simethicone to placebo, however, found no difference in effects on colic symptoms. Although it's available over the counter, we recommend that you try simpler strategies first and also check with your physician before giving it to your baby. Some doctors recommend diphenhydramine (Benadryl) for colicky babies, but this works as a sedative to help the baby sleep. It doesn't relieve colic symptoms.

Remember: Colic Is Temporary

If all our natural treatments failed, and we felt totally frazzled by our baby's colic, we would not head to the drugstore for something else. Instead, we'd entrust the baby to his grandparents or a kindly sitter, take a long nap, and dream of peace and quiet. It's good to take a break—a short, refreshing one just long enough for you to begin to miss your wonderful baby. Maybe Rip Van Winkle had a colicky infant at home.

Sometimes, when Linda felt vexed or puzzled by something one of her children was doing, she watched him sleep and a couple of times drew his peaceful little face. It helped her realize how small and helpless he was, how much in need of her protection, and how much she wanted to love and nurture him. This may help if you feel frustrated with your child's colic—or other health problems of any kind.

Chapter 20

BLADDER INFECTIONS

These infections aren't as common as ear infections or sore throats, but they can be just as troublesome. If your child is younger than two years, the only initial symptoms of a bladder infection may be fever and vomiting. What's important to remember about children's urinary tract infections is that they require medical attention. Untreated, they can ascend to the kidneys, where they can do permanent damage. Luckily, urinary tract infections are not contagious.

Bladder infections afflict approximately 1 to 2 percent of infants. During the school years, about 5 percent of girls and 0.5 percent of boys suffer from at least one urinary tract infection. After the immediate new-born period, girls are much more likely to get these infections than boys. Sometimes your child won't exhibit symptoms until the infection is full-blown. Then, she may complain of pain and burning on urination, and tenderness or heaviness above the pubic bone.

Doctors divide the urinary tract, including the urethra, bladder, and kidneys, into lower and upper sections. Lower urinary tract infections, sometimes called cystitis, involve the bladder. Upper urinary tract infections involve the kidney. Bladder infections are more common and generally less dangerous than kidney infections. Left untreated, kidney infections can cause per-manent scarring of the kidneys and lead to impaired kidney function and high blood pressure.

Why do girls have a greater risk of urinary infections than boys? The explanation has to do with anatomical differences. Girls have a shorter urethra (the tube that connects the blader to the outside) than boys. For this reason, bacteria have a shorter distance to travel from the bodily sur-face up to the bladder.

Bacteria, most commonly *Escherichia coli,* also known as *E. coli,* cause bladder infections. How do they get there? Wiping the wrong way— back to front—after going to the bathroom can transfer fecal bacteria to the urinary tract. Bubble bath, soap, and detergent residue on underclothes can irritate the opening of the urethra and cause a burning sensation on urination. If this is your child's only symptom, try having her soak in warm water, or, better yet, warm water plus a half cup of distilled vinegar. If this trick clears up symptoms within a day, then you'll know the culprit was chemical, not bacterial.

Signs and Symptoms

These will depend upon the child's age. Symptoms in infants are not specific to the urinary tract and include vomiting, fever, and, with chronic infection, failure to grow properly. Kids over two years old will probably be able to tell you about such localized symptoms as pain and burning on urination, tenderness or heaviness just above the pubic bone, or pain in the legs or lower back. With toilet-trained children, you may

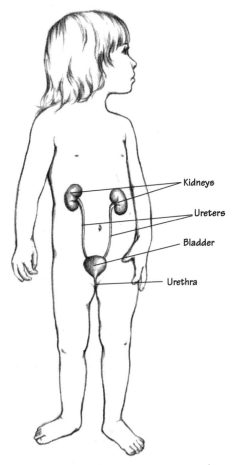

Inside the urinary tract

notice an urgency and increased frequency of urination. Or a previously "dry" child may begin to wet the bed at night. If you see her urine, you may notice it is cloudy, foul-smelling, and may even contain blood. Fever and sweating can accompany more severe bladder and kidney infections; so can pain in the middle back, right around the kidneys.

Diagnosis of a urinary tract infection involves physical examination and urine tests. Under the microscope, urine from an infected bladder contains lots of white blood cells and bacteria. Urine cultures often yield *E. coli* as the culprit. The trick here is collecting an uncontaminated urine sample. In the absence of infection, urine remains sterile until it hits the urethra. To reduce bacterial contamination as the urine leaves the body, a doctor or nurse may wash the area surrounding the urethral opening with an antimicrobial solution. Toilet-trained children should be able to produce a "midstream clean-catch specimen," which means the child, or you, must catch some urine after the child has begun urinating.

The only way to get a truly clean urine specimen is to insert a catheter (tiny tube) into the bladder or, if anatomic obstacles prevent catheterization, to insert a needle through the skin just above the pubic bone and into the bladder. Most pediatricians, particularly when faced with a feverish infant or toddler and no obvious source of infection, prefer to obtain a specimen via catheter.

After the infection is gone, your doctor may recommend studies such as an ultrasound of the kidneys, X-ray studies of the urinary tract, or less commonly the insertion of a cystoscope (an instrument akin to a tiny periscope) into the bladder. The objective is to find out if your child has any structural abnormalities that are causing the infection. Typical reasons for doing these tests include kidney infection, any urinary tract infection in a boy, second bladder infection in a girl under three years old, or a first infection in a child with a family history of recurrent infections or abnormalities of the urinary tract.

Conventional Treatment

Doctors will usually recommend two steps for bladder infections.

Eliminate bacteria with antibiotics. Usually this means oral antibiotics. Feverish infants with urinary tract infections are often, but not always, hospitalized for twenty-four to forty-eight hours of intravenous antibiotic therapy. Kids with kidney infections are also usually admitted. Antibiotics quickly and readily eliminate most bladder infections. Recurrent infections are typically treated with preventive oral antibiotics for twelve months.

Increase your child's fluid intake. Drinking lots of fluids dilutes the bacteria in the urinary tract and the resultant frequent urination flushes them out. Reducing the number of bacteria gives the urinary tract's natural defense team the upper hand. This strategy works in people with normally functioning urinary tracts. If you know that your child has a structural abnormality, do not encourage extra fluids without consulting your doctor.

Herbal Treatment

Before discussing individual herbs, we want to stress the importance of using them under the supervision of a health-care professional knowledgeable in both pediatrics and herbal medicine. Because bladder infections can progress to more serious conditions, proper diagnosis and appropriate treatment are essential. It's also important to follow up with your doctor after treatment—whether it's herbal, antibiotic or both—to make sure your child is no longer infected. This usually means an additional urine test.

Antimicrobial Herbs

Cranberries possess a well-known ability to prevent and treat urinary tract infections. Their juice acidifies the urine, although research says that an adult has to consume a large amount, about 1.5 liters or a little over a quart a day, to create this result. Two cups (1/2 liter) should be effective for a 50-pound child. More importantly,

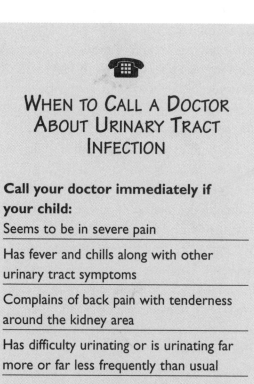

WHEN TO CALL A DOCTOR ABOUT URINARY TRACT INFECTION

Call your doctor immediately if your child:

Seems to be in severe pain

Has fever and chills along with other urinary tract symptoms

Complains of back pain with tenderness around the kidney area

Has difficulty urinating or is urinating far more or far less frequently than usual

Passes bloody or brownish urine

Cannot pass urine or, if in diapers, hasn't wet them for eight hours

Has had strep throat, impetigo, or scarlet fever within the last three weeks (nephritis, a rare complication of strep, can produce fever, bloody urine, swelling, and sometimes high blood pressure)

In any other way acts very sick

cranberries have antibacterial properties, chiefly an ability to inhibit bacteria from sticking to the lining of the urethra and bladder.

However, we recommend avoiding cranberry juice sweetened with sugar, because sugar tends to decrease immune function. Instead, look for juice sweetened with other fruit juices. Fruit sugars are still sugars, but at least they aren't refined. (Ideally, you'd serve straight cranberry juice, but we haven't found a kid yet who will drink it.)

Cranberry's close relatives blueberries and bilberries also contain the substance that prevents bacterial adherence. Eating plenty of blueberries is a delectable way to take medicine, and may be a good strategy for kids whose bladder infections tend to recur.

Berberine-containing plants such as Oregon graperoot have a long history of use in eradicating urinary tract infection. Test-tube studies show that berberine kills microbes, including *E. coli,* and prevents bacteria from adhering to the bladder lining. The usual adult dosage is one teaspoon of tincture (about three droppersful) three times a day. Using Clark's rule, give a 50-pound child one dropperful. Look for a glycerine extract or capsule for kids, but let us forewarn you that extracts of the berberine-containing plants taste bitter. You can disguise them in juice or a good-tasting herbal tea blend.

Caution: Berberine-containing herbs are not for use during pregnancy.

Acidophilus supplements can help sustain the bacterial colonies that normally keep our bodies healthy. While your child is using antimicrobial herbs and for four days afterward, give her daily doses of yogurt with live cultures or children's acidophilus. (It's a good idea to do this if she is on antibiotics, as well.)

Uva ursi. The leaves of this plant contain arbutin, which has urinary antiseptic properties. Uva ursi works against *E. coli;* it also increases urination. Researchers have yet to study the effectiveness of this herb in childhood bladder infections. However, the German Commission E lists it as okay for kids. In *Phytotherapy in Pediatrics,* Heinz Schilcher, a member of the German Commission E, recommends uva ursi tea in combination with birch leaves for an analgesic effect, goldenrod to increase urine output, and peppermint to disinfect the bladder and improve its muscle tone. His only concern is that parents need to make the tea taste good without adding too much sugar.

Caution: Stay within recommended dosage guidelines when using uva ursi, because overdose has reportedly caused nausea, vomiting, ringing in the ears, and shortness of breath. A reasonable dose of uva ursi tea for a 50-pound child is one cup three times a day, sweetened with honey. Limit use to one week. Do not use during pregnancy.

Garlic has activity against *E. coli.* It has anti-inflammatory and antibacterial abilities as well. It contains several sulfur compounds with antibiotic activity. You can cook with a lot of fresh garlic, adding it at the end of cooking to preserve its active ingredients. Raw garlic works well in salad dressings, dips, salsas, and bread spreads. Children can take garlic oil capsules; deodorized versions are available. You can also make a tea from garlic and honey. Simply steep a couple of chopped cloves in just-boiled water for ten minutes, sweeten to taste, and serve.

Other urinary antiseptic herbs include yarrow, thyme, echinacea, wild indigo, and goldenrod. Children can take them as teas, capsules, or extracts.

Herbs to Increase Urine Flow

Many plants can help flush bacteria from the urinary tract simply by increasing urine flow. These foods and herbs, unlike pharmaceutical diuretics, help support the proper balance of sodium and potassium in the body. Foods such as parsley, celery, and carrots fall into this category.

Dandelion. Both the leaf and root of this common plant are reliable diuretics. Dandelion is especially popular among herbalists because it contains potassium, an essential mineral. Most kids can drink several cups a day of tea made from the root or leaf.

Quack grass (*Elymus repens*), also known in European herbals as couch grass, is a well-known herbal diuretic with little or no toxicity. If you're harvesting it from your backyard, be sure to have a garden specialist help you properly identify it, and, of course, avoid areas that may have been sprayed with pesticides. Make an infusion from one to two teaspoons of fresh quack grass root per cup of water, and serve your child a half cup three times a day to increase urine flow.

Horsetail makes for a reliable diuretic that works without upsetting the natural balance of blood chemicals. European doctors specifically use it for blood in the urine and urinary stones. Horsetail is also known as shavegrass and contains natural silica, plus bioflavonoids including quercetin, which has anti-inflammatory effects.

If you plan on gathering fresh horsetail, make sure to properly identify it. This genus has both sterile and fertile plants. The sterile form grows into a horse-tail shape and is the preferred form of herbalists, although both are used medicinally. Harvest only in the early spring, before the plant gets tough and fibrous.

Fresh horsetail must be boiled or cooked before use to inactivate an enzyme that destroys vitamin B1 levels when eaten raw. Here's how Sunny does it: Lightly simmer several teaspoons of fresh or dried horsetail in an equal number of cups of water for five minutes. Cover, allow to steep for 15 minutes more, strain and serve. The resulting tea has a pleasant, grassy taste.

Caution: Pregnant women and those with kidney or heart disease should not take horsetail due to its selenium content, which can be high if the herb is harvested from polluted ground, or if the soil is naturally high in selenium.

Soothing Herbs

The demulcent herbs are essential components of any urinary tract herbal blend. They coat the urinary tract and prevent further inflammation. Herbs to choose from include marshmallow, cheese-weed, corn silk, and cleavers.

Marshmallow root is an effective urinary demulcent and an immune-system stimulant, but it has a weird, sickly-sweet flavor. Sunny uses it regularly in capsule form for people with urinary and digestive tract inflammations. The American Herbal Products Association points out that marshmallow may mildly delay the absorption time of other medications, so take marshmallow root and any prescriptions several hours apart.

Cheeseweed (*Malva neglecta*) is a pesky weed you may have growing all over your yard. Some folks call it common mallow. Don't pull it all out of your garden—it's a great edible and medicinal plant. The leaves and root are filled with mucilaginous material that makes an excellent soothing tea for bladder irritations. Cheeseweed tastes better than marshmallow root, too. Infuse the leaves or decoct the roots, sweeten if necessary, and serve this slippery tea to your child several times a day to ease urinary tract irritation. It's very safe for children.

Corn silk is the translucent collection of hairs or tassels at the top of an ear of corn. Most Americans discard corn silk. We invite you to try eating it. Just steam it right alongside your corn on the cob. Topped with a little pasta sauce or toasted sesame oil, it's a great side dish. Or simply steep a handful of very fresh corn silk in hot water to make a simple, nontoxic tea.

Cleavers helps comfort an irritated urinary

PREVENTING URINARY TRACT INFECTIONS

Your child's body possesses natural defenses against bladder infection. Beneficial bacteria stand guard at the external opening of the urethra. Repeated antibiotic use, however, can thin the ranks of these guards. Urine flow provides another defense; it tends to flush out bacteria ascending from the urethra. The bladder's surface also is coated with substances that, in a healthy child, prevent bacteria from sticking to it. Under normal conditions, urine itself is hostile to bacteria because it's acidic. Finally, when infection does occur, the body delivers white blood cells to the bladder to help it fight the microbes.

There are several strategies you can use to support these natural disease-fighting mechanisms.

Give your child plenty of fluids. We both use water filters to purify our local water supplies.

Encourage your child to urinate whenever he feels the urge. Most kids have to pee at least every three or four hours. Find tricks to overcome reluctance to use restrooms at child care or school. Kids can be motivated to urinate on targets; a piece of toilet tissue works fine.

Teach your child, especially your daughter, to wipe from front to back after using the toilet. This simple hygiene measure will reduce contamination of the urethra with intestinal bacteria.

Avoid the use of potentially irritating scented or colored toilet paper. Unbleached tissue is best. And while you're reducing household chemical use, switch to an unscented detergent and fabric softener as well.

If your child seems sensitive to chemical irritation, keep bath time short or have her shower instead. Don't use bubble bath or harsh soap. Make sure she rinses her bottom with plenty of water after using soap.

If your child has recently taken antibiotics, giving acidophilus supplements (usually *Lactobacillus acidophilus* and/or *Bifidobacterium bifidus*) can help recolonize beneficial bacteria. Follow package instructions for children's dosage. Also, lab studies suggest that lactobacilli help prevent urinary tract infection and have a positive effect on treatment when used in conjunction with an antibiotic. These "good" bacteria seem to prevent the bacterial enemies from sticking to the urethra (a first step in establishing an infection).

See an acupuncturist. Traditional Chinese Medicine excels at therapies for strengthening the kidneys and bladder. If possible, find an acupuncturist who specializes in treating children.

Let your child sleep without underpants to let her bottom air out. Make sure underwear or tights are made of cotton.

If your child has recurrent symptoms, but no signs of actual infection, a food allergy may be to blame. See Chapter 7 for more information about these allergies and sensitivities.

If your child is plagued by urinary incontinence, reccurent urinary tract infections, and chronic constipation, aim to cure the constipation. A recent study found that relief of constipation helped clear up many incontinence problems and all urinary infections in the kids who had no anatomic abnormalities.

tract. Its herbal properties include demulcent, antiseptic, and mild diuretic actions. Like corn silk, the fresh plant has more medicinal value than the dried plant. But if you can only find this herb dried, go ahead and use it. Steep two teaspoons of the fresh, chopped herb (one teaspoon dried) in one cup of water for five minutes. Your child can drink several cups a day.

Pain-Relieving Herbs

Cramp bark and **black haw bark** help relieve any type of muscle cramps or spasms, including irritable bladder muscles. Both contain astringent tannins for shrinking swollen tissue, salicylic acid to relieve pain, and antispasmodic compounds. The typical 7-year-old, 50-pound child with a urinary tract infection can take a half cup of decoction or half a capsule of either herb up to four times a day as needed for bladder pain. In case you're wondering about the name cramp bark, yes, this herb does have a long history of use for relieving menstrual cramps.

Caution: Patients with kidney stones or a history of kidney disease should not use these plants.

Kava kava can relieve bladder discomfort. Like cramp bark and black haw, it relaxes smooth muscles. Actually, it relaxes the entire body, so you and your child may get some much-needed sleep! Drinking a half cup of kava kava tea three times a day should help.

Caution: Large doses of kava kava can induce a euphoric state and still higher doses, muscle weakness and dizziness. Pregnant and nursing women should avoid the use of this herb, and adults should abstain from mixing it with alcohol or other central nervous system depressants.

A Parent's Dilemma: To Give or Not to Give Antibiotics

Neither of us have had to cope with urinary tract infections in our children. But here's what we'd do if we faced a decision about whether to turn to antibiotics for our own kids.

Linda's Approach

If my child had a first-time bladder infection, I would opt for antibiotic treatment, especially if she were still under age two. If my child were older, I'd add supportive herbal therapies. Afterward, I would give her acidophilus/bifidus supplements to recolonize beneficial bacteria and then I'd work on preventing further infections. If infections became recurrent, I would have my pediatrician investigate whether an anatomical problem could be the cause. I would also use herbal medicines and other preventive strategies to keep infections at bay or to nip them in the bud.

Sunny's Approach

Urinary tract infections are tricky. Sometimes you won't even realize that your child has one until symptoms are fairly significant. A child under two will almost always need antibiotics for a urinary tract infection.

If my child over age two had a minor urinary tract infection, without severe pain or fever, I would give her generous amounts of echinacea and the antibacterial and demulcent herbs mentioned above. I'd serve fruit-juice-sweetened cranberry juice several times a day. And, just to be sure that we'd eliminated the infection, I'd take her back to our health practitioner for another urine test in two weeks.

Chapter 21

SKIN PROBLEMS

Cradle cap. Diaper rash. Eczema. Warts. Poison Ivy. Acne. Ah, the things that can mar the perfection of your child's skin. Some produce no symptoms (other than an urge to hide the affected area under a paper bag). Some cause discomfort. Natural health practitioners often view the skin as a barometer of overall health, a reflection of deeper currents. And let's face it: when a child's skin is clear and glowing, there's nothing more attractive. When it's troubled, natural remedies can often provide relief. Sometimes topical treatment is all that's necessary; other conditions require an in-depth analysis of the child's health.

The skin has many functions. It is one of our primary defenses, sort of a Great Wall of China, a barrier between our bodies and marauding microorganisms. It keeps damaging light rays and many chemicals from harming more fragile, deeper tissues. It helps regulate our body temperature, receives sensory information from the outside world, secretes water and salt, and manufactures vitamin D.

The layer of skin closest to the outside, the epidermis, is a band of tough cells stacked one atop the other. The cells nearer the surface contain keratin, the same protein that exists in hair and nails. These cells are dead, and are continuously being shed and replaced by cells pushed up from deeper in the epidermis.

Below the epidermis is a thicker layer called the dermis. It contains collagen and elastic fibers, which make skin strong and able to stretch as your child grows. Embedded within the dermis are blood vessels, nerves, hair follicles, and sweat and oil glands.

To remain healthy, the skin depends upon many things; some we can control and some we can't. For instance, the skin's blood supply isn't easy to manipulate. But drinking plenty of fluids can assure the skin a rich moisture supply. A nutrient-rich diet nourishes skin. Vitamin A, for instance, helps sustain strong, smooth skin. Carotenes, which the body converts to vitamin A, do the same. Vitamin C maintains collagen. It and other antioxidants such as vitamin E and selenium help repair damage caused by insults such as ultraviolet radiation.

Essential fatty acids also play a role in skin health. Among other functions, they form essential components of cell membranes. When we eat a diet with a good balance of fats, our bodies generally incorporate the types of fatty acids that will create optimal cell membranes. Because skin cells are constantly dying and being replaced, we need to eat the right fats regularly.

Many Western European and American diets tend to be top-heavy in saturated fats, such as those present in many animal products, and omega-6 fatty acids, the kind contained in cooking oils such as corn, soy, sesame, and safflower. These diets tend to be deficient in the omega-3 fatty acids found in flaxseed, hemp seeds, pumpkin seeds, cold-water fish, and green leafy vegetables such as collard greens, kale, and chard. Without the proper ratio of fatty acids, cell membranes become less fluid and don't function as well.

Fatty acids also are needed in a chemical reaction that ends in the production of hormone-like substances called prostaglandins. Prostaglandins regulate many bodily processes: inflammation, allergic response, blood clotting, hormone production, and nerve transmission. There are many types of prostaglandins; some increase inflammation, others suppress it. Omega-3 fatty acids tend to produce prostaglandins with desirable effects, including decreasing inflammation and allergic response. So in allergic skin conditions such as eczema, fatty acid supplementation is important.

Other organs influence the skin, most notably the liver. To help you picture the liver's function in keeping the skin healthy, consider this: the skin is the largest eliminative organ of the body; the liver is the body's biggest filter. If the body produces too many waste products due to stressors such as illness and food allergies, the liver can't screen out or detoxify these products completely. This increases the burden on the skin, and it may become inflamed.

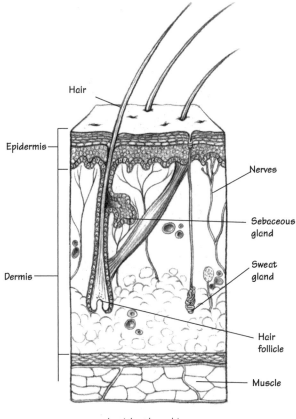

Inside the skin

Cradle Cap

It's such a lyrical name for an unsightly affliction. Too bad dandruff doesn't have such a euphemism. The flakes of infant cradle cap are heavier than dandruff. Not just the scalp is subject, but also a baby's eyebrows, skin behind the ears, forehead, sometimes even the armpits and groin.

What causes cradle cap, known medically as infantile seborrheic dermatitis? It is an inflammatory skin condition, but the reason it happens isn't known. Babies have immature oil glands, especially on their heads. In cradle cap, these glands produce excessive amounts of oil, which then dries into yellow, greasy-looking scales that can plug the oil glands' ducts—which causes them to secrete even more oil. Rest assured that your baby's cradle cap is not a reflection of hygiene or the quality of your breast milk.

Luckily, this quaintly-named condition does not itch, burn, or otherwise trouble the infant, unless the plugged oil glands become infected. Parents, on the other hand, may feel distressed or embarrassed about their baby's appearance and just wish the stuff would go away. And it will— usually, on its own. Some treatments, however, can hasten the disappearance.

Massage almond or olive oil into the scalp and leave it overnight. Even though this makes the skin look even more greasy, it's one of the best home remedies. You'll want to cover your infant's bottom sheet with an old towel. In the morning, gently comb the remaining oil and the loosened flakes through the hair with a fine-toothed comb. Then shampoo the oil out.

To make a cradle-cap oil for your baby, follow our directions for infused herbal oils in Chapter 12, Ear Infections. You may want to make antibacterial, anti-inflammatory oils such as calendula, St.-John's-wort, chamomile, or willow bark. Don't, however, confuse infused oils with *essential* oils. Infused oils are fine for skin; essential oils are usually too strong for babies unless they are diluted in a vegetable oil. You can also massage flaxseed oil directly into the baby's scalp.

Don't try to pry off flakes and crusts from the scalp. This can cause bleeding and irritation. Really, they'll loosen in their own time.

Nursing mothers can make sure they're getting a proper balance of fat. Specifically, they should try to decrease consumption of hydrogenated oils and increase intake of omega-3 fatty acids. If your baby drinks only formula, Dr. Michael A. Schmidt, author of *Smart Fats* (North Atlantic Books, 1997) says you can add one-half teaspoon of flaxseed oil a day to your infant's formula if she is younger than six months; 1 teaspoon if she's six months or over. Or you can use a supplement that contains a one-to-one ratio of omega-3 to omega-6 oils. Be sure to refrigerate flaxseed oil and toss it a month or two after it's opened. If it tastes bitter, it's rancid; don't use it.

Diaper Rash

Diaper rash is one of the most common skin problems of infancy. It's difficult to control and tends to wax and wane. The peak age for getting diaper rash is between nine and twelve months.

Diaper rash is a reaction to irritation by a diaper and its contents. It's diagnosed by the fact that it usually stops at the outer limits of the diaper, and that areas of skin that come into direct contact with the diaper generally look the worst.

People used to pin the blame for diaper rash on ammonia. Urine contains urea, and enzymes in it convert urea to ammonia. But when you put either urine or ammonia directly on skin and let it sit there a couple of days, it doesn't damage the skin.

WHEN TO CALL A DOCTOR ABOUT CRADLE CAP

The following symptoms may be signs of a secondary bacterial skin infection such as impetigo.

Raw, weepy skin and yellowish drainage

Sores that begin as small red bumps, then turn to blisters that burst, leaving honey-colored scabs

Skin that is already inflamed, however, may react to these chemicals. Best explanation: Through a series of chemical steps, urine, feces, moisture, and friction act in concert to produce a rash. Breast-fed babies, by virtue of a different mix of resident gut bacteria and enzymes, acquire serious diaper rash less often than formula-fed babies.

Home Remedies for Diaper Rash

First off, a few strategies can help prevent diaper rash.

Keep your baby's bottom dry and clean. The more often you change your baby's diaper (within reason, of course) the fewer his chances of getting a rash. In particular, you want to change soiled diapers as soon as possible. Whether you choose cloth or disposable diapers, the number one prevention factor is frequent diaper changes—so use the type that facilitates changing your baby. If you do choose cloth diapers, avoid waterproof plastic plants. Instead, look for a diaper wrap that contains a fabric that breathes. Back when our kids were in diapers, we had good luck with wool diaper wraps.

Don't get carried away with soaps and scrubs. After your baby pees, you don't need to wash her bottom. After a poop, you may want to wipe her down with warm water, then pat her bottom dry. When you bathe her, use a mild soap or no soap.

Protect your baby's skin with salve, cream, or ointment. When Linda's kids were in diapers, she successfully used Desitin or A and D ointment—not because she mistrusted herbs, but because she didn't have any herbal salves on hand. Sunny

WHEN TO CALL A DOCTOR FOR DIAPER RASH

The rash begins suddenly and covers a large proportion of your baby's bottom, particularly if it seems to cause your baby discomfort.

A mild to moderate rash seems to be getting worse or fails to improve despite three or four days of home care.

The rash becomes bright red, starting with small red patches that merge to form larger patches. This could be signs of a yeast infection. Although you can treat such a rash with over-the-counter antifungal creams (Monistat, Lotrimin, Mycelex) and topical antifungal herbs such as usnea or calendula, we feel that it's also wise to first get a diagnosis from a doctor.

Your child's bottom develops areas of bumps and blisters that burst to leave a honey-col-ored crust. This could be impetigo, a skin infection caused by strep or staph bacteria. Topical antibiotics and topical use of antibacterial herb teas (such as Oregon graperoot, yarrow, echinacea, oak leaves, or thyme) can clear mild cases, but you should get a diagnosis first. This is especially important if your child is a newborn. Extensive skin infection may require antibiotics.

Your baby also develops thrush, a yeast infection in the mouth, marked by white patches that don't wipe away easily. It's particularly important to consult a doctor if the infection seems to prevent him from feeding well.

You have any questions about the nature of your baby's rash and how best to treat it.

used an herbal salve containing beeswax, olive oil, and antimicrobial herbs such as calendula, comfrey, burdock, and yarrow. You can also use salves to treat diaper rash, but discontinue them if the rash becomes weepy or the baby develops a yeast infection.

Some people recommend powders to keep baby bottoms dry. One natural substance you can use is bentonite clay powder. Do not use talcum powder or products containing it, because inhaled particles can cause lung disease. And we advise care in using any powder, because inhaled particles will at the very least irritate the airways.

If your baby does develop a diaper rash, the following strategies can help you minimize her symptoms.

If you use cloth diapers and launder them yourself, make sure they're well-rinsed. If your water is hard and you don't have a water softener, try adding borax to your wash water. If the rash continues, your baby could be allergic to something in the soap. If this is true, you'll see irritated skin where his clothes contact him. Consider switching to a milder detergent. Dry diapers in sunlight or on high heat.

Give your baby a break from diapers, so that her bottom can get lots of fresh air. This makes particular sense when candida sets in. If you're feeling brave and don't mind clean-ups, try it. Putting your baby down on a blanket in warm sunlight is one approach.

Consider your baby's diet. Have you introduced

CANDIDA DIAPER RASH

Sometimes diaper rash shows signs of infection with the yeast-like fungus *Candida albicans*. Suspect it if patches of your baby's skin turn fiery-red with fine scales. The infection tends to spread in what's called "satellite lesions," meaning smaller red patches crop up a short distance from the mother lesion. Whereas routine diaper rash tends to spare the skin folds at the groin, yeast infection concentrates there and may infect the creases at the neck and armpit. You may also notice white, flaky-looking patches in the mouth. Called thrush, this is also caused by candida. Prior antibiotic use by you or your baby increases the chances of thrush in your baby, as well as yeast infection on your nipples.

With diaper candidiasis, you *don't* want to seal in water with ointments, as yeast thrive on moisture. You'll also want to avoid baby powders containing cornstarch. Instead, allow your baby's diaper area to dry out by leaving the diaper off for a while. Apply either plain yogurt (with live cultures) or liquid acidophilus, at room temperature, directly to her bottom several times per day. When you wash her bottom, try using a soap that contains grapefruit seed extract, a broad-spectrum antimicrobial with activity against candida. Three times a day, give the baby a little bifidus internally to help fight the candida, and if you're nursing, take doses of acidophilus yourself. Dr. Michael Schmidt suggests a daily dosage for infants of between one-fourth and one teaspoon. For oral thrush, some nursing mothers like to put a little acidophilus, bifidus, or yogurt directly on their nipples right before nursing. Be sure to clean your nipples thoroughly before and after each feeding. Several days of this routine, and your child's thrush usually disappears.

NATURAL BABY POWDER

For ages: Kids in diapers
Yields: About 1/2 cup

While corn starch is a great addition to baby powder, it can aggravate diaper rashes caused by yeast, so omit this ingredient if your child currently has a rash.

*1/4 cup corn starch
(soothing)*

*1/8 cup baking soda
(drying)*

*1/8 cup bentonite clay powder
(drying)*

*1 tablespoon dried rose petals
(antibacterial)*

*1 tablespoon yarrow leaves
(antibacterial, tissue toning)*

Grind the herbs finely in a clean coffee grinder. Combine all ingredients. Sift to remove coarse particles. Store in a small unbreakable shaker. Use at diaper changes to soothe and tone baby's tender skin.

a new food lately? Does one particular food seem to irritate your baby's digestive tract six to eight hours after eating? If so, he may have an allergy or intolerance to this food. If you're still nursing, review any new foods you've consumed recently.

Eczema

Kids with eczema (atopic dermatitis) have red patches of skin with dry flakes on the surface. Sometimes the patches are moist and oozing. Eczema itches, and over time, affected skin becomes scaly and thickened by the child's scratching. It most often affects the face, scalp, space behind the ears, and the creases at elbows, knees, and groin. A child with eczema typically has skin that tends to be dry and cracked.

Eczema is common, affecting around 10 percent of children in developed countries. Like other allergic diseases, its prevalence has risen over the past couple of decades. No one knows the exact reason. Medically, eczema is part of an inflammatory process. It tends to run in families, along with hay fever and asthma. It's persistent, and exposure to environmental or food allergens can aggravate the skin lesions. Eczema often begins in infancy. First symptoms often coincide with the introduction of certain foods, particularly cow's milk, wheat, or eggs. The child may also

WHEN TO CALL THE DOCTOR ABOUT ECZEMA

We advise seeing a naturopathic or medical doctor for initial diagnosis of eczema. After that, see your doctor if:

The condition worsens. If you see yellowish discharge or honey-like crusts, your child may have a bacterial infection on top of the eczema.

If your child gets a herpes infection. Generally, you want to keep a child with eczema away from anyone with herpes lesions, cold sores, or fever blisters. When the herpes virus infects eczematous skin, a serious condition called eczema herpeticum can develop.

have other signs of food allergies or sensitivities, such as intestinal cramping, gas, skin flushing, and a drippy nose. Eczema often begins to wane between the ages of three and five, although mild skin lesions may persist into middle age.

Medical and Complementary Treatment

Conventional medical treatment usually begins with what's called "hydration and occlusion". First the child hydrates his skin by bathing. Once out of the bath, he immediately applies cream, oil, or lotion to trap the moisture within his skin. Failing these simple measures, physicians may recommend low- to medium-strength topical steroids (nothing stronger than 1 percent hydrocortisone on the face or genitals) or oral antihistamines to relieve itching. Both of these treatments have side effects. Long-term use of topical steroids can literally thin the skin and cause acne and discoloration.

If your child has more than an occasional patch of eczema, we suggest that you consult an allergy specialist or naturopathic doctor for help in pinpointing potential allergens. Medical research supports a connection between the two. In one recent study, 60 percent of kids and teens with eczema had positive skin-prick tests to certain foods. Milk, eggs, peanuts, soy, wheat, catfish, cod, and cashews accounted for almost 90 percent of the allergies.

People of all ages with eczema often have fatty acid imbalances, with too much linoleic acid and not enough gamma-linolenic acid and omega-3 fatty acids. Fortunately, by changing the balance of fats your child eats, you can adjust these imbalances. Some clinical trials have found that supplements rich in gamma-linolenic acid, such as evening primrose oil and borage seed oil, improve eczema. A few of these studies looked at the effect of evening primrose oil on children with eczema and found positive effects. A more recent and larger study of sixty children between the ages of one and sixteen years found that evening primrose oil did not benefit either eczema or asthma.

Adult studies, on the other hand, have found benefits from fish oil. Dr. Schmidt, however, cautions that high doses of fish oil are not good for infants, particularly premature infants. It's safer and less expensive to increase your child's omega-3 fatty acid intake by supplementing his diet with flaxseed, pumpkin, chia seeds, and walnuts.

Flaxseed is the richest and most affordable source of concentrated omega-3 fatty acids. To get the oils from flaxseeds, grind them first. A clean coffee grinder works fine. You can also buy flax meal, powder, and oil. If your baby is formula fed, you may consider putting a few drops of flaxseed oil in her bottle. Teens can take the adult dosage of four teaspoons a day; for children over age two, Dr. Schmidt recommends one to two teaspoons a day when their eczema is under control, and three teaspoons a day during flare-ups.

You can also add ground flaxseed or flaxseed oil to foods. Linda blends the oil into salad dressings. Sunny takes 2,000 mg of flaxseed oil in capsules every day. Cold-water fish including salmon, herring, mackerel, sardines, anchovies, and bluefin, and dark green, leafy vegetables such as collards, chard, and kale also contain omega-3 fatty acids.

Home Care for Eczema

Warm, but not hot, baths are fine, but long soaks deplete skin oils and aggravate dry skin conditions. Show your child how to dry herself by patting rather than scrubbing with the towel. Afterward, apply almond oil to seal in moisture. Oatmeal and barley baths are soothing. Simply mix two handfuls of either grain into a pan of several quarts of hot water. Simmer ten minutes, turn off heat, and allow to steep for fifteen minutes. Strain and add the water to the bath.

Avoid harsh soaps and bubble baths. In fact, your child probably doesn't need to lather up, except on areas that get particularly dirty: hands, feet, armpits, crotch. Rinse well with clear water.

Research shows that chlorine in water seems to correlate with eczema. Some parents have reported that a dechlorinating water filter in the shower helps. See the Resource Directory for places to purchase these filters. You may also want to consider using a water softener; too many salts and chemicals can be irritating your child's skin. In fact, one study found that exposure to hard water significantly increased the prevalence of eczema.

Have your child use a moisturizer immediately after bathing and several times a day. Look for a product that contains natural oils, no synthetic fragrances or preservatives, and no alcohol. Avoid all mineral oil products, including most baby oils, because they deplete fat-soluble vitamins A, D, E, and K in the skin. We've heard that avocado oil or the mashed fruit itself applied directly to the skin helps relieve eczema and dry, irritated skin in general. Also avoid harsh laundry detergents and those that contain dyes and fragrances. Wash new clothes to remove chemicals. Try to avoid fabrics that irritate your child's skin.

Herbal Treatment for Eczema

Licorice root contains potent anti-inflammatory properties. It seems to act in a fashion similar to the body's anti-inflammatory hormone cortisone, but without the negative effects associated with long-term cortisone use. A study in the 1950s found that topical use of glycyrrhetinic acid, one of the key compounds in licorice, improved eczema even more than topical cortisone.

More recent studies have focused on the oral use of a decoction of ten Chinese herbs, including licorice. A British study of kids with eczema found that treatment with four weeks of this decoction produced improvement. A year later, eighteen of the original thirty-seven children continued to have at least a 90 percent reduction in eczema.

Caution: Long-term ingestion of licorice can upset the balance of sodium and potassium and cause water retention. Pregnant women and people with high blood pressure or adrenal gland disease should not take it. Do not give your child licorice tea or extracts internally for more than six weeks without a one-week break, unless you're under the supervision of a health professional.

Gotu kola. Herbalists recommend this herb's use for almost all skin inflammations, relying on its documented ability to stimulate the healing of connective tissue wounds, both with internal and external use. Studies have confirmed that gotu kola has strong anti-inflammatory and skin-healing mechanisms.

Those living in tropical regions such as Hawaii can make a soothing poultice for eczema out of fresh gotu kola leaves. The rest of us can find gotu kola in herbal creams and in capsules or glycerites. It is safe for children. Dosage is one capsule, one cup of tea, or twenty drops of extract per day for a 50-pound child.

Echinacea's lesser-known benefit is that it promotes tissue regeneration and reduces inflammation. You can apply a straight echinacea tea to an area of eczema, or give your child the capsules or glycerite internally. In order to best utilize echinacea's healing powers, use it for ten days, and then give your child a two-day break. You can also purchase manufactured echinacea creams or salve to apply directly to the inflamed area.

Comfrey. Comfrey lovers, unite! The U.S. Food and Drug Administration has recommended against the internal use of comfrey tea, due to an infrequent association with liver disease. But comfrey is still a powerful healing herb for external use. The major chemical constituent in comfrey is allantoin. It soothes the skin and speeds healing by promoting the growth of skin cells. Numerous studies show that allantoin helps heal torn tissue. Decocted comfrey root makes a gooey, soothing herbal wash to treat the itchiness of eczema.

Burdock should be in every herbal formula and salve for eczema. This plant's foot-long tap-root inhibits microorganisms such as bacteria and fungi. Its use in a salve prevents irritation and secondary infection of sensitive skin. Taken internally, it acts to help the liver keep filtering internal toxins. It's also safe for children: Use one cup of tea (simmer the chopped root for ten minutes) or one capsule per day for a 50-pound child. Continue for two weeks, take a one-week break, and resume the two-week regimen.

Adrenal support herbs. Herbalists and other holistic healers are trained to look beyond a skin inflammation to potential internal causes for the irritation. Eczema's allergic origin suggests support for the adrenal glands. Adrenal support herbs to consider are the above-mentioned licorice, plus schisandra and Siberian ginseng.

Liver-support herbs. The traditional liver herb for eczema is Oregon graperoot, which is also antibacterial. Other herbs to consider are milk thistle, turmeric, yellow dock, and dandelion root or leaf. One or more of these herbs can be added

---

HERBAL SALVE

For ages: Any
Yields: 3 to 4 quarter-cup jars of salve

Salves are easy to make, portable, and extremely handy to have around. Basically, they are infused oils with a little beeswax added to make them a solid. The more beeswax you add relative to the amount of oil, the harder the salve becomes. Softer salves are easier to spread on a baby's skin (for diaper rash, for example), but if you live in a warm climate, you'll want to add more beeswax, otherwise your salve will be too soupy.

1 cup olive or almond oil

1/6 to 1/4 cup grated beeswax

1/4 cup coarsely ground or crumbled herbs: burdock root or leaves, willow bark, echinacea root or herb, calendula flowers, comfrey leaf or root, singly or in any combination

Mix oil and herbs together in a pot. (If you have more than 1/4 cup of herbs, add as many as the oil will cover.) Warm on very low heat for 30 to 60 minutes, stirring occasionally. Keep a close eye on your salve, as it tends to burn. Remove from heat; pour through a fine straining cloth into second saucepan. Squeeze your cloth to get as much oil as you can out of the herbs. Strain again if necessary to remove herbs. Return the oil to very low heat, and stir in the beeswax until melted. Pour into clean, small jars. Cool until hard in the middle, and label.

To use: Apply to any dry skin condition, such as scabs, scars, eczema, mosquito bites, or diaper rash. Don't use a salve on moist, oozing skin conditions such as wet psoriasis, oozing poison oak or ivy, or on rashes with secondary infections, such as candida diaper rash.

to a homemade salve or to a tea or glycerite blend for eczema.

Warts

Warts are caused by a virus known as the human papilloma virus. The so-called common warts are those rounded, rough-surfaced, generally harmless growths that usually occur on the hands, but can appear on the knees, elbows, and face. Plantar warts occur on the soles of the feet and sometimes the palms of the hands, and can cause pain. Plane or flat warts grow in clumps, usually on the face, neck, chest, backs of hands, forearms, or shins, are flesh-colored and, as their name implies, flat.

Genital warts, on the other hand, are often, but not always, transmitted sexually. They are very contagious and can lead to cervical disease. Take your child or teen to the doctor if you think genital warts are present.

Conventional Therapy for Warts

There's a 50 percent chance that warts will disappear within two years without treatment. However, treatment does reduce the risk of the warts spreading. Because of the discomfort they cause, plantar warts should be eradicated. Genital warts also should be treated by a doctor.

Common warts can often be dealt with at home. Doctors typically recommend topical applications of acid solutions such as salicylic acid or lactic acid, available in over-the-counter products such as Wart-Off. Acid-containing plasters such as Mediplast work on the same principle. This is a slow but painless way to lose warts. We don't recommend this treatment for warts on the face, however, because it can result in scarring.

For stubborn warts, those on the face or neck, and any kind of wart other than the common ones, procedures performed in a doctor's office are more effective. Be forewarned that, no matter how they are treated, warts have an annoying tendency to recur.

Herbal and Complementary Treatments

Banana peel. We know this sounds a bit strange, but Sunny knows several tales of success using this kitchen cure. Cut one square inch from the peel of an organic banana. Center the inside of the peel directly over the wart. Tape it on with first aid tape or an adhesive bandage. If the wart is in a hidden place, you may be able to persuade your child to wear the banana peel all day. Otherwise, you'll have to settle for night-time treatment. Repeat with a fresh piece of peel daily for twenty-one days, and the wart should disappear. Discontinue if irritation occurs.

Dandelion juice. Dandelions produce a milky latex in their stems, a sort of rubberized wart killer. Simply pick large, juicy dandelion stem and squeeze out the white juice onto a wart. Do several times a day for several weeks to get rid of unsightly warts. We don't know exactly why this works, but the fact that the latex deprives the wart of oxygen probably helps.

Castor oil is for external use only. Apply a few drops to the wart every day. Castor oil has great drawing powers to "pull out" stubborn infections and soothe sore muscles. It's reputed to be particularly effective for plantar warts, although it may take months of dabbing the castor oil on the wart twice a day. Store castor oil away from toddlers; ingestion could be toxic.

Antiviral herbs for warts. Numerous herbs have antiviral properties, including lemon balm, licorice, skullcap, lemon thyme, lemon grass and chaparral. You could include any of them in an antiwart salve.

Homeopathic thuja (*Thuja occidentalis*) from the arbor vitae tree is often the remedy of choice for warts. It's a nontoxic way of working to kill warts from the inside out. Follow package directions for dosage. A naturopathic doctor prescribed thuja for one of Sunny's children's facial warts. Three weeks later, they were gone for good. Consult a qualified homeopathic practitioner if you want to try these remedies, as your child's symptoms may indicate a different approach is needed.

Poison Ivy, Oak, and Sumac

In sensitive people, these three plants produce a similar rash—reddened, itchy skin, then blisters, then oozing and crusting. The source of the reaction? A resin called urushiol causes cells to release histamines and other inflammatory chemicals into the skin. Mucous membranes that contact the resins can swell. Inhaling smoke from burning plants can trigger allergic reaction in the respiratory linings. For some people, only a tiny amount of resin will trigger the rash; others seem virtually immune.

A clue to diagnosing poison ivy, oak, or sumac as the source of your child's rash is that the blisters run in lines where the leaves brushed the skin. The rash can appear anywhere from a few hours to a few days after exposure, so tracking its source can be difficult.

Home Remedies for Poison Itchies

Rub a dub, but don't scrub. Right after exposure, wash the skin thoroughly to remove the irritating oil. Use soap and lots of water. Doing so within five to ten minutes may avert the rash. On the way to water, tell your child not to touch herself anywhere, especially around the eyes, to avoid spreading the resin. Try dissolving a half-cup of baking soda into a tepid or cool bath; this is believed to help remove plant residue and will also soothe irritated skin.

Meanwhile, wash all the clothing your child was wearing, especially her shoes, and any toys you think she may have dragged through the offending plant with her.

If a rash does appear, cut your child's fingernails short and ask her to try really hard not to scratch. Although some people think the fluid within the blisters can spread the rash, this isn't so. Nevertheless, you do want to discourage your child from scratching to avoid causing an infection or injuring fragile skin.

For itch relief, you can apply a baking soda paste or calamine lotion. Or you can let your child soak in a tepid baking soda bath. Rubbing the rash with an ice cube can soothe, too. Doctors often recommend over-the-counter antihistamines (Benadryl, Chlor-Trimeton); in severe cases, they prescribe topical or oral corticosteroids.

Herbs that Relieve Itching

Green clay is one of Sunny's favorite remedies. Clay has a natural ability to draw oils from the skin and works well for relieving the itch of poison oak or ivy. Clay powder comes in many colors and is available in the bulk jars at natural foods stores, and as an ingredient in clay-based toothpaste or facial masks. Either make a paste with water or help your child to finger-paint the mask directly onto the irritated areas. Your child may look like a polka-dotted avocado, but he'll likely feel better.

Oak or **willow bark** (*Quercus* spp. or *Salix* spp.) can be great astringents. According to Joy Gardner in *The New Healing Yourself* (Crossing Press, 1989), a strong decoction of white oak added to her bath worked on poison ivy "when all else failed." She suggests simmering one-half cup of chopped oak bark in one quart of water for twenty minutes, straining and adding the liquid to a cool or tepid bath. Bathe in the fresh tea for twenty minutes daily for several days.

Jewelweed (*Impatiens capensis*) has acquired a reputation for quelling the rash caused by poison plants. If jewelweed grows in your area, just apply the fresh, crushed leaves or a leaf tea. You can also purchase a variety of liquid extracts at health-food stores and apply them externally.

Grindelia (*Grindelia squarosa, G. robusta*), also known as gumweed, exudes a gummy resin that apparently has anti-inflammatory properties. Unless you'd like your child to be covered with this sticky resin, purchase an alcohol-based tincture made for this purpose at a health-food store and apply it externally to the rash.

Black tea bags work well for itches. Just dunk the bag in a scant cup of hot water for several minutes, cool, then apply the teabag or a tea compress to the rash. The tannic acid will contract inflamed tissue and relieve itching.

Other plant medicines that help include plantain, chickweed (*Stellaria media*), and cucumber slices. Apply a mash of any of these directly to a recent poison oak or ivy rash. Or you can make a strong infusion, let it cool, and apply cool compresses to your child's skin. Witch hazel lotion can be very effective in soothing and tightening swollen, irritated tissue.

Homeopathic treatment often involves the use of *Rhus toxicodendron*, one of the Latin names for poison oak. Natural food stores and many pharmacies carry Rhus tox and other homeopathic medicines. Follow package directions for dosage.

Preventing Exposure

Learn what poison plants look like and where they grow. Teach your children. Poison ivy (*Rhus radicans, Toxicodendron radicans*) and poison oak (*Rhus diversiloba*) have three leaflets, but often the leaves' shape varies slightly from plant to plant. Poison sumac (*Rhus vernix, Toxicodendron vernix*) has many-toothed leaflets.

Wash objects, such as garden tools, that have come in contact with these plants in soap and hot water to remove the oils. Pets usually won't get a rash from the oils, but they can carry the resin on their fur; when your kids stroke or hug them, bingo, they're exposed. If you suspect the family dog or cat has been playing in poison plants, get your veterinarian's advice on how to bathe them before they come inside. Wear gloves so you don't expose yourself to the oils, and be aware that the smoke from burning these plants can severly irritate some people.

Acne

The most common skin problem, acne, afflicts most people some time between the ages of eleven and thirty, but sometimes even later in life. It can be mild or severe and persistent. And it shows up right when kids are reaching the peak of their self-consciousness—as if coping with the other aspects of adolescence weren't challenge enough.

Issues of justice aside, here's what happens. Beginning in preadolescence, hormones secreted by the adrenal glands of both girls and boys stimulate the skin's oil glands. Excess oil, combined with sloughed skin cells, clogs the outlet from the oil glands. Voila, you have a zit, or in medical lingo, a comedo, plural comedones. These plugged pores are commonly called whiteheads, until or unless the plug reaches the surface and its fats and cells oxidize, turning dark. Then it's a blackhead. If a species of bacteria (*Propionibacterium acnes*) proliferates inside the blocked oil gland, the bump becomes inflamed, swelling and turning into a red bump or pimple. If the oil gland cavity breaks open inside the skin, acne nodules or cysts can develop. Cystic acne is the type most likely to leave scars.

Conventional Medical Treatment for Acne

Benzoyl peroxide helps slough dead skin cells so they don't clog pores. It also acts as an antiseptic to inhibit bacteria on the skin. It's available in several over-the-counter products. In order to be effective, it must be used daily. The problem with benzoyl peroxide preparations is that they can irritate the skin. Their advertisements make it sound as though teens need these products. We're skeptical.

If skin lesions become inflamed, some doctors prescribe antibiotics for either external or internal use. If your child takes or has taken oral antibiotics, supplementing the diet with acidophilus/bifidius bacteria can recolonize the bowel with "friendly" bacteria. Because of the potential drawbacks of antibiotics, we recommend reserving them for severe cases of acne, particularly cystic acne.

Tretinoin (Retin-A and other products) is a prescription cream or gel effective for both acne and the fine wrinkles associated with aging. It can cause the skin to redden, peel, and become more sensitive to the sun. For severe acne, some doctors prescribe oral isotretinoin (Accutane) which, like tretinoin, is related to vitamin A. It reduces skin oil production and usually clears acne. However, this drug can cause side effects such as painful joints, tendinitis, and elevated blood fats. It can also cause birth defects. Although physicians warn people who take it not to get pregnant, many pregnancies are not planned; a fair amount happen even while a woman is using contraceptives. If one of our teens had acne, we'd try all other remedies before resorting to such a potentially toxic treatment.

Oral contraceptives are sometimes prescribed to help control acne and other problems in menstruating teens. Again, we would explore natural therapies before trying such treatment for acne.

Natural Remedies

Guide your preteen or teen in the use of gentle cleansers. His skin is oily, not dirty. No matter what your teen puts on his skin, he will not change how much oil it produces. Using lots of soaps and astringents will not clear up his skin. In fact, vigorous scrubbing and abrasive cleansers can actually worsen acne. This does not mean your teen shouldn't wash his face, but that he should do so with gentle cleansers.

Tell your teen to try to keep her hands off her face. Unless just scrubbed, hands carry germs. Hands that have raked through hair carry oil. Most teenaged faces don't need any more of either ingredient.

Urge your teen not to squeeze her pimples. Such manipulation can increase inflammation, cause infection, and lead to scarring. If your child has a pimple that has come to a head, and the urge to pop it becomes irresistible, show her how to wrap tissue around both index fingers to protect the skin from fingernail scratches. She should wash hands and face before and after.

If your teen wears foundation, she should toss it every few months to avoid applying contaminated goo to her face. Suggest that she pour it into her hand, rather than stick her fingers into the bottle. Washing makeup off with a gentle cleanser at day's end will help offset the tendency of these products to block pores.

Encourage your teen to drink lots of water. Water helps clean the entire body. Depending upon humidity, temperature, and activity level, eight to twelve big glasses a day are ideal for teens and grownups. The water contained in carbonated beverages, particularly caffeinated or sugared ones, doesn't count because caffeine increases water loss from the kidneys. Herbal teas and diluted juices do.

Boost fiber intake. Healthy, regular bowels are important for skin health. Make sure your teenager is getting plenty of fiber every day. Whole grains, vegetables, and fruits are great sources.

Provide healthy snacks and meals. So far, no particular diet has been shown to cause or cure acne. Nonetheless, we advocate a diet that contains whole grains, fresh vegetables, fruits, nuts, and (if your family isn't vegetarian) seafood, poultry, and meat. Getting the right vitamins contributes to healthy skin: vitamin A, B vitamins (especially B6 in girls who get premenstrual break-outs) carotenes, vitamin E, selenium, and zinc.

Because eating hydrogenated oils depletes the fatty acids the body needs, teach your teen to read labels and avoid hydrogenated fats. Chips and crackers often contain these oils.

Consider essential fatty acid supplements. Fatty acid deficiencies have been linked with acne. Apparently this deficiency causes more skin cells to slough, meaning there's more stuff available to clog pores. Although no studies show that fatty acid supplementation helps acne, these essential fats generally reduce inflammation and contribute to the skin's health.

Do what you can to keep the air clean. Humid environments and air pollution can aggravate acne. Moving may not be an option, but keeping tobacco smoke out of your house is.

Herbal Support for Acne

Tea tree oil acts as an antiseptic and antifungal and has activity against the bacteria associated with acne. It is used externally. One study found that a 5-percent tea tree oil preparation worked as well as 5-percent benzoyl peroxide in treating acne, but with fewer side effects, except for the smell.

Lavender essential oil, which is antimicrobial and smoothing, is a tried and true remedy. Just dot it onto individual blemishes. It dries out pimples almost overnight, and with a far more pleasant scent than tea tree oil.

Fruit acids, or alpha-hydroxy acids, get rid of dead skin cells. You can spend a lot buying products containing these acids, but you can also have some fun in the kitchen making them with your teen. Pineapple husks can be applied directly to the face, or whirred in a blender to make a poultice. Grapes contain alpha-hydroxy acids, too; strawberries contain these acids and salicylic acid, just like some commercial acne products.

Borage seed oil. We're starting to hear more about topical uses of seed oils that contain essential fatty acids. Given that such oils also contain natural anti-inflammatory compounds, this makes sense. We haven't tried it yet ourselves, but you can grind up flax or borage seeds and make them into a poultice/mask. Or puncture a capsule of borage, evening primrose, or flaxseed oil and apply it directly to the affected skin.

Burdock, taken internally, may also help. We know of one woman in her twenties who cleared up a severe case of pimples by taking one dropperful of burdock seed and root tincture, twice a day. And she didn't change her diet or lifestyle one iota. Burdock tones the liver and boosts digestion, so that may be why it helped.

One study has shown that burdock has anti-inflammatory and free-radical scavenging ability and that it helps prevent liver damage—all properties that benefit skin health.

Lactobacillus acidophilus. Here we go again, promoting that beneficial bacteria. According to Derrick DeSilva, M.D., in *Ask the Doctor* (Interweave Press, 1997), acidophilus can help promote healthy functioning of the bowel, with more efficient elimination of toxins. He writes, "Thus the skin's job becomes easier, and it heals faster." We couldn't have said it better ourselves.

Chapter 22

CHICKEN POX AND HERPES

"She's bound to get it sooner or later."

"We may as well get it over with."

"We won't be able to go anywhere for days!"

"An illness with spots—how medieval!"

Chicken pox seems almost a rite of passage for kids and parents alike. Herpes, though we may think of it as an adult disease, afflicts children with fever blisters and systemic infections. In fact, most first-time infections with herpes simplex 1 occur before age ten. We've grouped chicken pox and herpes together because the viruses that cause them both belong to the herpes family and both produce similar symptoms.

The herpes virus family includes *Herpesvirus varicellae,* which causes chicken pox, and types of *Herpesvirus hominis* (herpes simplex) that cause herpes infections of the mouth and genitals. Both viruses produce malaise, fever, and blister-like skin lesions.

When the illness seems to be over, both viruses can retreat up the nerves to lie dormant along the spine. Later, the virus can reactivate. With herpes, the result is recurrent fever blisters or genital sores. Less commonly and usually not until adulthood, the chicken pox virus can reactivate to produce shingles, an intensely painful rash that parallels the course of a nerve. Herpes tends to reactivate repeatedly. Shingles usually crop up once or not at all.

Who can get chicken pox? Anyone—child or adult—who hasn't had the disease. Once your child gets it, her immunity is lifelong and repeat infections are highly unlikely. Although 90 percent of chicken pox cases occur in children under age ten, the virus can strike at any age. Pregnant women who have never had chicken pox must be especially careful, as unborn children are vulnerable to the disease. Chicken pox is usually more severe when it occurs in teens or adults, so it's actually desirable for your children to encounter it while young.

Outbreaks of chicken pox typically occur in the late winter and early spring. Direct contact with the skin lesions spreads it, although early sneezing and coughing may send the virus into the air from its primary residence in the nose and throat. The disease is contagious from a day or two before the rash appears until the lesions crust over. That kids are contagious before the rash appears facilitates spread of chicken pox through schools and day-care facilities. Once your child has been exposed, it takes about fourteen days, with outside limits of ten to twenty days, before the illness sets in.

Symptoms of Chicken Pox

Signs and symptoms of this ailment unfold gradually. Your child may complain of miseries such as fever, headache, mild sore throat, and poor appetite. Then comes the rash: small pink spots that quickly progress to bumps, then fragile blisters, then crusts. The blister stage usually itches. Crusts typically fall off within five days.

The rash tends to be most dense on the trunk, but can appear anywhere—the mouth, genitals, the membrane that lines the inner eyelids and front of the eye. The spots come out in crops, usually three crops over a period of three days. Some children develop only one crop of a few lesions, while others might have five crops of up to 500 lesions each . . . ouch! Fever often parallels the rash, both peaking at about day three. When the rash is sparse, a child's temperature can vary from normal to slightly elevated; with more severe eruptions, it can hit 105°F (40.5°C).

If you have more than one child, it's common for the first child to get a relatively mild case of chicken pox and her siblings to become sicker, with higher fever and a rash that is more intense and takes longer to heal. Apparently, children who catch the disease from siblings (rather than casual friends and classmates) come in contact with a greater number of viruses.

Complications of Chicken Pox

Although complications are uncommon, you should know about them. If your child develops these symptoms, call your doctor.

WHEN TO CALL A DOCTOR ABOUT CHICKEN POX

Your infant three months old or younger develops chicken pox.

Your child has a chronic illness, particularly one that compromises her immunity, such as AIDS or leukemia, or takes such immunosuppressant medications as corticosteroids or chemotherapy drugs.

You are pregnant, haven't had chicken pox, and have been exposed.

Your child develops blisters on his eyeball or complains of eye pain.

Your child's lesions show signs of bacterial infection: redness, swelling, yellow discharge.

Your child's fever exceeds 104°F.

Your child develops a bad cough or difficulty breathing.

Your child effortlessly vomits three or more times.

Your child becomes confused, extremely irritable, delirious, very lethargic, has a seizure, or difficulty walking.

Your child complains of stiff neck and can't bring his chin to his chest.

Your child acts very ill in any way.

Secondary bacterial infection means the chicken pox lesions have become infected with bacteria such as strep or staph; untreated, these bacteria can enter the bloodstream and cause pneumonia, arthritis, and bone infections. If the normally clear fluid of a blister becomes yellowish, or a crust goes from dry to weepy, call your doctor, who may prescribe topical or oral antibiotics. You may be able to avoid this complication by washing the pox with a decoction of Oregon graperoot. This yellow tea contains berberine, one of the most effective antibacterial agents in the herbal repertoire. (Be aware, however, that it will stain towels and washcloths.)

Chicken pox pneumonia, although more common in adults and particularly pregnant women, can afflict children. Call your doctor if your child develops a bad cough, chest pain, rapid or difficult breathing, blue-tinged lips, or coughs up blood. Recovery is usually prompt.

Encephalitis, or **brain inflammation,** occurs in fewer than one in 1,000 cases of chicken pox. Signs include fever, repeated vomiting, headache, stiff neck, confusion, poor coordination, and stupor.

Risk Factors for Developing Complications

Immunosuppressed people, including children who have leukemia or are taking corticosteroids or chemotherapy, can become seriously, even fatally, ill with chicken pox. If your child has a chronic disease and has been exposed to chicken pox, check with your doctor.

Teenagers and adults, particularly pregnant women, tend to have more severe cases. Fortunately, the vast majority of chicken pox infections occur in children.

Managing Chicken Pox at Home

First, reassure your child that the spots are not serious. Tell him the crusty scabs will fall off on their own, often leaving a shallow pink depression that should fade within six to twelve months. Unless the scabs are picked or become infected, scars are rare.

Tell your child not to scratch or pick at the pox. Keep her nails short and her hands clean. If your baby has chicken pox, you can try putting her hands in light gloves for a day or two. These won't inhibit her ability to explore the world, but they may prevent scars.

Keep your child cool. Overdressing her, piling on the blankets, and giving her hot baths may actually lead to increased itching and more spots.

Wash bed sheets and all other linens daily in hot water, and keep your child in clean, fresh pajamas, preferably cotton ones so the skin can breathe.

Give your child a daily bath. If it relieves the itching, bathe your child up to once every four hours, but protect her skin from dryness and aggravated itching. Tepid baths relieve skin symptoms better than very warm baths. Pat skin dry—don't rub—then launder the towel.

Wait until the scabs fall off before putting oil, beeswax-based salves, or ointments on your child's skin. Such treatments can keep the skin from breathing and may also lift off the scabs prematurely. Calamine and other light lotions are fine.

Encourage fluids and healing foods. Your child's appetite may flag, particularly if she has sores in her mouth. Offer her lots of fluids and soft foods. Also give your child plenty of raw garlic, which boosts the immune system and fights viruses. You can mix raw garlic into salads or smoothies, give your child deodorized garlic tablets, or, if she can't swallow a pill, slip liquid garlic extract into her juice or pureed foods.

Vitamin therapy. Several vitamins (including A, beta carotene, the Bs, C, and zinc) are important for optimal immune function and tissue healing, and the body requires increased amounts when

TIME-HONORED CHICKEN POX BATHS

The oatmeal bath. Don't repeat Sunny's long-ago mistake and pour oatmeal directly into your bath water; cleaning up afterward is a chore! Colloidal oatmeal flakes such as Aveeno are less messy. Or you can bind raw or partially cooked whole-grain (not instant) oatmeal in a washcloth or a clean sweat sock, which you can then use to gently pat your child's skin in the bathtub.

The baking soda bath. Simply add a quarter to a half cup of baking soda to the running bath water. Our kids liked making a paste of baking soda and water and finger painting each chicken pox spot with it. Adding a little pink beet powder or food coloring makes it into a game.

The herb bath. Yarrow is both anti-inflammatory and antiseptic. Make a strong infusion as follows: Boil a pint of water and steep in it an ounce (about a handful) of yarrow for ten minutes. Strain out the herb and add the liquid to the bath.

fighting off and healing from an infection. Feeding your child foods rich in vegetables (especially the dark green leafies), fruits, and grains will probably ensure that he gets enough of these vitamins. Replace depleted carotenes by serving apricots, squash, carrots, sweet potatoes, and cantaloupe.

What to Do About Fever

Because moderately elevated body temperature has beneficial effects, you don't need to treat a fever unless your child feels uncomfortable. Call your doctor if your feverish child is under three months old or if your older child's fever exceeds 104°F (40°C).

Because of the association with Reye's syndrome, **do not give aspirin to a child who has chicken pox.** Although the exact cause of Reye's syndrome is unknown, it is strongly associated with taking aspirin during viral illness. This serious syndrome damages the brain and liver; its symptoms include confusion, sleepiness, and persistent vomiting.

Many physicians recommend acetaminophen to relieve fever and discomfort during chicken pox, but this routine practice may do more harm than good. In a study of children with chicken pox, acetaminophen prolonged itching and the time to scabbing compared to placebo treatment. It increased the sick children's activity by the second day, but whether or not that's good depends on whether you think sick kids should rest. The study authors concluded that acetaminophen didn't help with symptoms, and actually prolonged the bout with the virus.

Holistic management of mild fever—less than 102°F (38.8°C)—often includes a hot bath to "break" or ease the fever and encourage sweating. But in chicken pox or other skin rashes, this can make the child more uncomfortable. We suggest that you avoid hot baths and temperature-increasing herbs such as hyssop, ginger, cayenne, cinnamon, and the traditional children's fever-tea blend of peppermint, elder, and yarrow.

Infants and Chicken Pox

If a pregnant woman comes down with chicken pox before the twentieth week of gestation, her fetus has a remote chance of developing a serious illness, congenital varicella syndrome, that leads to growth retardation and severe developmental defects. The condition is extremely rare; only forty cases have been reported in the last fifty years.

If a mother develops chicken pox later in the pregnancy, the infant receives protective maternal antibodies from the disease. If the mother contracts chicken pox three or more days after the delivery, the infant is still at risk, but the infection is transmitted via the respiratory tract (the usual route) rather than the bloodstream, so the infection tends to be less serious.

Newborns are at greatest risk of suffering from chicken pox when their mothers get it between four days before and two days after delivery. In this case, the baby receives the virus via the bloodstream, but

without the benefit of the mother's antibodies, which have not yet been manufactured in abundance. About 20 percent of infants exposed during this critical period get the disease. Although older figures show a 30 percent mortality rate for these newborns, a 1990 study of 240 infants born to women with chicken pox failed to report a single death.

When newborns go home to siblings with chicken pox, few problems occur if the infant is otherwise healthy and the mother is immune. If, on the other hand, the mother does not have chicken pox antibodies, doctors often recommend that both mother and infant get a shot of varicella-zoster immune globulin, described on the following page, before going home.

What about chicken pox in older infants? Most pediatricians want to see any infant less than three months old who develops chicken pox (and any child who acts very sick). If an infant is otherwise healthy and older than three months, don't worry.

Treatment for People at High Risk

Acyclovir is an antiviral medicine that, when given intravenously, has prevented complications of chicken pox in children with compromised immune systems and has shown some clinical benefit in otherwise healthy adults. When given to normally healthy children, it resolves fever sooner, decreases the number of skin lesions, and hastens the onset of healing of those lesions. It does not seem to change the rate of complications.

Recently, oral acyclovir has been used to shorten the duration and severity of chicken pox in children with normal immune systems. Other than modestly reducing children's suffering, the main goal of such therapy seems to be getting children back to school.

Varicella-zoster immune globulin, or VZIG, given as an injection, loads an exposed, susceptible person with chicken pox antibodies. People who may benefit include those with compromised immune systems, susceptible pregnant women, and newborns exposed to chicken pox. If given within seventy-two to ninety-six hours of exposure, VZIG can shorten and perhaps prevent the disease.

The varicella vaccine, or Varivax, is currently recommended for all healthy children who have not had chicken pox. One dose of the vaccine is recommended between age twelve and eighteen months, at the time of the measles, mumps, and rubella vaccination. Immunization is also recommended for kids over eighteen months who have not had chicken pox, and for susceptible adults who come in contact with children who have leukemia or AIDS or who take immune-suppressive drugs.

Whether or not all healthy children should get this vaccine remains controversial. Vaccination provides 70 to 90 percent protection against infection and 95 percent protection against severe disease. Universal vaccination would lower the risk of those people to whom chicken pox is dangerous. Perhaps kids would miss less school, and parents would miss less work.

The vaccine is far from perfect, however. The immune response it produces isn't as strong or enduring as that resulting from actual infection. Kids who receive the single dose of the chicken pox vaccine face a 15-percent risk of losing immunity sometime during their lives, perhaps during adulthood or pregnancy, when their symptoms would be much worse. Some authorities, then, advocate booster vaccinations, presuming that older people will show up for the shot.

Neither of us has vaccinated our kids against chicken pox. We're more comfortable with the idea of their getting lifetime immunity from the actual illness. Then again, our children are normally healthy and not at risk for serious chicken pox complications. Also, by the time the vaccine became widely available, Linda's kids had already had blessedly uneventful chicken pox.

Herpes

The herpes simplex virus (*Herpes hominis*) comes in two varieties that produce different symptoms. Type 1 (HSV-1) causes cold sores, also called fever blisters, although neither colds nor fevers are to blame. Cold sores are not the same as canker sores, those tiny ulcers on the inside of lips and cheeks. Usually herpes sores occur on one side of the mouth; canker sores can be scattered on both sides.

Herpes simplex type 2 (HSV-2) causes genital herpes, a sexually transmitted disease characterized by recurrent, painful genital ulcers. Since the mid 1970s, the occurrence of HSV-2 has increased by 30 percent in the United States and is now detectable in about one in five people 12 years old and up.

HSV-1: Cold Sores

By the time they are ten years old, 30 to 60 percent of children have been infected with HSV-1, the virus that causes cold sores. The initial infection with HSV-1 often goes unnoticed. When symptoms do appear, they include fretfulness, fever as high as 105°F (40.5°), enlarged and tender lymph nodes in the neck, and refusal to eat. Several days later, the child's gums become reddened and painful, and his breath may smell bad. The child may complain of tingling, burning, or itching around the mouth or nostrils.

The small, red pimples that soon appear on and around the lips, gums, tongue, and roof of the mouth rapidly grow to small blisters, then ulcers. The lesions itch and hurt. The mouth sores make some children so uncomfortable that they refuse to eat or drink, thereby risking dehydration. Crusting sores signify that the illness is turning around.

The time from exposure to symptoms ranges from two to twelve days, and the illness typically lasts between four and ten days. Pain tends to disappear two to four days before the lesions heal. Rarely, the herpes virus can cause serious illness by infecting the membranes enveloping the central nervous system, the brain, or the eye.

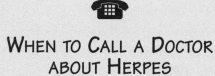

WHEN TO CALL A DOCTOR ABOUT HERPES

Your child develops genital lesions.

Your child has eczema and develops herpes, too. This can result in a serious illness.

Lesions seem to be spreading.

Lesions appear on or near the eye, or the white of the eye becomes pink.

The sores persist beyond two weeks.

Fever exceeds 104°F (40°C).

Your child refuses to drink or appears dehydrated. Look for dry lips and skin, crying without tears, no urination within eight hours, and, in infants, a sunken soft spot (fontanel).

Your child complains of stiff neck or can't bring his neck to his chest.

Your child becomes very irritable, difficult to awaken, delirious, or has a seizure or difficulty walking.

Your child otherwise acts very ill.

After the initial infection, the herpes virus remains dormant near the spinal cord. It can hang out there for days, months, even years, until something triggers its migration back down the nerve to cause another outbreak in the same general location where it first appeared. A variety of stressors (sunburn, sun exposure, fever, injury to the area, menstruation, gastrointestinal upsets, emotional upheavals) can reactivate the virus. The HSV-1 travels down the nerve and causes another outbreak in the same general location where it first appeared.

HSV 2–Genital Herpes

Genital herpes usually begins with tingling, burning, or itching in the genital area. The first episode produces the most symptoms: fever, swollen lymph nodes in the groin, muscle aches, headache, and burning on urination. The affected area first becomes reddened, then breaks out in small, painful blisters that ulcerate. A person without obvious symptoms can be contagious and spread the infection.

HSV-2 is a sexually transmitted disease. If your child is too young to engage in voluntary sexual activity, ask if anyone has touched his or her genitals. If the answer is yes or you suspect it could be yes, contact your doctor.

Conventional Treatment

No cure exists for either kind of herpes. You can relieve and reduce symptoms, but the pesky virus continues to recur. Doctors often recommend acetaminophen (Tylenol and others) and sometimes prescribe Viscous Xylocaine, a topical anesthetic, to paint on the lesions. Use the lowest effective dose; too much can cause serious side effects. Also, a numb mouth can cause kids to accidentally bite their tongues or the inside of their cheeks, so don't give them food or chewing gum until the anesthetic effects wear off.

The antiviral drug acyclovir (Zovirax) effectively suppresses or prevents herpes outbreaks and reduces symptoms during an outbreak. Oral treatment, started within the first three days of illness, significantly shortens the duration of symptoms and infectiousness of mouth herpes. Acyclovir and a newer, similar drug, valacyclovir significantly hasten healing of genital herpes, too. When daily treatments are stopped, symptoms can reappear. Side effects include confusion, loss of appetite, nausea and vomiting, constipation or diarrhea, excessive sweating, dizziness, malaise, and headache. Acyclovir ointment can be applied to the lesions. Side effects include local irritation and rash.

Home Care for Herpes

Herpes cold sores are very contagious. If someone in the house has cold sores, make sure each person uses a separate cup, utensils, and lip balm. And, sorry, but take a rain check on kisses from your sick child until the lesions disappear. Go for hugs instead.

Encourage fluids. Often kids with mouth herpes find cool beverages comforting. Frozen foods may provide numbing relief. Try iced herbal tea or herbsicles made from lemon balm and lemon grass tea. Some people report that ice sometimes stops a repeat infection when directly applied at the first signs of tingling. To avoid tissue damage, don't leave ice on for more than a couple of minutes at a time.

Avoid ointments or salves. Drying helps speed healing, and ointments only trap moisture. The only exception is the external use of St.-John's-wort oil. It's strongly antiviral and keeps the cold sores moist so they don't crack and bleed. It does not seem to slow down the healing.

Herbal Relief for Herpes and Chicken Pox

A first step toward quelling viral outbreaks (especially the initial infection of herpes) is to strengthen natural immunity with antiviral herbs such as echinacea, astragalus, and schisandra. Preventing herpes recurrence is the best medicine, so keep your child healthy with a good diet, plenty of rest, low sugar intake, and avoidance of food allergens. Good health will lower susceptibility to these viral illnesses.

We haven't seen specific research on the use of these teas during chicken pox, but their antiviral effects on cold sores are so clear that we would not hesitate to have our kids with chicken pox take baths in them and drink copious amounts.

Lemon balm inhibits the spread of a variety of viruses, including the herpes virus. A German study showed that cream containing lemon balm extract, applied soon after herpes symptoms begin, eased symptoms and reduced the size of the outbreak, apparently by protecting healthy cells from infection. Swelling and redness were decreased and there were few side effects. Another study concluded that lemon balm extracts lengthened the time between outbreaks and helped cold sores heal quickly.

To use lemon balm, give your child several cups of lemon balm tea or several doses of extract per day, and look for lip cremes at natural products stores. You may want to mix echinacea, lemon balm, and lemon grass herbs together for a tasty tea. Simmer the echinacea roots for ten minutes, remove the pan from heat, and add the lemon grass and lemon balm. Steep the tea for ten minutes, strain out the herbs, and serve the warm tea to your child.

Licorice root contains a component that, in test-tube studies, inactivates the herpes simplex virus. Licorice tea, when used as a skin wash, is mildly pain-relieving, soothing, and has anti-inflammatory powers on a par with hydro-cortisone. We like to use it during the early throbbing, itching stages of chicken pox or a herpes outbreak.

Caution: Do not use for more than six weeks. Not for use with hypertension, kidney or liver disease or diabetes, or while pregnant or nursing.

Mullein flowers and **leaves** soothe irritated skin. An infusion of flowers and leaves is best if made from the fresh herb, but de-bug the flowers first. You can have your child drink the tea and use it to wash the skin, too. An alternative we haven't tried is to use mullein-flower ear oil externally on cold sores. If the ear oil contains garlic, that's fine: Garlic fights viruses, too.

St.-John's-wort. Laboratory tests show that hypericin, an active ingredient in St.-John's-wort, kills both types of the herpes virus. We've found that the oil gives almost instant relief to painful or itchy cold sores or chicken pox blisters. But be careful: In rare cases, it can cause photosensitivity. Since sun exposure appears to activate the herpes virus in some people, this would be the last herb you'd want to use while vacationing at the

DO THE BURDOCK MASH

Burdock, whose huge leaves are used by some people to ease the itching and burning of poison oak, may also help chicken pox. Mash up a bit of clean burdock leaf with a blender or mortar and pestle and apply a test patch to your child's skin. If it still feels good ten to fifteen minutes later, let your child smear burdock mash all over the spots. Fresh leaf is best, but you could try soaking some dried leaf until it feels plump and moist again and use it the same way.

ANTIVIRAL GLYCERITE FOR CHICKEN POX

For ages: Over one year
Yields: 2 cups

*1/4 cup echinacea root
    (immune stimulant, antiviral)*
*2 tablespoons astragalus root
    (immune support, adaptogen)*
*2 tablespoons hyssop leaves
    (antiviral)*
*2 tablespoons lemon balm leaves
    (antiviral, calming)*
*1 teaspoon skullcap leaves
    (nerve support, antiviral)*
1½ cup vegetable glycerine
1 cup distilled water
*3,000 mg vitamin C powder or ground
    tablets (optional)*

Directions: Grind all herbs together in a blender or clean coffee grinder until coarsely powdered. Set aside. Mix vegetable glycerine and distilled water in a 1-quart canning jar. Stir in herbs until all are moist. Cover tightly, and shake well once a day for 2 weeks. Strain once through loosely woven cheesecloth to remove herbs, and a second time through a tightly woven cloth or coffee filter to catch the fine particles. Add vitamin C powder to preserve if necessary. Shake well before each use. Refrigerate for up to one year.

Dosage: 30 drops, 3 times a day for a 50-pound child. Use at the first signs and for several days after viral illness, including herpes and chicken pox.

COLD SORE AND CHICKEN POX GEL

For ages: All
Yields: 3/4 to 1 cup

If you have access to fresh St.-John's-wort flowers, wonderful; they're more potent than the dried version. Simply substitute twice the amount.

*1 cup aloe vera gel
    (soothing, antiviral, drying)*

*1/8 cup dried licorice root
    (anti-inflammatory, analgesic,
    antiviral)*

*1/8 cup dried St.-John's-wort flowering
    tops
    (anti-inflammatory, antiviral)*

*4 500-mg lysine capsules
    (antiviral)*

*3 drops lavender essential oil
    (anti-inflammatory)*

Mix all ingredients in a clean pint- or quart-sized jar. Allow to sit at room temperature for 12 to 24 hours. Strain through a tightly woven cloth, such as an old T-shirt or bandanna. Store in refrigerator between each use; keeps several months.

Apply as needed on herpes and chicken pox blisters. Shake well and apply with a clean cotton swab directly to herpes and chicken pox sores.

Caution: Keep away from small children; drinking this mix could be very laxative.

beach or a ski area. If you must go out in the sun, our compromise suggestion for cold sores is to use St.-John's-wort oil at night, and keep your child's lips slathered with a strong sun block or zinc oxide during the day.

Tea tree oil is a strongly antiseptic essential oil with antifungal properties. While mostly studied for its antimicrobial effects, it contains several antiviral components. To prevent bacterial infection in chicken pox and herpes, we dilute one drop of concentrated tea tree oil in one teaspoon of cooking oil and apply with a cotton swab to affected areas. Some parents have reported that their kids with chicken pox have received relief from this technique.

Tea tree can be mildly irritating to the skin, so we'd suggest trying it on a small spot first. Wait several hours before applying elsewhere.

Echinacea inhibits herpes virus in test-tube studies. Although internal use of echinacea can boost the immune system—and we do recommend its use during chicken pox and those miserable first-time herpes outbreaks—it probably kills the virus only when applied directly to the skin lesions. You can try poultices, compresses, or a lotion/salve formula that contains echinacea; a bit of tea on a cotton swab, dabbed directly on the sore, may help, too.

Nervine herbs such as chamomile, hawthorn, catnip, lavender, hops, and fennel are essential during chicken pox and herpes. The irritation of the cold sores or chicken pox blisters can antagonize a normally calm child. A good-tasting glycerite made from one or more of these herbs can restore calm. To help your child sleep, try hops, passionflower, and valerian.

Skullcap is a particularly appropriate nervine herb during chicken pox and cold-sore outbreaks because it fights viruses, too. The taste is quite bitter, so look for it in extract or capsule form. Don't forget that parents and caretakers of a sick child usually need some calming herbs themselves.

Flower essences for chicken pox. Linda knows a pediatrician who advises parents to add ten drops of Rescue Remedy to their child's bath during chicken pox and/or give a few drops by mouth. Another way to use the flower remedy is to soak the child's cotton pajamas (or a sheet) in a basin containing warm water and ten drops of Rescue Remedy, wring the pajamas out, and put them on the feverish child; the wet coolness helps relieve the itching. Make sure your child doesn't become chilled, however; wrap her in a warm blanket (a non-electric one!) and remove the damp pajamas as necessary.

Dietary Support During Herpes Infections

Reduce arginine-rich foods such as brown rice, wheat products, cereals, dairy products, carob, chocolate, corn, peanuts, beans, soy products, nuts, and seeds when herpes infection becomes evident. Adults should restrict or avoid alcohol as well. Sorry, but chocolate seems to be another common activator of the dormant virus. You can resume your normal diet after the outbreak.

Emphasize lysine-rich foods such as legumes, poultry, fish, high-lysine corn, eggs, high-quality meats, and most vegetables. This amino acid inhibits herpes replication by blocking arginine. Although a low-arginine, high-lysine environment inhibits herpes virus in test-tube studies, clinical trials have yielded mixed results.

Check with a naturopath or other health professional with expertise in nutritional supplements about giving your child lysine. Adults with herpes report that taking 500 mg of lysine three times a day at the first sign and throughout the herpes infection tends to help reduce symptoms. Ask your practitioner about children's doses.

Boost vitamin C-rich foods including guavas, sweet peppers, green leafy vegetables, broccoli, cauliflower, cabbage, citrus, strawberries, mangoes, and kiwi. Vitamin C, used topically and taken internally, has been shown to hasten healing.

Zinc, used both orally and on the skin, has helped stave off and heal herpes. Vitamin and mineral treatments work best if begun soon after the onset of symptoms. Again, check with your practitioner about children's doses.

Chapter 23

HEADACHES

If you think headaches fall into the category of adult illnesses, think again. Some studies have found that up to 82 percent of children suffer headaches. Most headaches in children are benign and respond to gentle therapies or simple preventive strategies. When they recur, however, parents may need to look deeper for a cause. Some types of headaches require medical attention.

Headaches can be categorized by their cause: tension headaches, caused by muscle contraction in the shoulders, neck, and scalp; migraine headaches, which follow constriction and dilation in the arteries in and around the brain; injury-related headaches, the kind that normally result from a head bonk or other mishap; infection-related headaches, which are exactly that; psychologically related headaches, such as those induced by stress or depression; and those rare ones caused by increased pressure within the skull, as can happen with brain tumors.

Tension Headaches

Also called muscle contraction headaches, these are by far the most common kind. More than a third of Americans get tension headaches, and more than two-thirds of all headaches fall within this category. Muscle tightness in the shoulder, neck, and scalp is to blame. This tension creeps over the scalp to the forehead, resulting in pain that's usually generalized, meaning that it's not limited to one side of the head. Your child may describe the pain as feeling like a headband or hat that's too tight. Often these headaches come on over the course of the day and go away after a nap or a good night's sleep. Given sufficient stress, however, tension headaches can persist several days.

One of the ways to prevent tension headaches is to avoid common triggers: muscle strains, hunger, poor sleep, inadequate diet, poor posture, eyestrain, emotional stress, dehydration, and constipation. Of course, to completely avoid all these things, your child would have to live in a bubble. But if one of these triggers causes headaches repeatedly, the solution is sometimes as basic as making sure your child drinks enough fluids.

Migraine Headaches

This type of headache strikes some 4.5 percent of children and often runs in families. If both parents have migraines, their offspring may face a 75 percent chance of having them, too. If only one parent is affected, the odds go down to 50 percent. Kids as young as two have been diagnosed, but more commonly, children who suffer migraines are hitting puberty.

If your child has a true migraine, he'll look ill and the attack will stop him in his tracks. These headaches usually entail more pain than a tension headache. The pain often, but not always, occurs on one side of the head, and can be throbbing. In 60 to 85 percent of children's migraines, the headache happens without warning signs other than withdrawal from activity or mood changes. Other kids experience a group of symptoms that precedes the actual headache, called an aura or prodrome. These symptoms can include moodiness, sweating, sensitivity to light, pale or flushed appearance, loss of appetite, nausea, or vomiting. In young children, stomach upset can be especially prominent. Older kids and teens may also share adult symptoms of blind spots, flashing lights, or other visual disturbances, transient numbness or weakness in one side of the body, or difficulty speaking.

Migraines usually last two to three hours, but can persist for a few days. Often, vomiting breaks the headache. Drowsiness typically follows, and sleeping often relieves the pain. Fortunately, most kids with a tendency toward migraines don't get them often.

Here's what is believed to happen during a migraine: something causes an initial narrowing of the arteries in and around the brain. The insufficient blood flow produces the aura symptoms. Then the arteries dilate, which produces the pain.

Migraine-headache triggers include stress, insufficient sleep, too much sleep (possibly because blood sugar levels get too low), poor nutrition, menstrual periods or premenstrual syndrome, oral contraceptives, excessive noise, bright lights, smells, and food sensitivities. Stress-related migraines usually don't occur during the heat of a stressful event, but after the conflict has been resolved.

Diet can contribute to migraines in three ways. Some people get migraines when they allow themselves to become very hungry and their blood sugar drops. Nutrient deficiencies can be at fault; low magnesium levels have been linked to both migraine and tension headaches. Finally, foods high in substances that influence blood vessel diameter can trigger migraines in susceptible people. Typical culprits include red wine, chocolate, nuts, aged cheeses, fermented soy products such as tempeh and miso, brewer's yeast, diet drinks, and caffeine. Smoked fish, hot dogs, sausages, and luncheon meats often contain migraine-provoking nitrates. Food additives such as monosodium glutamate and aspartame (Nutrasweet) can trigger headaches for some people. Sensitivities to foods such as wheat, eggs, citrus, corn, and dairy can also precipitate headaches.

Injury-Related Headaches

No great surprise here. After a minor injury, the resultant headache usually resolves within a day. With a more severe head injury, especially one that leads to loss of consciousness, your child's headache can persist for months. If your child loses consciousness for any reason, he should see a doctor. If he has hit his head and has persistent headaches, also take him to the doctor. (See Chapter 5, First Aid, for herbal remedies to use for headaches that result from minor head bonks.)

Infection-Related Headaches

Many common childhood illnesses can result in headache, notably strep throat, influenza, and sinusitis. Unfortunately, more serious but less common infections can cause headaches, too. In meningitis, an infection of the membranes that envelop the brain and spinal cord, a child will also have fever, stiff neck, vomiting, lethargy, and extreme sensitivity to light. Encephalitis, an infection of brain tissue, causes headache but also delirium, stupor, and, eventually, coma. A brain abscess, or localized brain infection, can cause lethargy, fever, progressive weakness on one side of the body, localized seizures, or loss of vision.

In any of these cases, your child will act very ill. You won't confuse a run-of-the-mill headache due to muscle tension with one caused by infection of the central nervous system.

Depression can also give your child a headache. If this is the cause, you may also see symptoms of loss of interest in activities and changes in appetite, weight, and sleep. If you suspect that your child is sad or angry, talk to

her about her feelings and get professional help. Counseling can often shorten the duration of a problem by getting to the heart of it. You may be surprised how much your child enjoys having someone other than a parent listen to her.

Conventional Treatment of Headaches

Medical treatment of a headache depends on the cause. Those associated with infections such as influenza will resolve after a day or two; relief of symptoms is all that's needed. Kids with suspected strep throat and sinusitis need to be seen by a doctor. Serious infections such as meningitis make a child so obviously ill that parents will doubtless know to seek emergency care. The

WHEN TO CALL A DOCTOR ABOUT HEADACHES

Call a doctor if your child has any of the following symptoms:

Recent onset of migraine or frequent headaches of any kind

Severe pain

Pain that worsens in the morning

Pain associated with recurrent morning vomiting

Pain that's aggravated by sneezing, coughing, or straining

Pain that is always in the same place, particularly the back of the head

Pain that is chronic and not alleviated by pain medications

You suspect your child is depressed

If your child experiences the following problems, get medical help right away. Call your doctor to find out whether you should proceed to the office, or straight to the emergency room.

Headache comes with seizures, delirium, troubles with balance and gait, slurred speech, or visual disturbances other than the usual beginning symptoms of a migraine

Your child has fever, lethargy, or irritability and a stiff neck

GRANDMA'S HEADACHE REMEDIES THAT WORK

Foot baths. One of the sweetest moments Sunny remembers from herb school was when a friend offered to give her a foot bath to relieve a headache. Laura, a trained massage therapist, knelt next to Sunny and gently placed her feet in a bowl of hot water lightly scented with floating rock rose flowers. For several minutes, she lightly massaged Sunny's entire foot—toes, instep, rough calluses and all. Even though it was a very warm day, Sunny still remembers the sense of peace and acquiescence she felt with the heated water drawing blood to her toes. Within ten minutes, her headache was gone, but the memory has remained for years. If you want to try a foot bath for your child, ask him whether he wants the temperature hot or cold. Some kids will actually gain the most relief from an ice-cold foot bath. Or you can try five minutes of a hot soak, followed by two minutes of cold.

Hot towel, cold towel. As with foot baths, some kids like it hot and some like it cold. You can alternate five minutes of a hot towel on your child's forehead and shoulders with two minutes of a cold towel. (Always check the temperature yourself; microwaved towels can get especially hot!)

Hot water bottles. If you don't have a hot water bottle, you can use a glass canning jar filled with hot water and wrapped in a towel. The heat will stimulate blood flow to cramped capillaries. Start by holding the jar against your child's forehead, and later move it to his shoulders. Microwaveable heat bags or a microwaved sock filled with dried legumes or rice also work for this technique.

Frozen peas. These frozen veggies are a first aid kit all by themselves; we like them because they're so flexible and wrap well around little knees and elbows. They're just as gentle to little foreheads. Take straight out of the freezer and apply the entire bag if your child craves coolness.

Bitter makes better. Sometimes kids and adults get simple headaches from indigestion. Referred to as "bilious headaches" in turn-of-the-last-century medical texts, this type of

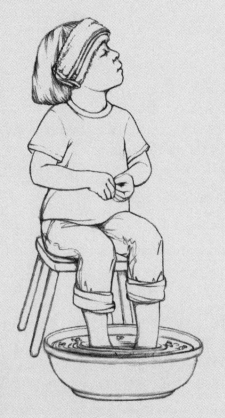

Herbal foot baths and compresses can ease many minor headaches.

headache often responds well to bitter substances. Feverfew extract is the perfect solution, because its bitterness on the tongue stimulates liver and gall bladder secretions, and it is anti-inflammatory as well. In Germany, people use a strong brew of artichoke leaves for a similar effect.

Regular relief. Constipation can result in headaches. Encourage your child to sip one to two tablespoons of prune juice every two hours all day long, and you should have relief for two problems.

Alkalinity helps. Sometimes all you need to turn the tide of a minor headache is a temporary switch from an acid-based diet to an alkaline one. You don't have to be a chemist to do it; you just have to know a few alkaline foods. Alkaline foods include dark green leafy veggies, almonds, carrots, figs, miso, seaweed, turnips, tamari, salt, and umeboshi plums or plum paste.

Sour saves some. Some kids love the sour tastes of life; if yours is one, she'll enjoy lemons, pickles, sauerkraut, and vinegar-based salad dressings. With these kids, try a little fresh lemon juice in water to relieve headaches. Traditional natural health lore says that the sour taste stimulates the liver and generates healthy digestion, which in turn can soothe headache pain.

headache of a brain tumor or other structural problems produces symptoms that don't fit with the pattern of common headaches, and usually will alert a parent to the need for medical intervention.

Pseudo headaches such as those invented to avoid school are usually resolved by talking them out. Participants in this discussion will include you, your child, and his teacher, plus or minus a mental health professional. Headaches caused by depression or other mental causes often respond to therapy and, if needed, drugs.

Tension headaches are often treated with pain-relieving medications including acetaminophen, ibuprofen, or naproxen. Because of the risk of liver toxicity, acetaminophen shouldn't be taken more than five times a day and for no more than five consecutive days. Aspirin, ibuprofen, and naproxen can cause gastrointestinal upsets. Also, because chronic use can cause rebound headaches, analgesics should not be used long-term. With our kids, particularly if the headache is mild, we prefer to try other remedies first. Sometimes just lying down and relaxing goes a long way toward relieving a tension headache. So do warm baths and head, neck, and shoulder massages.

Migraine treatment depends upon the frequency and severity of the attacks. Ideally, parents and doctors try to identify triggers and help the child avoid them. If your child has infrequent, mild-to-moderate migraines, most doctors usually recommend symptomatic treatment with the same over-the-counter pain relievers used for tension headaches. When given at the first sign of a migraine, these medicines may abort the attack or at least minimize the pain. If the headache does break through, the child should rest in a dark, quiet room. Caffeine, because it constricts arteries, can help tame a headache, but it doesn't work for habitual users. Also, chronic, heavy use of caffeinated beverages can lead to migraines. And the usual caffeine vehicles for children are carbonated colas, which are packed with sugar and detract from bone health. Some pediatric patients use an over-the-counter caffeine product to avoid sodas.

Heavier-duty drugs are usually reserved for children who have frequent and/or severe migraines. Some drugs are given to abort impending headaches. Most commonly prescribed is ergotamine tartrate, which goes by several trade names, including Cafergot. This drug causes constriction of the blood vessels. A newer medication with similar actions is sumatriptan, sold under the trade name Imitrex. It works better when injected under the skin than when taken by mouth. A nasal spray will soon be available.

Both drugs can produce significant side effects; you should ask your doctor for complete information on them. Pregnant women and anyone with heart disease or high blood pressure should not take either drug.

If migraines are so frequent and severe that they interfere with a child's activities, doctors may then go on to recommend daily use of a medication to prevent migraines. Choices include the antidepressant amitriptyline (Elavil), which works by influencing serotonin, and propanolol, (Inderal), which dilates blood vessels. All the preventative drugs have significant side effects, so make sure your doctor knows your child well and considers the risks.

Migraines are a good example of a problem for which both natural and pharmaceutical treatment can work; sometimes a combination of both is best. Both Linda and her son get migraines, but not often enough to take feverfew every day. When Linda's son feels a migraine coming, she gives him ibuprofen and feverfew and has him lie down in a darkened room. Feverfew alone isn't enough to block his pain. Ideally, your child's doctor will support you and work with you in trying natural remedies first, or in combination with pharmaceuticals.

Dietary Changes for Migraine Prevention

Studies in both adults and children have found that many migraine sufferers have food allergies and that withdrawal of offending foods reduces headaches. In a study of 88 children with severe and frequent migraines, 98 percent recovered on diets designed to eliminate food allergens. Among the trigger foods: cow's milk, wheat, chocolate, eggs, oranges, benzoic acid, cheese, tomatoes, tartrazine (a food additive), and rye.

Many other foods and additives can, in sensitive people, cause headaches: sugar, monosodium glutamate, aspartame (Nutrasweet), excessive salt, excessive fat, fish, citrus, and strawberries, to name a few. Sugar is a common culprit, according to Jaqueline Krohn, M.D., author of *The Whole Way to Allergy Relief and Prevention* (1991, Hartley and Marks, Inc.) You may want to compare your child's headaches with her sugar consumption over a day to two days to see whether a connection exists. For more information on food allergies, see Chapter 7, Allergies and Intolerances.

Key dietary supplements may help with your child's headaches. Studies that have investigated the effect of magnesium supplements have found either some benefits or no effect. According to Leo Galland, M.D., author of *Super Immunity for Kids*, children should have 6 mg of magnesium per pound of body weight each day. Taking large doses of magnesium citrate supplements, however, can cause diarrhea and stomach irritation in some children, so we advise starting with a low dose and working your way up. A safe bet is boosting your child's intake of foods rich in magnesium: dark green leafy vegetables, grains, potatoes, nuts, seeds, figs, grapefruit, yellow corn, apples, and seaweed. Herbs that contain small amounts of magnesium include oatstraw, licorice, nettles, burdock, sage, yellow dock, dandelion, parsley, and red clover. Parents of children with special medical conditions such as diabetes should consult with a qualified nutritionist before supplementing with magnesium.

One of the theories of the genesis of migraines involves a chemical in the body called serotonin. Many migraine sufferers have low tissue levels of serotonin. These individuals can raise their levels by taking a modified form of the amino acid tryptophan called 5-hydroxytryptophan, or 5-HTP.

This substance also increases endorphins, the body's natural opium-like painkillers.

This nutritional supplement has actually been studied in children, with good results. One study found no effect; in at least three others, the subjects saw significant benefits. The results aren't immediate, however; your child will need at least a couple of months for the supplement to take effect. A 50-pound child will take about 114 mg. If 5-HTP is not available at your natural foods store, try contacting a naturopathic or chiropractic physician—a good idea before you begin any nutritional supplement.

Because of the presence of inflammation during headache, it makes sense that essential fatty

HEADACHE RELIEF GLYCERITE

For ages: Over one year
Yields: 2½ cups, or 20 one-ounce dropper bottles

*1/4 cup ginkgo leaves
    (boosts cerebral circulation)*
*1/4 cup feverfew leaves and flowers
    (headache preventive)*
*1 teaspoon rosemary leaves
    (circulation booster,
    anti-inflammatory)*
*1 tablespoon chamomile flowers
    (anti-inflammatory, calming)*
*A pinch of fresh grated ginger
    (anti-inflammatory)*
*1 tablespoon peppermint leaf
    (aromatic, digestive)*
*1 teaspoon skullcap herb
    (calming)*
2½ cups vegetable glycerine
1½ cups distilled water

*3,000 mg vitamin C powder or three
    1,000-mg tablets, ground*
*5 drops natural food flavoring: blackberry,
    raspberry, or orange (optional)*

Grind all dried herbs into a coarse powder in a blender or clean coffee grinder. Mix vegetable glycerine and distilled water together in a one-quart or larger canning jar. Stir in herbs until all are moist. Cover tightly, and shake well once a day for 2 weeks. Strain once through loosely-woven cheesecloth to remove herbs, and a second time through a tightly woven cloth or coffee filter to catch the fine particles. Add Vitamin C powder; add optional flavorings to taste. Use a clean funnel to measure out into dropper bottles. Shake well before each use. Keep refrigerated. This batch of glycerite should last at least one year.

HEADACHE RELIEF MASSAGE OIL

For ages: Over one year
Yields: 3 ounces, or almost 1/4 cup

*6 drops peppermint essential oil
(anti-inflammatory, digestive)*

*3 drops eucalyptus essential oil
(analgesic, anti-inflammatory)*

*3 drops lavender essential oil
(relaxant)*

*2 drops Roman chamomile essential oil
(anti-inflammatory)*

*3 ounces almond, apricot kernel,
safflower, or canola oil*

Directions: Blend all oils together and mix well. If your child has delicate skin, do a test patch on his arm and wait two hours. If no symptoms of reaction appear, your child should be able to use the oil. If a rash does appear, wash the area with soap, and then apply a plain vegetable oil to the area.

To use this massage oil for your child's headache, have him relax face down in a darkened room and gently massage his scalp, neck, and shoulders. If you don't feel him begin to relax, try working on his arms, hands, or feet.

Store the oil in a tightly sealed container, away from heat. It's not necessary to refrigerate the oil, although refrigeration will extend its shelf life.

Caution: Do not use near the eyes.

acids may help. Sources include cold-water fish such as salmon, flaxseed and flaxseed oil, and the oils of other plants such as borage, black currant, and evening primrose. Two small studies, one using two omega-3 fatty acids found in fish and one using fish oil itself, reported a significant reduction in migraine intensity and frequency.

Complementary Approaches for Headaches

If your child has recurrent headaches and your doctor has already ruled out serious underlying causes, you may want to consult some other trained practitioners—perhaps an allergy specialist, naturopathic doctor, ophthalmologist or optician, psychologist or psychiatrist, nutritionist, acupuncturist, or homeopath. Your child's headache may be a symptom of allergies, especially if she has had other ailments such as eczema, gastrointestinal problems, or ear infections.

Traditional Chinese Medicine is another possible avenue. Several small studies have shown acupuncture to be effective in relieving migraine and tension headaches and reducing their subsequent occurrence. In one study involving adults with chronic tension headaches, acupuncture reduced pain by 31 percent. Relaxation techniques and biofeedback have been shown to reduce headaches. Some area hospitals offer classes in these techniques for children.

You may also want to explore various types of body work. We're not sure what the studies say, but we know chiropractic care and massage have helped relieve many of our own headaches.

Herbal Remedies for Headaches

Feverfew has developed quite a reputation as a migraine preventive. Since the 1980s, several studies have shown benefits for this herb; one showed no effect. Controversy surrounds the issue of the best way to use feverfew and which of its compounds is responsible for its effects. However, we've used the whole plant successfully for headaches; it's probable that many different forms are effective.

Until recently, scientists chalked up feverfew's migraine-prevention capability to the constituent parthenolide. And many of the highly advertised feverfew products on the market today are processed in order to deliver a certain, standardized amount of parthenolide in each dose. But recent study results indicate that taking the whole herb is probably the most effective way of using feverfew. Whether a tincture or glycerite comes from dried or fresh leaves does make a difference. In lab studies, fresh leaf extracts dropped onto blood vessels blocked their constriction (which is desirable in preventing migraines). Extracts made from dried leaves brought on constriction in that study.

Bottom line: If you're shopping for feverfew, we suggest you look for whole-herb products and avoid the standardized extracts that concentrate on only one of this plant's constituents. You'll generally pay less for the whole plant products, too, because standardization is often an expensive process. If you're buying tincture or glycerite, choose a product made from fresh leaves.

Cayenne pepper contains capsaicin, which lab studies have shown blocks a chemical involved in nerve transmission of pain. Repeated intranasal applications of a preparation containing capsaicin have prevented the occurrence of cluster headaches, migraine-like headaches that are brief, but recurrent and excruciating. These headaches don't trouble young children, but cayenne cream may be helpful for easing older children's migraine-like headaches. Consult a naturopathic physician about using topical preparations of capsaicin.

Your child can also take cayenne internally. At the first sign of pain, give an eighth to a half capsule of cayenne powder with food. To administer a fraction of a capsule dose, open the capsule, dump the amount of powder you don't want, and put it back together. You can give cayenne to your child every three hours with food, as long as she can reliably swallow capsules all the way down (usually at about age seven). Follow with a glass of water and thoroughly wash your hands with soap after touching the powder. If you make your own capsules at home, beware of the varying strengths of the herb available in bulk: African bird-pepper type is three times hotter than the regular cooking cayenne and can cause severe stomach irritation

ROSEMARY INHALER

For ages: Over one year
Yields: One inhaler

1 drop rosemary essential oil
1 teaspoon salt

Mix one drop of pure rosemary essential oil with one teaspoon of salt in a small bottle with a tight cap. To ease headache, open the bottle and inhale deeply. Other essential oils work well, too: grapefruit, orange, peppermint, and lemon balm, to name a few.

Caution: Don't apply these oils to the nasal area or inside the nose, as one such use has been reported to trigger respiratory arrest. Don't apply undiluted essential oils to your child's skin, and don't take them internally. Store them safely out of your kid's reach.

to children. Most pre-made capsules use the milder cayenne. You can also massage a cayenne-containing balm into your child's temples.

Caution: Don't apply topical cayenne products to open wounds or get them near the eyes, as even the fumes cause a burning sensation and tearing. Don't use them for more than a few days without a break, either; they can cause minor nerve irritation with long-term use.

Ginger hasn't yet been studied in clinical trials for headaches. It does, however, have a long history of use, complete with lots of anecdotes of its effectiveness, and it is safe. Lab studies have shown that it acts as an anti-inflammatory substance and decreases the tendency of platelets to clump together. Both attributes help ease headaches, including migraines. Ginger also contains a substance called 6-shogaol that seems to act like the capsaicin in cayenne to decrease pain.

Ginger is also wonderful for easing nausea associated with some headaches. We both keep natural ginger ale on hand at all times; you never know when you're going to need it for an upset tummy or headache. Just read the label before you buy to make sure that the bottle contains real ginger, not artificial flavoring. A ginger tea or candied ginger also work well.

Peppermint is a great headache reliever. Menthol, its primary aromatic ingredient, helps relieve pain externally and internally. In a recent study of people with tension headaches, a blend containing peppermint essential oil provided significant relief compared to placebo treatment.

Willow bark is a useful but somewhat controversial pain reliever. Considered the "original aspirin," willow bark is full of naturally occurring salicylates, which are the chemical sisters to the acetylsalicylic acid in aspirin. However, due to the concern about the use of aspirin during viral illnesses contributing to Reye's syndrome (a serious illness characterized by liver damage and brain swelling), many prominent herbalists are suggesting that children avoid the use of willow bark during viral illnesses. However, no cases have connected salicylate-containing herbs to Reye's, and many common foods also contain salicylates. To be safe, we don't use this herb when the child's headache accompanies a viral illness. Sunny has, however, used willow bark numerous times to relieve her own headaches. Other herbs with salicylates include poplar, aspen, meadowsweet, and spirea. Any would make a great analgesic contribution to an herbal salve.

Passionflower is a great herbal sedative for kids. Small doses will relax your child; larger doses will sedate her. Either will relieve headache pain. The tea isn't the best tasting beverage on the planet, but you can make it more palatable by adding a little juice. Or give passionflower in a glycerite.

More herbs for headaches. We just have to mention a few other great-tasting headache relievers: lemon balm, chamomile, lavender flowers, catnip, thyme, and fennel. Each of these herbs has been used traditionally for hundreds of years, and some have current clinical research to verify their effects. Fennel and chamomile are great for headaches that go with tummy aches; if tension is the cause, try lemon balm, lavender, or catnip. All make great glycerites or teas.

Chapter 24

SLEEP

In terms of survival, not to mention optimal well-being, sleep ranks right alongside food and water in the hierarchy of human needs. When insufficient sleep becomes the norm, most of us grow irritable, moody, inattentive, and less creative. We don't cope with stress as well, which in small children may manifest as a temper tantrum. Our immune systems weaken, and we have more accidents.

And as we all know: If baby doesn't sleep, nobody sleeps.

We suspect that many a parent would gladly forego a gourmet dinner, a dance in the moonlight, and four-star sex for eight hours of uninterrupted sleep. Even in times B.C. (before children), sleep can be elusive. You can tuck yourself in bed and shut your eyes, but sleep, in its own feline way, will either come or it won't. Add a baby to the equation and the likelihood of satisfying sleep plummets. In fact, parents of young children rank alongside long-haul truck drivers for being at risk for chronic sleep deprivation. Parents, as well as children, often need help to develop healthy sleep patterns.

All kinds of things can temporarily interrupt the sleep of infants and children. Discomfort such as hunger, colic, teething, illness, physical injury, milk allergy, or wet or soiled diapers can disrupt sleep for babies. Additional bugaboos can disturb the sleep of older children: things that go bump in the night, emotional trauma, nightmares, being in a strange place, pinworms, or anxiety about recent or upcoming events. When children of any age ingest stimulants, for example caffeine and, for some children, sugar, they may well have trouble sleeping.

Some problems can cause habitual poor sleep in children. A partial list follows.

Separation anxiety in small children can produce reluctance to fall asleep, setting the stage for stubborn, perpetual bedtime resistance. Infants and small children experience going to sleep each night as a parting from you, and each morning as a reunion. Some anxiety is normal, but habits can turn this molehill into a mountain. For example, a baby may get used to falling asleep while in an adult's arms. When she wakes in the night, as babies often do, she cries out because she needs to be held as a bridge to sleep. This sort of dependency progresses as the child cries for her parent at intervals during the night. For most of us mortals, getting up to comfort a child back to sleep every few hours is difficult to intolerable.

Bedtime resistance is probably the most common sleep problem. In a survey of 987 parents of elementary school children, resistance topped the list—27 percent of parents admitted their children have this problem. These kids generally do not soothe themselves to sleep, but instead require an adult to be present (and often a parent in bed with them) to go to sleep.

Habitual night-time awakening is generally limited to infants, thank heavens. Some 10 to 25 percent of babies between 4 and 24 months wake up and cry one or more times during the night. Generally, they want to be fed or comforted by a parent. Newborns need a night-time feeding.

Normal babies over four months can theoretically go the night without a feeding, but habit comes into play. A baby who is always nursed or rocked to sleep doesn't learn to comfort herself back to sleep.

Morning wake-up problems usually stem from undesirable bedtime habits. In small children, the typical pattern is this: A child has bedtime resistance, awakens in the night, and crawls into his

THE SLEEP TRAP

Linda and her firstborn fell into this trap. A child prodigy in this regard, her son devised elaborate schemes to keep Mom with him. He wouldn't sleep on his own, and the family bed didn't work; no one slept. After living like zombies for a couple of years, Linda and her husband steeled their hearts and closed their bedroom door. "You can come into our room in the morning, when it's light outside," Linda said as she tucked her little boy into bed.

Many a dawn, she was awakened by a small person in footed pajamas climbing into her bed, his stubby finger pointed at the feeble light creeping through the window: "Look, Mommy. Dark's all gone."

parents' bed. Lacking either physical energy or emotional resolve, his parents let him stay. Nobody sleeps well—except the child, who can't awaken in time for child care or school. Kind-hearted parents who let him sleep in only perpetuate this late-to-bed, late-to-rise rhythm.

The sleep cycles of teens, however, naturally shift toward later bedtimes. They're just not drowsy till later at night, although they still need lots of sleep. Thus, it's really hard to drag them out of bed in the morning. We think high schools would better make use of the teenage brain if classes began at 10 A.M.

Night terrors and sleepwalking both stem from a nervous-system arousal at the transition from deep sleep to the dreaming stage. Night terrors are most common in two- to five-year-olds; sleepwalking in slightly older children. Night terrors usually occur between one to three hours after falling asleep. Parents find their child screaming, staring without seeing, sweating, thrashing, and inconsolable. It's as though the poor child can't awaken from a nightmare. Indeed, although his eyes maybe be open, he is otherwise asleep.

The episode resolves within five minutes. For the anxious parent, however, it can seem like an eternity. We know—Linda's son had night terrors. In the morning, the child usually remembers nothing of the event. Factors that increase the likelihood of a night terror include illness, emotional stress, and sleep deprivation.

Sleepwalking can be dangerous. Parents may need to lock doors and windows, cover sharp corners, shut bathroom doors, and set up gates to block the child from leaving his room or tumbling down a stairway. It may be helpful to set up a motion alarm that will go off when the child wanders from bed.

Transient upper airway obstructions during sleep can cause periodic awakening. The tissues of the throat collapse momentarily, causing the child to awaken briefly to restore adequate breathing. Most people with this disorder—the medical term is obstructive sleep apnea—don't realize they awaken many times during the night. Clues are snoring during sleep, punctuated by spells of breath-holding. See your doctor if you think your child may have this problem. Enlarged adenoids or tonsils can cause snoring, sleep apnea, and daytime mouth breathing.

Other medical problems can interfere with sleep. Acute illnesses, especially painful ones like rip-roaring middle-ear infections, will awaken a child. Chronic illnesses such as asthma and allergies or food intolerances can perpetually fragment sleep, as can night-time coughs. Allergies also can make nose breathing difficult, and associated itchy skin can periodically awaken a child.

How to Help Your Child Sleep

Parents can make bedtime easier, especially if they start early in the day by managing their kids' activities and diet and continuing to make bedtime mellow and reassuring for the child.

Limit nap time. Two naps a day is enough for infants (once they're on a schedule) and toddlers. Most kids outgrow the morning nap at eighteen months to two years of age. If your child snoozes for more than two hours at a stretch, wake him.

Parents can make up for lost night-time sleep by napping, too. But don't start that afternoon snooze after 3 P.M. or you'll both have trouble getting to sleep that night.

A varied, whole-foods diet can help your child sleep; poor nutrition can disrupt it. Deficiencies that can interfere with sleep include those of B vitamins, calcium, and magnesium. We give our children their calcium/magnesium supplements at night, because these minerals can be gently relaxing.

Avoid foods containing caffeine such as chocolate, tea, or soda within a few hours of bedtime.

A light meal before bedtime, however, can tide over infants and small children who awaken from hunger. Please don't put your baby to bed with a bottle, however; this will predispose him to cavities and middle-ear infections.

Create a mellow bedroom ambience. Make it a dark, quiet, warm, and well-ventilated sanctuary for sleep. If your child likes stuffed animals, dolls,

When to Call a Doctor About Sleep Problems

Call during office hours to schedule an appointment if:

You think that nighttime crying may have a physical cause such as illness or pain.

Your child snores loudly and constantly, especially if punctuated by periods of breath-holding.

Your child has frequent sleep terrors or sleepwalks. You may need help coping with the former and safety-proofing your child's bedroom for the latter.

Your child routinely resists bedtime or, when he awakens in the night, won't go back to sleep on his own.

You suspect allergies from food or airborne sources contribute to your child's poor sleep. Tip-offs include ongoing physical symptoms such as runny nose, ear infections, stomachaches, diarrhea, gas, and eczema.

Your child's sleep is restless, and she scratches at her anus. Your doctor may want to rule out pinworms.

special blankets, or the like, let him snuggle with them in bed.

Reduce your child's stress. If you suspect that anxiety is troubling your child's sleep, try to discover what's causing it: an overly busy schedule, apprehensions about separating from you, worries about homework, fear of the dark. This is not a conversation for bedtime, however, but for earlier in the day, when there's plenty of time to talk and find solutions to the anxiety.

After identifying sources of anxiety, brainstorm with your child about ways to minimize these concerns. A night light may reduce her fear of the dark, or playing a tape of soft classical music or nature sounds may relax her. Leaving the door ajar may also help your child feel less separated from the rest of the family. If she dreads nighttime separation from you, reassure her you'll spend lots of time together during the day—more if you get a good sleep—and just as importantly, follow through. A few visits to a skilled children's counselor may be valuable, too.

Bedtime Strategies

Just before bedtime, avoid stimulating activities such as vigorous play. Although watching television seems passive, it can agitate a child's mind, particularly if the content is action-packed, violent, or frightening. Find a quiet show, or avoid the television entirely.

If you have a baby or toddler, go ahead and rock, sing, cuddle, nurse—just before she goes to sleep. If your baby habitually cries for you in the middle of the night, you may have become a bridge to sleep. Many experts recommend that you respond to her cries and comfort her, then put her to bed while she's quiet, but still awake, so that she learns to fall asleep on her own. This doesn't mean that you can't stand by her bed or

respond to her cries in the night. Just don't hang around too long.

Establish a bedtime routine, and stick with it. This nightly pattern may include tooth-brushing, face-washing, putting on pajamas, massage, hair-braiding, reading, singing lullabies—activities that create a peaceful ambience. For little kids, simple repetition and habit are comforting. A favorite stuffed toy or blanket can help your child make the transition to sleep. Whatever your routine, start it about the same time every night and don't vary it much.

If your child awakens with a night terror, don't try to wake him up. Normally, you can't. Sometimes trying to soothe him will only increase his agitation. Of course you can't ignore a child who seems so terrified; we choose to stay by the bedside until the episode passes.

If a nightmare awakens your child, reassure her that these bad dreams are not real, but sort of like a scary movie. Sometimes you can help your child ease back to sleep by encouraging her to conjure happy thoughts to replace the frightening ones. Books on meditating with children may offer other helpful techniques.

Herbs to Bring Sleep

A nervine is a calming, relaxing herb that gently but effectively takes the edge off when your child needs to slow down. Safe and effective for children over twelve months old, these include the world-wide favorite, chamomile, along with catnip, oats, linden flower (sometimes hard to obtain in the United States), skullcap, passionflower, and many others.

The relaxation effect is generally dependent on the size of the child and the size of the dose: the smaller the child or the larger the dose, the greater the calming effect. We start with a quarter cup of tea for children over twelve months, and increase to approximately one cup for kids sixty pounds and up. Follow package instructions for store-bought remedies, because strength may vary from product to product. Generally, start with one small dose in the evening as needed for difficulty getting to sleep. Increase to a double dose if needed.

Herbal sedatives on the other hand, are sleep-inducing. In general, they produce sleepiness and minor muscle relaxation; they are safe for children over age two. Herbal sedatives include hops, California poppy, kava kava root, and valerian root. Again, start with a small dose and work your way up. For children two and up, you can start with a quarter cup of tea and increase to 1 cup for a 50-pound child. These herbs can be used as needed for occasional sleep problems. Get help if your child has nightly problems getting to sleep.

Nervines

Chamomile and **passionflower** both reduce anxiety and induce sleep. Several million cups of chamomile tea are consumed around the world each day. Many herb books caution patients with ragweed allergies to avoid chamomile, but we've never heard of an allergic reaction to this herb.

Catnip is considered gentle enough for babies. Purchase food-grade catnip from a natural foods store, not from a pet store, or grow your own; catnip is quite hardy. Prepare an infusion using one teaspoon of herb per cup of water. A few ounces of lightly sweetened catnip tea in a fussy baby's bottle or a cup of catnip tea for toddlers and older kids should do the trick.

Hawthorn is well-studied for the curative effects of the leaves, flowers, and berries on the cardiovascular system. This herb can also reduce anxiety, often in only minutes. The leaves, flowers, and tasty berries make a delicious tea or syrup that kids will drink readily. Hawthorn berries are safe, nontoxic, nonaddictive, and deli-cious. With hundreds of hawthorn species in the United States alone, we encourage you to take an identification class from your local native plant society to correctly identify and harvest these juicy gems.

Lemon balm, also known as balm or melissa, is lemony, musty, and minty. Kids like it. Lemon balm tea has been traditionally used for hundreds, if not thousands, of years to calm spirited kids.

You can also use the essential oil of lemon balm externally. We find the undiluted essential oil a bit strong for children's skin in a bath, but diluted it's fine for use as a massage oil. Use 2 or 3 drops per tablespoon of carrier oil.

Herbal Sedatives

Valerian is the best-studied sleep-inducing herb. Extracts of the root shorten the time need-ed to fall asleep and improve sleep quality without side effects. One study in adults compared a product containing extracts of both valerian root and lemon balm with the commonly prescribed hypnotic drug Halcion. Both groups slept better, but the Halcion group was troubled by morning hangover and impaired day-time coordination. Those who took the lemon balm/valerian prepa-ration had no such side effects. Participants in these studies were adults, but we've given valer-ian to our kids thirty minutes before bedtime with reliable, soothing results. Kids who can swallow capsules may prefer to take valerian in that form; younger kids can take it as a glycerite blended with more palatable herbs.

Valerian is not physiologically addictive, but we don't suggest you use it every single night, as it can be mentally habit forming. Chronic use of any herbal sedative can keep kids from developing their own healthy approach to falling asleep. For a very small percentage of children, valerian pro-duces a stimulating rather than a sedating effect. If this occurs, discontinue use.

HERBAL NERVINES AND SEDATIVES

The following herbs are listed weakest to strongest—kids will have individual reactions.

Lemon balm

St.-John's-wort

Hawthorn

Oats

Catnip

Chamomile

Linden

Passionflower

Skullcap

Hops

California poppy

Kava kava

Valerian

Kava kava can also help bring sleep, particularly when anxiety causes insomnia. Clinical trials show that it promotes sleep by modulating the brain's emotion centers and by relaxing muscles.

We have given our older kids a few drops of tincture with good, mellowing results. Start with just a few drops of tincture (or a small cup of tea) for a few nights before increasing dosage to label instruction levels.

Caution: Large doses of kava kava can induce a euphoric state and still higher doses, muscle weakness and dizziness. Pregnant and nursing women should avoid kava kava. Do not mix kava kava and alcohol or other central nervous system depressants.

California poppy plant and roots are used widely in Europe for the treatment of insomnia. Native Americans in California and Oregon once used the whole plant as a gentle sedative for babies. Lower doses reduce anxiety; higher doses sedate. California poppy is a good choice for active kids who have trouble getting to sleep each night.

Caution: Check with your doctor if your child is taking antidepressants or other central nervous system medications.

Essential Oils and Baths

Calming essential oils include neroli (orange blossom), Roman chamomile, lavender, rose, geranium, marjoram, and ylang ylang. You can add three to five drops to your child's warm bath, place a few drops on a small cloth next to his pillow, or slip the cloth under the pillowcase. You can also make a simple massage oil by mixing three to five drops into one tablespoon of a high-quality massage oil, such as almond or apricot-kernel oil. If your child has sensitive skin, do a patch test on her inner arm. Wait two hours. Unless the skin looks irritated, you can then give your child a relaxing, full-body massage.

Herb baths can become a nice evening ritual for mellowing high-strung kids. To make an herb bath, boil 2 to 3 quarts of water in a large pot. Turn off the heat and toss in a handful (about a half-ounce) each of dried herbs: lavender, chamomile, and old-fashioned oatmeal. Cover the pot and steep for 10 to 15 minutes. Strain to remove herbs. Add to bath water.

Recommended Reading

Ferber, R. *Solve Your Child's Sleep Problems.* New York: Fireside/Simon & Schuster, 1985.

Hobbs, C. *Stress and Natural Healing.* Loveland, CO: Botanica Press, 1997.

Schmidt, B. *Your Child's Health* (revised). New York: Bantam Books, 1991.

Chapter 25

ATTENTION DISORDERS

Humans show an astonishing range of ability to learn and concentrate. Some require absolute silence for reading; others can read (and understand) Nietzsche while listening to The Mighty Mighty Bosstones at full volume. Some kids and adults comprehend quickly when they see pictures, text, diagrams, charts, and the like. Others learn best when they hear a lecture, radio broadcast, or the lyrics of a song. Still others need to move and touch things in order to learn.

Some children, however, respond to none of these approaches to learning. They have trouble sitting still, listening, and taking directions. Their tasks remain unfinished; they're easily distracted. These impatient kids may talk too much, behave impulsively and unpredictably, and have explosive tempers; they may have trouble forming friendships. Yet these children are often very intelligent and talented.

Some kids are more kinetic or more inattentive than others, even from birth. They seem exceptionally active and distractable, and they're still entirely normal. When a child's behavior is significantly more rambunctious, impulsive, and unfocused than that of his peers and results in impaired schoolwork and social relationships, however, that child may have crossed into the realm of hyperactivity. Three to five percent of school-aged kids, most of them boys, manifest what's known as attention-deficit disorder (ADD) or attention-deficit-hyperactivity-disorder (ADHD). The acronym ADHD refers to both disorders and indicates that hyperactivity may or may not be a factor.

ADHD probably ranks as the fastest growing children's behavior diagnosis in America. Unfortunately, the cause of ADHD isn't completely understood. It apparently arises from an interplay of physical factors influenced by genetics, biochemistry, and brain function. Psychosocial factors, such as stress and family conflicts, may play a role. Natural health practitioners believe that the disorder is influenced by environmental factors including food allergies and intolerances, nutrient deficiencies, exposure to lead, and overexposure to food additives and dietary sugar, although no one factor has been proven beyond doubt. Each child or adult diagnosed with ADHD presents a unique brew of contributing factors, leading conventional and natural practitioners to tailor treatment with a variety of methods.

When diagnosed with ADHD, many kids are promptly started on prescription medications. If such a diagnosis occurred in our own families, we would prefer to first try an integrated approach to this health challenge, employing whatever complementary practices seem appropriate. Herbal medicine alone may not overcome ADHD, but a program that includes analysis of the child's diet, herbs, counseling, and educational planning may help.

Signs and Symptoms of ADHD

ADHD usually begins by the age of three years, but often remains undiagnosed until the child reaches elementary school. It manifests in three general types.

1 Attention deficit disorder (ADD). The child is inattentive and easily distracted but doesn't have much hyperactive or impulsive behavior; this type is most typically associated with learning disorders.

2 Hyperactivity disorder (HD). The child is hyperactive and impulsive, but can pay attention appropriately. This is the least common type.

3 Attention deficit hyperactivity disorder

WARNING SIGNS OF ADHD

If most kids are active, and young children often have short attention spans, how do you sort out abnormal behavior? Here are some tip-offs to the possibility that your child may have ADHD.

Your preschooler is not just constantly on the go, but also aggressive and emotionally volatile. He has lots of temper tantrums, argues frequently, hits other kids, and takes their toys.

Your young child seems unusually fearless. His noisy, boisterous, reckless behavior often leads to accidents and injuries.

Your child just can't—or won't—obey rules.

Your child fails to pay attention to details and makes careless mistakes.

Your child doesn't seem to listen when spoken to.

Your child fidgets, picks at things, squirms, can't remain seated when required to do so, or runs about and climbs things when such behavior is inappropriate.

Your child has difficulty awaiting his turn, talks excessively, interrupts, and blurts out answers in class.

Your child has trouble getting organized to start a task, shifts restlessly from one activity to the next, or never quite finishes anything.

Your child forgets what she's supposed to be doing and constantly loses possessions.

In addition to these problems, your child has trouble sleeping.

(ADHD). The child is inattentive, hyperactive, and impulsive. This combined type occurs most frequently.

Seeking Help for ADHD

If you or your child's teacher suspects ADHD, you'll need a proper evaluation, usually from a psychiatrist or psychologist. School systems typically provide professionals who are capable of this evaluation. Network with everyone involved in the process. You may discover a person whose job is to guide parents and guardians through this evaluation process, or a team of school psychologists, teachers, and knowledgeable volunteers who are called together to evaluate your child.

Diagnosis

Mental health workers generally diagnose ADHD from the histories given by parents and teachers and by observing the child. Physical exams and lab work are aimed at excluding diseases that can produce similar symptoms. The evaluation will also search for learning disabilities, impairments of speech, language, or hearing, or other behavioral disorders. In addition, a qualified nutritional practitioner can rule out dietary deficiencies and food allergies or intolerances.

Medical Treatment for ADHD

Stimulant drugs, psychological therapies for the child and other family members, and sometimes behavioral strategies for the teachers form the foundation of medical treatment for ADHD. The drugs include methylphenidate (Ritalin) and dextroamphetamine (Dexedrine). When combined with behavior-modification techniques, these drugs relieve ADHD symptoms quite effectively. They should not be prescribed until a child is properly evaluated, however. Many specialists feel that medication without educational

programs and behavioral therapy has no long-term benefit. The medication can cause insomnia, drowsiness, irritability, headache, and sadness. Loss of appetite may bring on weight loss and even impaired growth. But these symptoms often accompany ADHD, meaning that kids have them before they start medication. In some cases, stimulant drugs actually decrease these pre-existing symptoms. A very few children develop temporary tics—twitchy, repetitive movements. Pemoline (Cylert) has caused liver failure in a few patients. Too much of these drugs can induce a "zombie-like" state, which is why your physician should see your child for regular checkups.

The current thinking among professionals is that because the disease probably has multiple causes, the treatment should be multifaceted. The child needs to learn how to replace disruptive behaviors with desirable and appropriate ones. He needs to learn skills to replace negative thoughts about himself with positive ones. He needs focusing skills. Parents need to learn effective coping strategies. Teachers need tools for rewarding desirable behavior and decreasing unwanted behavior so the child can feel successful.

If Your Child Seems to Fit the Diagnosis of ADHD

First, don't blame yourself or your child. ADHD is not caused by poor parenting or "bad" teachers. These disorders have a biologic basis. Get help promptly—your child needs and deserves it. She probably does not enjoy teachers' perception of her as difficult, nor the social ostracism kids inflict upon anyone seen as weird. Instead of blame and anger, your child needs a boost of self-esteem that will help get her out from under the cloud of this negative label.

Your child also needs to acquire some tools to help her capitalize on her strengths and gradually extinguish her less desirable habits so that she can fit in. This can be a long process, so be patient. Because a child with ADHD can sometimes feel like a failure, reward her good behavior and positive achievements—even the smallest ones.

As a parent coping with your child's disorder, you may benefit from meeting regularly with a mental-health professional who can reassure you, help you learn ways to support and encourage your child, and improve your skills for coping with her behavior. A key concept is setting behavioral limits while remaining tender, compassionate, and consistent. Such training can help reaffirm your effectiveness as a parent.

Check out the school environment closely. Some kids with ADHD generally do best with a predictable schedule and structured environment, but others thrive on a less-structured school day. Regardless, keep your child's teacher informed and ask the teacher to do the same for you; some therapists advocate that teachers send home a daily report card. It can also help your child to keep his home environment organized and his activities on a regular schedule. Make sure that he gets plenty of exercise to release all that energy. To diminish distractibility, try to help him play with only a few toys at a time. And make sure he gets plenty of rest, because fatigue will only aggravate symptoms.

Above all, remember you are your child's advocate, even when teachers complain about him and other adults raise their eyebrows as he twirls in his seat or thrashes in rage on the supermarket floor. Sometimes being a parent is not an easy job—and you may feel like quitting. Please don't. Take a break, take a vacation, but don't ever quit loving and supporting your child.

ADHD and the Food-Intolerance Connection

Disagreement and controversy swirl in the medical world about whether true food allergies create ADHD symptoms. Research has not yet fully explored food intolerances, food-related symptoms that cannot be detected by the classic allergy tests. Because a food-intolerance reaction may occur hours or days after the food is ingested, the problem may remain undetected.

One study has documented that 73 percent of 26 children with confirmed ADHD showed improvement in symptoms and behavior when classic food-intolerance items (dairy, soy, peanuts, wheat, chocolate, artificial colors, and preservatives) were removed from their diet for two weeks. Researchers concluded that it's better to remove the underlying cause of the problem than to medicate symptoms.

Another study found similar results. Researchers placed 76 children with ADHD on a standard antiallergy diet. Eighty-two percent showed significant improvement. Forty-eight foods were found to cause symptoms, with food additives triggering significant behavior problems. The researchers found that many kids' chronic digestive and allergy-related problems improved as well. Accordingly, the researchers devised an allergy-densensitization program for children.

Eliminating possible dietary offenders, then gradually returning them, one by one, into your child's diet and observing her reactions may identify food intolerances. See Chapter 7, Allergies and Intolerances, for more information about elimination diets.

Does Sugar Cause ADHD?

Almost any teacher will tell you that sugar consumption doesn't help kids concentrate, but most research shows no correlation between sugar and candy intake and the typical hyperactive or impulsive behaviors associated with ADHD. Recent research, however, has produced some insight into kids with ADHD. Normal children and those with ADHD were given a high-sugar, high-carbohydrate breakfast; no protein was included. The ADHD kids showed more hyperactive behavior than the others, and researchers theorized that hyperactivity may arise from eating sugar in the absence of a well-balanced meal.

Another study has found that children with ADHD don't have the usual hormonal response to a high-sugar meal. Usually, the pancreas releases insulin, which drives sugar into the cells. Then, the adrenal glands stabilize blood sugar. ADHD kids' blood sugar levels did not stabilize efficiently; their blood sugar dropped, which reduced their brain activity but increased physical activity.

Antibiotic use may also affect sensitivity to sugar by destroying beneficial intestinal flora and allowing yeast (*Candida alibicans*) to proliferate. Indeed, one study found that children with repeated ear infections—and repeated rounds of antibiotics—were 3.5 times more likely to develop hyperactivity. Whether or not scientific investigation will hold up this yeast theory remains to be seen.

In the absence of definitive research, we can only say that refined sugar may have a negative effect on children diagnosed with ADHD. If you suspect sugar worsens your child's behavior, try keeping him sugar-free for at least two weeks. Read labels carefully. Avoid fruit juice and drinks sweetened with high-fructose corn syrup, because the high fruit-sugar content can also create problems. Keep a journal of your child's behavior, making careful notes about what happens when sugar is removed, then later reintroduced into his diet. You may be surprised by the results.

On the other hand, if you don't think sugar is a major trigger for your child's hyperactivity and don't wish to remove it, try balancing high-carbohydrate meals with protein, particularly at breakfast; this will help your child start the school day with a more even blood sugar level. Scramble an egg or some tofu to accompany cereal and toast. If you're packing a lunch box, make sure to add protein such as string cheese or a container of milk or soy milk.

Herbs for ADHD

Two classifications of herbs are especially helpful for children with ADHD. The first, calming herbs, helps settle jangled nerves. The second, adaptogens, helps the body cope with or adapt to stress—and kids with ADHD have plenty of stress in their lives. So do their parents; some of the following herbs may help you, too.

Calming Herbs

Lemon balm offers sedative and antispasmodic properties. The German Commission E rates lemon balm as useful in "problems going to sleep that are nervous in origin." The commission recommends an infant dose of a quarter cup of tea three times a day. Young children up to 50 pounds can have up to five ounces, three times per day.

We find that a cup of regular-strength lemon balm tea (one teaspoon of dried herb infused in one cup of water) has a calming effect on kids during the day, and a double-strength tea is more sleep-inducing, especially at bedtime. For reducing the symptoms of ADHD, we suggest you try the lower dose first. Lemon balm makes a fantastic-tasting glycerite.

Chamomile and **skullcap** are two of Sunny's favorite herbs for calming overactive kids, particularly when the two herbs are blended. Chamomile is the tastier of the two, but both are safe for children in reasonable doses: a cup of tea or a dropperful of extract for the average 50-pound child.

Hawthorn. In Traditional Chinese Medicine, hawthorn is believed to nourish the "shen," an intangible quality we Westerners might call the spirit or the personality. A child with a shen disorder may show a flat, colorless complexion, dull eyes, or chaotic personality patterns. The concept of shen disharmony seems a beautiful—and apt—way of describing ADHD.

Hawthorn is often included in ADHD remedies for its calming actions on the nervous system and the heart, the symbolic holder of spirit. The fresh berries are juicy and delicious, and two teaspoons of dried berries make a sweet tea. Glycerite or syrup can be given in 10- to 15-drop doses several times per day. Children of any age can sip hawthorn tea. Two cups of tea per day is a typical medicinal dose for a 50-pound child. Follow package directions when using tinctures or glycerites.

Oats, good old cooking oats, are a calming remedy for children and adults. Feed your child oatmeal without sugar for breakfast, and start adding a small amount of oat flour (purchased or made by grinding oats in your blender or coffee grinder) to your baking recipes.

Oatstraw and **oat seeds** harvested at the "milky flower juice" stage are widely used in Europe and North America for the treatment of anxiety, tension, and overexcitement. A 50-pound child can drink several cups of mild-tasting oatstraw tea per day. You can also find oat seed in many herbal nervine formulas.

Adaptogens

Schisandra, called *wu-wei-zi* in Chinese, has an age-old tradition of safe use. Herbalists regularly use it to treat insomnia, calm the spirit, and relieve stress.

Chinese herb shops and natural food stores usually carry schisandra. Try giving these raisin-like dried fruits to your kids as a snack.

TURNING DOWN THE TENSION

One night Sunny's 2½-year-old had a particularly frenzied evening, so Sunny decided to host a bedtime tea party. She brewed chamomile tea, turned off the lights, lit a candle, and settled down with her daughter. In the calm and drowsy atmosphere, the chamomile did its magic: Her child was sleepy in no time at all.

Siberian ginseng, also called eleuthero, has been studied in Russia for its tonic effect. The most famous study involved 2,100 Russian adults. An extract of the herb helped improve mental alertness and the ability to cope with both physical and emotional stress. In very rare circumstances, insomnia has been associated with lavish use of Siberian ginseng. Otherwise, however, the herb is generally considered safe when used with moderation.

Use this herb only for children over five years. A 50-pound child can start with half a capsule once a day and increase to half a capsule morning and evening for up to one month if well tolerated. Take a one-week break and repeat the two doses for four weeks.

Caution: Please note that Siberian ginseng is not a true ginseng of the *Panax* genus. Please DO NOT give your children real *Panax* ginseng without professional guidance.

Licorice root has been used medicinally for thousands of years in cultures around the world. Its tonic activity likely comes from its ability to mimic the adrenal glands' own corticosteroids.

Give your child plain licorice tea before incorporating it into an herbal blend to make sure your child tolerates the tea.

Caution: Limit licorice use to six weeks because long-term doses of this otherwise safe herb may aggravate high blood pressure.

Pregnant women and anyone with high blood pressure, kidney or heart disease, or diabetes should avoid licorice.

Nutritional Supplements for ADHD

Essential fatty acids are just that: essential. Only in recent history have humans developed a diet that ignores the basic human need for small but critical amounts of these nerve- and skin-nourishing oils. Hydrogenated oil in margarine and many other modern food interferes with the absorption of essential fatty acids.

Essential fatty acid metabolism affects ADHD. Our bodies require but cannot produce two fatty acids: linoleic acid (LA, an omega-6 fatty acid) and alpha-linolenic acid (ALA, an omega-3 fatty acid). These acids help mediate inflammation and immune responses and regulate bodily secretions, hormone production, and nerve transmission. They supply the building blocks for cell membranes. The brain and retina need fatty acids to function properly.

When researchers compared 52 boys with ADHD to 42 normally active boys, they found that a significant number of the hyperactive boys had signs of essential fatty acid deficiency—thirst, frequent urination, dry skin and hair, dandruff, brittle nails, frequent colds. A subgroup of twenty-one ADHD boys also had significantly lower blood levels of various fatty acids. The authors speculated that either low dietary intake or poor metabolic conversion of one or more essential fatty acids might be to blame and suggested that ADHD patients undergo blood tests to identify fatty acid deficiencies that supplements could correct.

Without doing any tests, however, you can improve the quality of fats your child eats by reducing intake of fried and processed foods made with saturated fats and hydrogenated oils, while boosting intake of high-quality omega-6 and omega-3 oils. Food sources of GLA (an omega-6 oil) include evening primrose, black currant, and borage oils. ALA, an omega-3 oil, is abundant in flaxseed oil, our favorite and the least expensive medicinal oil. Look for essential fatty acid oils and capsules in the refrigerator of your natural foods store, and stick with daily doses for six to eight weeks before expecting results. A typical children's dose is one teaspoon

GIVE YOURSELF A BREAK

Natural remedies are but one part of a whole-child treatment plan for ADHD. While herbs can support a child's nervous system during times of stress and hyperactivity, sometimes prescription medication is needed to tame symptoms quickly so that you can begin to work with gentler, slower-acting therapies. Don't criticize yourself if you decide to use Ritalin or other prescription medications to get you and your child through difficulties.

This point was driven home by a 10-year-old child whose busy mother hated the idea of using drugs to subdue her hyperactive daughter. After months of inconsistent herbal treatment, the daughter finally said, "Mom, please let me try Ritalin. You just don't know what it feels like to be me." Mom gave in, and after a successful year of Ritalin, herbs, and other complementary therapies, she is working with the pediatrician to wean her daughter off the prescription, with good results. For that family, at that time, Ritalin was the right choice.

of flaxseed oil per 33 pounds of body weight. Follow package instructions for capsules. Flaxseed and other nutritional oils blend well into uncooked foods, such as smoothies, salsa, bean spreads, bread spreads, and salad dressings. Keep the oils refrigerated.

Magnesium is needed to convert carbohydrates, fats, and proteins to energy. It plays an important role in nerve transmission, muscle contraction, and relaxation. When researchers tested magnesium levels in the blood and hair of 116 children with ADHD, they found that 95 percent were deficient. The same researchers then gave 200 mg of magnesium daily for six months to fifty children with documented ADHD and magnesium deficiency; they showed a significant decrease in hyperactivity and increased tissue levels of the mineral. This research is preliminary, but you may wish to ask your practitioner whether your child's magnesium level should be measured.

Massage may help unwind a hyperactive child. Twenty-eight adolescents with ADHD received either massage therapy or relaxation therapy for ten consecutive school days. The massage group, but not the relaxation-therapy group, reported feeling happier, and observers judged them less fidgety following sessions. After that two-week period, teachers noted that the kids who had massages were more "on task" and less hyperactive than before treatment began.

YUMMY FLAXSEED OIL SALAD DRESSING

This dressing, high in omega-3 and omega-6 essential fatty acids, may help kids with ADHD.

Yields: about one cup of dressing.

1/8 cup flaxseed oil

1/8 cup cold-pressed safflower oil

1/8 cup extra virgin olive oil

1/8 cup balsamic vinegar

1 teaspoon honey

1/4 teaspoon fresh lemon juice

Fresh herbs to taste, such as rosemary, garlic, thyme, basil

(Optional: 1 teaspoon Dijon mustard, salt to taste, pinch of freshly ground pepper)

Mix all ingredients and serve over fresh green salads. Keep refrigerated. Delicious!

For Further Reading

Armstrong, T. *The Myth of the ADD Child.* New York: Plume, 1997.

Block, M. *No More Ritalin.* New York: Kensington Publications, 1996.

Garber, S., M. Garber, and R. Spizman. *Beyond Ritalin.* New York: HarperCollins, 1996.

Ingersoll, B. and S. Goldstein. *Attention Deficit Disorder and Learning Disabilities.* New York: Main Street/Doubleday, 1993.

Taylor, John F. *Helping Your Hyperactive/ADD Child* (2nd ed.). Rocklin, Calif: Prima, 1997.

Zimmerman, M. *The ADD Nutrition Solution: A Drug-Free 30-Day Plan.* New York: Henry Holt/Owl Books, 1999.

Chapter 26

PSYCHOLOGICAL DISORDERS

It's natural for parents to have an idealistic view of childhood as a happy, carefree time of life. But the truth is, in the United States, at least 12 percent of children and teens experience some form of mental illness. We decided to discuss the most prevalent psychological disorders of children and teens because of the likelihood that some parents may encounter them, and because these illnesses often affect a child's overall health .

Children are works in progress—they change quickly as they grow. So changes in their behavior, especially gradual ones, can be hard for parents to catch, and easy to chalk up to a child's transition into another phase of his growth. Mental maladies can go not only underdiagnosed, but undertreated. The good news: Once properly diagnosed, your child has a lot of opportunities for successful treatment. Psychological therapies, pharmaceutical medications, herbs, and other complementary medicines can all help relieve symptoms.

We'd like to make three important points about psychiatric disturbances.

• **It's essential to get professional help for a thorough evaluation and proper treatment.** Your pediatrician's office or school counselor should be able to recommend competent professionals in your area. Don't assume that such treatment won't be covered by your health insurer; some now have provisions that at least cover psychiatric evaluation and short-term counseling. The earlier treatment is begun, the earlier symptoms tend to be relieved.

• **The family of an afflicted child also needs support.** Stress has a tendency to be shared. Your own depression, sadness, or anxiety can and will affect your children and your partner. We don't say this to make you feel guilty, but to encourage you to take care of yourself and your child.

• **Your child may need drugs.** While both of us believe in natural remedies, we also know that researchers have traced many psychological illnesses to physical origins, usually imbalances in the brain's chemical neurotransmitters. Particularly in the acute stages, medicating your child may do a world of good. Once things have stabilized and she feels better, she may be able to participate in counseling and complementary therapies. Please don't sacrifice your child's well-being because you're hung up about putting her on, for example, Prozac. Finding a psychiatric professional whom you and your child trust, and who is willing to work with you as a partner in your child's care, is crucial. Once you've made that step, follow the guidance you're given and, as always, look to your child for answers.

Diagnosing Mental Illness in Children

The most common psychological illnesses among kids are depression, anxiety, and obsessive-compulsive disorder. Psychological disorders can overlap; for example, a child may feel both anxious and depressed. Bipolar disorder also occurs in children; usually, however, their only symptom is the manic phase—the giddy, hyperactive "high" of this illness.

Depression

As much as parents would wish their children to lead completely happy lives, reality seldom fulfills that wish. Like you, your child will experience disappointment, failure, and loss. Sadness is a normal response to these types of events. What's not normal is prolonged sadness, a depressed mood that interferes with a child's ability to engage in the activities he usually enjoys. Sometimes a child becomes depressed because of a traumatic event in her life; sometimes a chemical imbalance in the brain triggers the depression. Sometimes both occur.

Symptoms of bona fide depression occur more frequently in adolescents than in children,

although even small children can experience profound sadness. Experts estimate that up to 2.5 percent of children and 8.3 percent of adolescents are depressed. An additional 10 to 14 percent of kids are *dysthymic,* meaning that they suffer from chronic sadness, irritability, negative thoughts, and low self-esteem, but the symptoms are not dramatic enough to qualify as major depression.

Conventional Treatment for Depression

Usually, depression is treated in several ways at once. Counseling and other cognitive therapy helps a child gain perspective and replace negative thoughts with positive ones. Sometimes this therapy takes place in groups or with the whole family. Behavioral strategies, on the other hand, reward changes in how your child acts.

If a psychiatrist determines that the depression is moderate or severe, or the child isn't responding to psychotherapy, antidepressant drugs may be an option. The new generation of antidepressants—the well-known Prozac and its lesser-known cousins Paxil, Zoloft, and Luvox—work with a chemical in the brain called serotonin. They can significantly relieve symptoms and have fewer side effects than the older drugs. Side effects can include nausea, diarrhea, constipation, sleepiness, insomnia, nervousness, and dry mouth; they are most pronounced when a patient is first put on the drugs. If your child is put on antidepressants, his reaction to the drugs will need careful watching. Prozac and related drugs usually take about two to six weeks to show effects.

Things Parents Can Do

Avoid blaming yourself or your child for depression. It is nobody's fault. Depression is not a personality flaw, nor a reflection of poor parenting. A mix of genes, neurobiology, diet and environmental stressors probably play roles, but no one can pinpoint a single cause.

That said, don't delay in seeking help for your child. Generally, the earlier treatment is begun, the shorter the depression. If your stress levels are high, or if you also feel sad and worthless, seek help as well (we know that's easily said, given the expense and the general lack of insurance coverage).

Be open-minded about antidepressants. If your child is very sick, these drugs may be necessary to help rebalance her brain chemistry. Depression has a biological basis. Simply urging your child to change her attitude won't cure it. Depression can be serious; it can even end in suicide.

At times like this, the whole family needs social support, love, and encouragement. Let your friends know you need them. Take part in activities that bring you pleasure. Get involved with your child's school, with religious organizations, or yoga classes, whatever makes you feel connected to humanity.

Encourage your child to gradually, steadily resume his normal schedule. Reward him for each step forward he takes. Look for the good in him. Punishing him for any failure to perform will only worsen his self-image.

WHEN TO CALL A DOCTOR ABOUT DEPRESSION

Anytime you suspect your child is depressed, take her to a psychiatrist, psychologist, or other mental health professional, preferably one who specializes in children and adolescents. The following symptoms are clues. Understand that substance abuse can also cause many of these symptoms; so can medical disorders such as mononucleosis and hypothyroidism.

Sad mood that persists beyond two months. A depressed child may cry often and easily, act lonely, or express hopelessness and unhappiness.

Irritability: more frequent temper tantrums in toddlers and pre-schoolers; hypersensitivity in older children

Low self-esteem

Agitation: restlessness, irritability, hostility

Apathy and withdrawal: a loss of interest in usually pleasurable activities and friendships

Changes in school performance and attitude toward school

Change in appetite and weight: Appetite and weight loss are more common, but weight gain can also occur

Sleep disturbance—either insomnia or excessive sleeping

Fatigue and general lack of energy

Difficulty concentrating or thinking clearly

Potty training relapses or constipation

Unexplained, vague physical complaints

If your child discusses hurting himself, take him seriously and get immediate professional help. If your child reports that a friend has discussed suicide, we urge you to contact the child's parents.

Anxiety

It would be nice if we could spare our children anxiety until they reached adulthood. But we can't. All kinds of things make children anxious: separation from those who care for them, the dark, the loss of a favorite cuddly toy, new environments, bullies, overly strict teachers, excessive homework, demanding parents, athletic events, recitals, driving tests, first dates.

Although kids commonly experience fear and anxiety, some are more easily flummoxed than others. Some children handle minor amounts of stress and change with equanimity; others fall apart at seemingly trifling events.

An adult with normal coping skills may still find that her freak-out threshold drops when she hasn't had enough sleep, fun, or nutritious food—or when her menstrual period draws near. But a child with an anxiety disorder feels anxious most of the time, and this emotion and its attendant behavior interfere with healthy functioning. Nearly three percent of children and adolescents suffer from anxiety.

Helping Your Child Cope with Anxiety

We can't eliminate worry from our kid's lives, but we can look for opportunities to increase their sense of security and self-confidence. Strategies differ, depending upon the child's personality and age.

If you're the parent of an infant, do your best to respond to your baby's cries, hold her often, and basically become a fairly constant fixture in her life. Of course, you'll need to get out on your own—we're not advocating martyrdom—but when you do leave, find a good surrogate and try to use this same caregiver most of the time. If you use day care, find a safe, nurturing situation. Some therapists believe that young children are often best off in very small groups, with only one or two other children.

WHEN TO CALL A DOCTOR ABOUT ANXIETY

The following symptoms can mean that your child needs professional help. Your pediatrician may be able to help you establish whether your child's fears are within the realm of normality.

Your child worries and feels anxious more days than not, can't control her fears, and seems to constantly need reassurance.

Your child is restless, tense, and irritable, or has emotional outbursts, poor appetite, or poor sleep.

These feelings and behaviors significantly distress your child and interfere with his ability to make friends or do well in school.

Your child pleads with you not to leave him, cries excessively or has a tantrum when you do leave, acts apathetic and listless when you're away, or expresses unrealistic worries about what could befall you while you're gone. Many small children cry when a parent first leaves, only to perk up a few minutes later. A child whose anxiety needs treatment worries that you may not come back, balks at going anywhere without you, follows you everywhere, or has nightmares about losing you.

Your child frequently uses complaints of physical malady or other excuses to avoid school.

Know that some children easily pick up on a parent's moods and fears. If you feel anxious, your child may well feel your concern and suspect that perhaps he should worry, too. On the other hand, reassurance goes a long way. Let's say your preschooler doesn't like to walk down a certain street because of a barking dog. You can take his hand and say in a calm voice, "I'll bet that dog looks huge to you. But he's behind a big, strong fence. We'll be fine. Oh, did you see that butterfly? Let's follow it."

When your child becomes old enough to engage you in conversation, help him identify his feelings. Ask if he wants to talk about what's worrying him. If he opens up, allow him to have his feelings. Instead of saying, "That's silly. That shouldn't bother you," try, "That sounds like it really upset you," or "You sound like you're feeling really scared."

Parents can, however, help children sort out whether their worries are realistic. Let's say your child frets that he doesn't understand math. You can say, "Well, maybe that math test didn't go well, but wasn't that you who aced last week's spelling test?"

Once you find out what worries your child, try to help her brainstorm ways to remedy the situation. The trick is allowing children to work out their own problems, so that they learn coping skills. This boosts feelings of competence and, hence, self-esteem.

If your child feels anxious about academic pressures, you may need to help by providing a good environment for study, giving examples for how to budget time after school, talking to the teacher, hiring a tutor, or maybe even switching schools. You may wish to have your child tested for learning disabilities. Remember that you are your child's advocate for obtaining special services; if you believe she needs them, speak up.

Help your child and yourself find ways to relax. Children of all ages can benefit from a warm bath or a massage. Spend time outdoors, just sitting or going for walks. Any kind of exercise usually helps reduce stress. An older child or teen may be open to a yoga class.

Reward yourself for modeling good coping skills for your child. Kids learn by imitation. If you freak out because missing that green light caused you to get the carpool to soccer late, you may want to think about learning some relaxation skills yourself.

Conventional Treatment for Anxiety

Although doctors do sometimes prescribe anxiety-reducing drugs to children, most prefer first to try to find the cause of the anxiety and use various types of non-drug therapy to treat it. Most therapists will want to combine talking with your child and having him try certain behavioral techniques. Relaxation training can help minimize the resultant anxiety. If medication becomes necessary, commonly used drugs include tranquilizers and antidepressants.

Obsessive-Compulsive Disorder

People with obsessive-compulsive disorders have unwanted, recurrent, disturbing thoughts that they can't suppress. To relieve the anxiety these obsessions cause, they may repeatedly perform ritualized behaviors. For example, an irrational fear of germs may lead to repetitive hand washing. Some people suffer more from intrusive thoughts without a lot of behavioral symptoms. For others, senseless rituals dominate the picture. In the extreme, these behaviors can interfere with day-to-day functioning.

Some five million Americans suffer from this disorder, and at least one in two hundred adolescents has it. Because this disease often goes unrecognized and undiagnosed, the actual figure may be higher. A recent study of middle-school kids has found that 3 percent have obsessive-compulsive disorder and 19 percent have a subclinical form—symptoms too mild to meet the criteria for diagnosis. Although symptoms often first appear in childhood or early adolescence, many people successfully hide their symptoms for years.

The cause seems to be a biologic one involving an imbalance of brain chemicals, most likely a serotonin deficit. Brain scans of obsessive-compulsive patients have actually shown abnormalities in certain nerve circuits. New data suggests that an autoimmune reaction to strep bacteria may play a role, meaning that antibodies directed against strep also attack normal brain tissue.

Some physicians recommend antibiotic treatment in children whose pre-existing obsessive-compulsive behavior flares up with upper respiratory tract infection.

Diagnosing Obsessive-Compulsive Disorder

Young children often go through phases where they repeat words or phrases and prefer things "just so." It's part of their need to master certain skills. But in obsessive-compulsive disorder, the distressing thoughts and rituals cause the child to lose all sense of proportion and interfere with his enjoyment of life. If you suspect that your child may have this disorder,

ABOUT LEARNING DISABILITIES

This term means that a child has difficulty acquiring or performing such skills as reading, writing, speech, or math. They have trouble interpreting what they see or hear, or a problem linking this information from the outside world with different parts of their brains. Sometimes affected individuals also have problems with coordination and self-control.

The frustration and stress that an unaddressed learning disability causes can affect a child's mental and emotional state. Children with learning disabilities aren't slow learners; their difficulty is independent from environmental deprivation, vision or hearing impairment, or other neurological problems. In fact, people with learning disabilities are by definition of average or above average intelligence; many are gifted learners in areas unaffected by the disability. According to the National

Institutes of Health, 12 to 20 percent of people in the United States have some form of learning disability.

Diagnosis is usually made during grade school, when parents and teachers notice that a child is having trouble in a particular area, despite good effort and normal intelligence. There are many types and variations of learning disabilities, so the process of testing for them may require a lot of patience.

Your school should be able to help you find out about testing for learning disabilities. Some public school districts have departments that serve this need; others refer to outside professionals. For more information, contact the National Center for Learning Disabilities, 381 Park Ave. South, New York NY 10016; (212) 545-7510. The center's website is www.ncld.org.

consult your child's doctor for a referral to a psychiatrist or psychologist.

Conventional Treatment

Psychotherapy, with or without medication, can help children with obsessive-compulsive disorder. John March, M.D., director of the program in child and adolescent anxiety disorders at Duke University Medical Center, has developed a therapy method for these children. In a nutshell, the child exposes himself to progressively more difficult situations (say, touching the toilet seat for a kid who fears germs)—without performing the ritualistic behavior afterward. About 80 to 90 percent of kids who follow his technique are at least 50 percent better within six months.

Often people with obsessive-compulsive disorder also need the help of a pharmaceutical, at least while they're learning cognitive and behavioral therapies. Fortunately, antidepressants can greatly relieve symptoms. The new generation of antidepressants—Prozac, Paxil, Luvox, and the like—are generally well tolerated. Combining therapy with antidepressants reduces the risk of relapse once the medication is withdrawn.

Bipolar Disease

When children have this disorder, also known as manic depression, it can be marked by mostly manic symptoms. It is uncommon in childhood, but can surface in adolescence. During manic episodes, the child will exhibit an abnormally elevated mood, will act grandiose and expansive, and may become irritable and combative. The inflated mood and agitation interfere with school, work, and relationships. Manic symptoms come on quickly, and persist for a week or longer. People with episodic mania often also experience the flip side—depression.

Conventional Treatment for Bipolar Disease

This disorder requires expert medical and psychiatric treatment. You'll want a doctor to rule out non-psychiatric causes: drug abuse, hyperthyroidism, side effects from other medications, head trauma, or neurologic disorders.

Once these other causes are ruled out, bipolar disease usually requires treatment with drugs known as mood stabilizers (for example, lithium, carbamazepine, or valproate) and may necessitate initial hospitalization until symptoms abate.

WHEN TO CALL A DOCTOR ABOUT OBSESSIVE-COMPULSIVE DISORDER

Here are some clues indicating that your child may need professional help from a psychiatrist.

Your child expresses irrational fears about germs, doing something wrong, or about something bad happening to those he loves.

Your child admits to persistent or recurrent troubling thoughts about sex, religious blasphemy, or violence.

Your child realizes these thoughts make no sense, but has no control over them or the anxiety they cause him.

Your child feels compelled to perform repetitive, senseless behaviors: washing her hands, checking door locks, hoarding or saving useless possessions, counting things, or redoing an entire page of homework each time she makes an error.

Often long-term drug treatment is recommended to prevent relapse. All these drugs have side effects, making compliance difficult.

Herbs for Mild Depression and Anxiety

We want to distinguish here between using these herbs for your child's occasional angst, sadness, or irritability, and substituting home care when a professional examination is needed. We think the first is fine—and the second is hazardous. We want to be clear that *true psychological illness requires professional diagnosis and treatment.* If your child's symptoms are persistent or recurrent, or if they alarm you in any way, discuss them with your doctor or your child's school counselor. They may be able to help you decide whether a specialist is needed. Once a practitioner is engaged, you'll need to be up front with him about your use of natural remedies. Some herbs can have negative interactions with prescription drugs; never substitute an herb for a medication without your doctor's consent.

Kava kava is commonly prescribed for anxiety and stress in Germany. Several trials in adults have found standardized kava extracts effective in reducing anxiety. The authors concluded that the kava extract was an effective alternative to conventional drugs and did not produce the side effects of the drugs.

Clinical studies, however, don't necessarily indicate a kid's dosage. Our suggestion is to try small amounts of a kava whole-root capsule for several days to test for allergic reaction. After a few days, gradually increase your child's dose; just don't go beyond the dosage you calculate from the adult dosage using Clark's Rule. We have occasionally given our kids small doses of kava with good relaxation results.

Caution: Not for use by pregnant or nursing women, or with drugs that act on the central

WHEN TO CALL A DOCTOR ABOUT BIPOLAR DISEASE

Seek help if your child exhibits these symptoms as a sudden change from his normal behavior.

Elevated or expansive mood out of proportion to the situation; inappropriate giddiness

Irritability: Your child becomes testy, angry, or belligerent

Grandiosity: Your child suddenly thinks he's Superman, for example, and boasts about his powers and abilities.

Rapid, constant speech, with a tendency to blurt out remarks in class

Racing thoughts: Your child may tell you that her ideas zip by so fast she can't express them all.

Distractibility, difficulty paying attention in school

Restlessness

Excessive pleasure-seeking: shopping binges; promiscuous, reckless, or thoughtless behavior

Note that abuse of stimulant drugs—amphetamines or cocaine—can cause many of these symptoms. Bipolar disease has also sometimes been misdiagnosed as attention deficit hyperactivity disorder (ADHD). The last thing a manic teen needs is the amphetamine-like drugs used to treat hyperactivity.

nervous system such as sedatives and antidepressants. Long-term use has occasionally been correlated with a yellow skin rash. Small doses of kava are relaxing; larger doses can induce a euphoric state and still higher doses, muscle weakness and dizziness.

Valerian in small doses such as a few drops of tincture or glycerite can also soothe anxiety, but at higher doses it will make most children sleepy. Long-term studies show that valerian is sedative, antispasmodic, and not habit forming.

Chamomile and **passionflower** have a long history of use for anxiety. Scientific data now shows that substances in these plants (apigenin in chamomile and chrysin in passionflower) bind to the same brain receptors as benzodiazepines—the class of tranquilizers that includes Valium. This means that they produce their effects in a like manner. Unlike Valium and other similar drugs, however, the herbal constituents do not interfere with memory. At low doses, chamomile and passionflower are calming; at higher doses, they have a mild sedative effect and relax muscle. So far, clinical trials haven't included children, but both herbs are safe for kids. Try starting out with one cup of tea or one-half capsule, two times a day, for a 50-pound child. If you see no side effects, double the dose. For tinctures and glycerites, follow the package directions.

California poppy has been shown to decrease anxiety and is widely used by German physicians for just this reason. Smaller doses of tea calm anxiety, while larger doses can induce sleep. We'd start a 50-pound child on 1/4 cup of tea, if she can stand the bitter taste. In the United States, California poppy is usually available for purchase only in liquid herbal blends.

Caution: Because preliminary research shows that this herb may influence brain chemicals involved in mood and may have an antidepressant effect, do not use it if your child is also taking an antidepressant medication.

Lavender. Bathe your child in an infusion of lavender flowers to unwind tense muscles and soothe frayed nerves. Five to ten drops of lavender essential oil can be added to a massage oil or bath. We also like to create an aromatherapy vial so that the peaceful essence of lavender oil is readily available.

St.-John's-wort. Over 25 double-blind studies (meaning neither the doctors nor the patients know who's getting which treatment) have shown that this herb eases mild and moderate depression as well as some pharmaceutical antidepressants do, with far fewer side effects. Patients taking St.-John's-wort reported they felt less anxious, less

---

CALMING INHALER

For ages: One year and older

This inhaler is portable, fragrant, and soothing to worn-out little ones.

1 teaspoon salt

5 drops essential oil—a blend of any two of the following: lavender, Roman chamomile, bergamot, lemon, rose, rosewood, orange, tangerine, grapefruit

Directions: Mix ingredients together in a small, clean glass vial with a tight-fitting lid. Cover. Can be sniffed at will for a gentle mood lifter and to calm mild anxiety.

Caution: Much as we'd like to think this will never happen, kids may try to eat this mixture. So don't let a child under five have an inhaler to keep themselves. Store all essential oils out of the reach of children.

sad, and more hopeful about life. Side effects of St.-John's-wort, though uncommon, can include gastrointestinal irritation, allergic reactions, restlessness, dry mouth, fatigue, and, very rarely, increased sensitivity to the sun.

Like most herbal research, none of these studies was conducted in the United States. At the time of this writing, the U.S. National Institutes of Health has announced that it is sponsoring a three-year study on the use of a standardized extract of St.-John's-wort in moderate depression. Researchers will compare the herb to a placebo and to Prozac.

The safety record of St.-John's-wort is good. Keep in mind that, as with prescription antidepressants, St.-John's-wort may take up to six weeks to produce an antidepressant effect. Increasing the dosage doesn't speed up its effects. There have been a few case reports of St.-John's-wort, combined with therapy, easing symptoms of obsessive-compulsive disorder.

Caution: No one yet knows if this herb can safely be used during pregnancy or nursing. Most practitioners advise that St.-John's-wort not be taken concurrently with synthetic antidepressants. Also, don't substitute it for prescription antidepressants without your doctor's consent and supervision. We recommend that you avoid the internal use of St.-John's-wort for children under two years of age.

Ginkgo is another well-studied herb for depression. One research project involved older adults from ages 51 to 78 years. All the patients suffered from mild to moderate depression and continued with their antidepression medications during the ginkgo trial. The result showed a significant decrease in depression.

Can we generalize this study to children? No. So far the studies have looked at ginkgo's effect on mood in people over the age of 50. However, it's safe to add ginkgo leaves to an herbal depression formula for kids. Ginkgo leaves are nontoxic, but do not take the seeds internally.

There is no research on using herbs to treat bipolar disease. However, nervines, or calmative herbs, do have a long traditional use in calming overwrought children. We are not suggesting that you try to treat bipolar disease solely with herbs. First take care of your child's safety and medical needs. Once his condition stabilizes, you can work with your mental-health practitioner to find an appropriate treatment plan for your child.

Skullcap is a wonderful calming herb. We find that a cup of skullcap tea induces a sense of peace and quiet. It's like turning the ringer off on the phone. Skullcap's components have sedative and antispasmodic activity. It tastes a little bitter, so your child may prefer it in extract form. If you want to make a tea, try adding a little organic orange peel or juice to improve the taste.

Caution: Not for children under one year.

In addition, you may want to mix these time-tested herbs together for a nerve-settling tea blend: catnip, hawthorn, kava, and valerian. You may find that you could use a cup yourself—we know that orchestrating treatment for these disorders can be exhausting and exasperating.

Other Complementary Techniques

Nutritional treatments. First off, make sure your child eats a healthy, well-balanced diet, and investigate nutritional deficiencies and food allergies, both of which have been linked with depression. Insufficient amounts of a single vitamin can cause mood to deteriorate. Examples include vitamin C and a host of B vitamins (thiamine, riboflavin, niacin, biotin, pantothenic acid, B6, folic acid, B12). Giving your child a good multivitamin may be wise.

High-dose inositol (a B-vitamin relative) has been shown to help depression, panic disorders, and obsessive-compulsive disorder. In one small study, thirteen adults who took inositol significantly reduced symptoms of obsessive-compulsive disorder. In another study, people with a variety of psychiatric illnesses benefited from inositol supplements. The adult dose was 18 grams a day; children's dose was 200 mg per 2.2 pounds of body weight—or about 4.5 grams for a 50-pound child. Fatty acid imbalances can also contribute to depression. Given that the brain is largely composed of fats, this makes sense.

Mindfulness. It's difficult to ruminate over anxious thoughts and simultaneously live in the present moment. Those of us who grew up in the 1960s fondly remember Ram Das's dictum: Be here now. See if your child can switch from worrisome, repetitive thoughts to something pleasant that is happening at that moment. Have him pet his cat, feel the fur under his fingers, watch his cat's whiskers twitch, listen to the purring.

FLOWER ESSENCES FOR EMOTIONAL DISTRESS

Flower essences were first created in the 1930s by Dr. Edward Bach, a well-known British bacteriologist who was disenchanted with the way modern medicine was developing. Bach wanted a system of healing to address emotional needs. The theory behind flower essences is a little "out there"—and is not, to our knowledge, supported by clinical or other research. There are respectable herbalists who think that these essences are not useful, and respectable herbalists, including Sunny, who believe they are. We have used flower essences on ourselves and our own children and found them to be helpful, as have many parents we know.

Flower essences are widely available. While we would never recommend that you use them instead of the advice of a qualified mental-health practitioner, you may wish to investigate the various essences that are designed for different areas of emotional healing.

Recommended Reading

Foster, C. H. *Polly's Magic Games: A Child's View of Obsessive-Compulsive Disorder.* Ellsworth, ME: Dilligaf, 1995.

Hobbs, C. *Stress and Natural Healing.* Loveland, CO: Botanica Press, 1998.

March, J. S. (ed.). *Anxiety Disorders in Children and Adolescents.* New York: Guilford, 1995.

Rapoport, J. *The Boy Who Couldn't Stop Washing: The Experience and Treatment of Obsessive-Compulsive Disorder.* New York: NAL-Dutton, 1990.

Schwartz, J. and B. Beyette. *Brain Lock: Free Yourself from Obsessive-Compulsive Disorder.* New York: HarperCollins, 1997.

Steketee, G. and K. White. *When Once is Not Enough: Help for Obsessive-Compulsives.* Oakland, CA: New Harbinger, 1990.

Glossary

Acute—having a sudden onset, sharp rise, and usually a short duration.

Adaptogen—an herb that enhances the body's ability to adapt to a wide variety of stressors.

Analgesic—a substance that relieves pain.

Antibacterial—able to destroy bacteria or inhibit their growth.

Antibiotic—drugs that eliminate infectious bacteria; literally, "destructive of life."

Antifungal—able to destroy or suppress the growth of fungi such as candida, the yeast that can cause diaper rash and thrush.

Antigen—a substance that the immune system identifies as foreign, and against which it mounts an immune response.

Antihistamine–able to counteract the action of histamine, a body chemical that dilates small blood vessels and constricts the airways.

Anti-inflammatory—able to counteract or suppress the body's production of inflammatory substances such as histamine.

Antioxidant—a substance that inhibits oxidation within the body. Everyday examples of oxidation outside the human body are rusted iron or butter gone rancid. Inside the body, oxidation processes can be caused by such stressors as radiation, pollutants, tobacco smoke, physical trauma, and fighting off infection.

Antiparasitic—able to destroy or inhibit the growth of parasites and protozoan infections.

Antipyretic—fever-reducing.

Antiseptic—a substance that inhibits the growth of microorganisms without necessarily killing them.

Antispasmodic—substances that relieve spasms or cramps by relaxing muscles, either the skeletal muscles that help the body move, or the smooth muscle that encircles the airways and intestines.

Antitussive—cough-relieving.

Antiviral—able to inhibit the reproduction of viruses.

Astringent—used to contract swollen tissue.

Bitter, bitters—an herb or herbal formula that stimulates digestion by increasing digestive fluids.

Bronchodilator—substance that opens up or enlarges the caliber of the airways.

Calmative—able to exert a mild sedative action.

Many herbal calmatives act as sedatives when used in large doses.

Carminative—able to dispel gas from the intestines to relieve flatulence.

Chiropractor—practitioner who attends four years of college, then four years in chiropractic college. Chiropracters specialize in treating structural problems via manipulation of the bones and deep tissues.

Chronic—used to describe an illness that is slow in onset, ongoing, or recurrent.

Contraindicated—not for use under certain circumstances or with particular other substances.

Decoction—water in which an herb or blend of herbs has been simmered for ten minutes or longer; usually for hard or woody plant parts such as roots, bark, or seeds. (Decoctions are often referred to as teas, although strictly speaking, only infusions are teas.)

Demulcent—a substance that soothes inflamed tissues and protects them from further irritation.

Diaphoretic—able to promote sweating.

Digestive—a substance that promotes or aids digestion, usually by increasing or decreasing the amount of digestive fluids.

Diuretic—a substance that increases urination.

Elimination/provocation test—a technique for identifying food allergies that involves removing potential allergens from the diet, then restoring them one by one and noting reactions.

Emetic—able to induce vomiting.

Emollient—a substance that soothes or moistens irritated skin.

Essential fatty acids—a group of fats that the body uses for many functions. Deficiencies or imbalances in these types of fats have been implicated in many illnesses, particularly inflammatory disorders such as asthma and eczema.

Expectorant—a substance that expels mucus from the respiratory tract.

Free radical—an unstable molecule that lacks an electron. In the body, free radicals attempt to stabilize themselves by stealing electrons from other molecules. Antioxidants neutralize free radicals by providing those missing electrons.

Galactogogue–a substance that encourages the production of breast milk.

Herbalist—practitioner who uses plant-based medicines. Training varies widely. In England, herbalists can practice after four years of training and earn the title MNIMH (Member, National Institute of Medical Herbalists). In the United States and Canada, some herbalists have been peer-reviewed by the American Herbalists Guild and use the title "Herbalist, AHG."

Histamine—a body chemical that dilates small blood vessels and increases their permeability, producing swelling. Histamine also causes the airways to constrict, making breathing more difficult.

Homeopathy—practice that treats disease by administering very minute amounts of substances that, in large doses, would produce similar symptoms in a healthy person. These minute doses are believed to stimulate the body's own healing response. Practitioners may have received formal training, independent study, or both; some medical doctors and naturopathic doctors use homeopathy.

Hypertension—high blood pressure.

Hypotension—low blood pressure.

Inflammation—the body's response to local tissue injury characterized by heat, redness, swelling, and tenderness.

Inflammatory disease—a disorder characterized by chronic inflammation of certain tissues—for example, in eczema, the skin is inflamed.

Infusion—hot water in which an herb or blend of herbs has been steeped; basically a tea.

Intolerance—a poor reaction to a substance that is similar to an allergy, but more subtle and seldom detected by standard allergy tests, possibly because it involves a different immune response.

Laxative—a substance that encourages a bowel movement. Emollient laxatives make the stool softer; bulk laxatives promote the digestive tract's muscle contractions; saline cathartics draw water into the intestines; and stimulant cathartics directly effect the bowel to speed the transit of its contents.

Licensed acupuncturist (L.Ac.)—a practitioner who trains for three to four years, learning the principles of Traditional Chinese Medicine.

Massage therapist—a health worker whose training and certification varies, based on state-by-state regulation.

Naturopathic doctor (N.D.)—a medical practitioner who does four years of post-graduate study at an accredited naturopathic medical school, studying many of the same subjects as a medical doctor, but focusing on complementary medicine. At this time, only eleven states confer licenses upon naturopathic doctors; some states allow lay people to obtain an unaccredited degree by mail.

Nervine—a substance that soothes nervous excitement, similar to a calmative.

Nurse practitioner (N.P.)—a nurse with four years of nursing school, plus a master's degree in nursing, who is licensed to diagnose and prescribe for most common childhood illnesses. In some areas, nurse practitioners may practice on their own. In others, they must work within the practice of a medical doctor.

Oriental medical doctor (O.M.D.)—a practitioner of acupuncture and other Traditional Chinese Medicine practices, including the use of Chinese herbs. Training varies; make sure you ask.

Osteopathic doctor (D.O.)—a medical practitioner whose training is similar to that of a medical doctor, but with schooling in spinal adjustment.

Physician assistant (P.A.)—a practitioner who functions similarly to a nurse practitioner, but whose training is different. Physician Assistants, after earning undergraduate degrees, undergo additional training at medical schools to earn either a second bachelor's degree or a master's degree in medicine. Like nurse practitioners, they are licensed to diagnose and prescribe under the supervision of a licensed physician.

Sedative—a substance that promotes sleep by lessening excitement and irritation.

Stimulant—a substance that quickens the activity of a system or physiologic process. Ephedra, for example, stimulates the central nervous system, producing alertness and, in excess, jitteriness. Echinacea stimulates portions of the immune system.

Tonic—a substance that, taken regularly over several months, gradually restores strength to an organ or body system; examples include astragalus and reishi.

Virus—very small infectious agents that replicate only within living host cells. Flu viruses undergo mutation frequently so immunity from exposure or flu shots lasts only for one year.

Volatile oil—the concentrated, unique chemicals that reside in a particular plant. Volatile oils are weakened or destroyed by heat and light; herbs should be purchased in whole form, stored out of heat and sunlight, and crumbled or ground immediately before use.

Vulnerary—a substance that aids in wound healing.

REFERENCES

Chapter 4: Keeping Kids Healthy

Abrams, S. A., M. A. Grusak, et al. "Calcium and Magnesium Balance in 9–14-year-old Children." *American Journal of Clinical Nutrition* 66:1172–77, 1997.

Aligne, C. A. and J. J. Stoddard. "Tobacco and Children: An Economic Evaluation of the Medical Effects of Parental Smoking." *Archives of Pediatric and Adolescent Medicine* 151:648–53, 1997.

Committee on Nutrition, American Academy of Pediatrics. "Cholesterol in Childhood." *Pediatrics* 101:1141–46, 1998.

Fischer, M., K. Hedberg, et al. "Tobacco Smoke as a Risk Factor for Meningococcal Disease." *Pediatric Infectious Disease Journal* 16:979–83, 1997.

Galland, L. *Superimmunity for Kids.* New York: Dell, 1988.

Garland, C. F., et al. "Could Sunscreens Increase Melanoma Risk?" *American Journal of Public Health* 82:614–15, 1992.

Howard, G., et al. "Cigarette Smoking and Progression of Atherosclerosis." *Journal of the American Medical Association* 279:119, 1998.

Louhiala, P. J., N. Jaakkola, et al. "Day-care Centers and Diarrhea: A Public-Health Perspective." *Journal of Pediatrics* 131:476–79, 1997.

Montagu, A. *Touching.* New York: Harper and Row, 1978.

New, S. A., C. Bolton-Smith, et al. "Nutritional Influences on Bone Mineral Density: A Cross-sectional Study in Premenopausal Women." *American Journal of Clinical Nutrition* 65:1831–39, 1997.

Pabst, H. F. "Immunomodulation by Breast-feeding." *Pediatric Infectious Disease Journal* 16:991–95, 1997.

Saarinen, U. M. and M. Kajosaari. "Breastfeeding as Prophylaxis Against Atopic Disease: Prospective Follow-up Study Until 17 Years Old." *Lancet* 346:1065–69, 1995.

Sanchez, A., J. Reeser, et al. "Role of Sugars in Human Neutrophilic Phagocytosis." *American Journal of Clinical Nutrition* 26:1180–84, 1973.

Steenland, K., et al. "Environmental Tobacco Smoke and Coronary Heart Disease in the American Cancer Society CPS-II Cohort." *Circulation* 94:622–28, 1996.

Teegarden, D. and C. M. Weaver. "Calcium Supplementation Increases Bone Density in Adolescent Girls." *Nutrition Research* 52:171–74, 1994.

Williams, S. R. *Nutrition and Diet Therapy* (8th ed.). St. Louis: Mosby, 1997.

Chapter 5: First Aid

Busing, K. "Hyaluronidasehemmung durch echinacin." *Arzneimittel-Forschung* 2:467–68, 1952.

Davis, R. H., et al. "Wound Healing: Oral and Topical Activity of *Aloe vera.*" *Journal of the American Pediatric Medical Association* 79:559–62, 1989.

Fulton Jr., J. E. "The Stimulation of Postdermabrasion Wound Healing with Stabilized *Aloe vera* Gel-Polyethylene Oxide Dressing." *Journal of Dermatologic Surgery and Oncology* 16:460–67, 1990.

Fusco, B. M. and M. Giacovazzo. "Peppers and Pain. The Promise of Capsaicin." *Drugs* 53:909–14, 1997.

Jamieson, D. D. and P. H. Duffield. "The Antinociceptive Actions of Kava Components in Mice." *Clinical and Experimental Pharmacology and Physiology* 17:495–507, 1990.

Knight, T. E. and House, B. M. "Malaleuca Oil (Tea Tree Oil) Dermatitis." *Journal of the American Academy of Dermatology* 30:423–27, 1994.

Krugman, S. and S. Katz. *Infectious Diseases of Children.* St. Louis: Mosby, 1981.

McGuffin, M., et al (eds.). *American Herbal Product Association's Botanical Safety Handbook.* Boca Raton: CRC Press, 1997.

Mukhopadhyay, A., et al. "Anti-inflammatory and Irritant Activities of Curcumin Analogues in Rats." *Agents and Actions* 12:508–15, 1982.

Rose, J. *Jeanne Rose's Modern Herbal.* New York: Perigee, 1987.

Schmitt, B. D. *Your Child's Health.* New York: Bantam, 1987.

Scott, J. *Natural Medicine for Children.* New York: Avon, 1990.

Suguna, L., et al. "Effects of *Centella asiatica* Extract on Dermal Wound Healing in Rats." *Indian Journal of Experimental Biology* 34:1208–11, 1996.

Watcher, M. A. and R. G. Wheeland. "The Role of Topical Agents in the Healing of Full-thickness Wounds." *Journal of Dermatologic Surgery and Oncology* 15: 1188–95, 1989.

Chapter 6: About Antibiotics

Boken, D. J., et al. "Colonization with Penicillin-resistant *Streptococcus pneumoniae* in a Child-care Center." *Pediatric Infectious Disease Journal* 14:879–84, 1995.

Gonzales, R., et al. "Antibiotic Prescribing for Adults with Colds, Upper Respiratory Tract Infections and Bronchitis by Ambulatory Care Physicians." *Journal of the American Medical Association* 278(11):901–04, 1997.

Green, M. "Appropriate Principles in the Use of Antibiotics in Children." *Clinical Pediatrics* No volume: 207–08, April, 1997.

Hamm, R. M., R. J. Ricks, et al. "Antibiotics and Respiratory Infections: Are Patients More Satisfied when Expectations are Met?" *Journal of Family Practice* 43:56–62, 1996.

Neu, H. C. "The Crisis in Antibiotic Resistance." *Science* 257:1036, 1992.

No author. "Drug-resistant. *Streptococcus pneumoniae*: Kentucky and Tennessee, 1993." *Morbidity and Mortality Weekly Report* 43:23–36, 1994.

Stephenson, J. "Icelandic Researchers Are Showing the Way to Bring Down Rates of Antibiotic-resistant Bacteria." *Journal of the American Medical Association* 275:175–76, 1996.

Wichtl, M., ed. Tr. N. G. Bisset. *Herbal Drugs and Phytopharmaceuticals: A Handbook for Practice on a Scientific Basis.* Stuttgart: Medpharm Scientific Publishers, 1989. Distr. Boca Raton, FL: CRC Press, 1994.

Chapter 7: Allergies and Intolerances

Aberg, N., et al. "Increase of Asthma, Allergic Rhinitis and Eczema in Swedish Schoolchildren between 1979 and 1991."*Clinical and Experimental Allergy* 25: 815–819, 1995.

Barrie, S. "Food Allergies." *Natural Medicine Journal* 1:6–17, Aug./Sept. 1998.

Bruno, G. et al. "Results of a Multicentric Study for the Prevention of Atopic Allergy." *Minerva Pediatrica* 48:413–19, 1996.

Ci Carlo, G., et al. "Effects of quercetin on the gastrointestinal tract in rats and mice." *Phytotherapy Research*, 8:42–45, 1994.

Fotherby, K. J. and J. O. Hunter. "Symptoms of Food Allergy." *Clinics in Gastroenterology* 14(3):615–29, July 1985.

Johnston, C. S. et al. "Antihistamine Effect of Supplemental Ascorbic Acid and Neutrophil Chemotaxis." *Journal of the American College of Nutrition* 11:172–76, 1992.

Levin, B. "Intestinal Permeability and Nutritional Support of Intestinal Integrity." *Quarterly Review of Natural Medicine*, 141–49, Summer 1994.

Lindahl, O. et al. "Vegan Regimen with Reduced Medication in the Treatment of Bronchial Asthma." *Journal of Asthma* 22(1):45–55, 1985.

Majamaa, H. and Isolauri, E. "Probiotics: A Novel Approach in the Management of Food Allergy." *Journal of Allergy and Clinical Immunology* 99:179–85, 1997.

Marini, A. et al. "Effects of a Dietary and Environmental Prevention Programme on the Incidence of Allergic Symptoms in High Atopic-Risk Infants." *Acta Pediatrica, Supplement* 414:1–21, 1996.

Satoskar, R. R. "Evaluation of Anti-Inflammatory Property of Curcumin (Diferuloyl Methane) in Patients with Postoperative Inflammation." *International Journal of Clinical Pharmacology, Therapy, and Toxicology.* 24(12):651–54, Dec. 1986.

Chapter 8: Fevers

Bass, L. W. "Fever Revisited." *Archives of Pediatric and Adolescent Medicine* 151:647, 1997

Berg, A. T., et al. "Predictors of Recurrent Febrile Seizures. A Prospective Cohort Study." *Archives of Pediatric and Adolescent Medicine* 151:371–78, 1997.

Delgado, D. G. and C. G. Cobbs. "Approach to the Management of Fever and Granulocytopenia." *Southern Medical Journal* 73:627–30, 1980.

Doran, T. F., et al. "Acetaminophen: More Harm Than Good for Chicken Pox?" *Journal of Pediatrics* 114:1045–48, 1989.

Downing, J. F. and M. W. Taylor. "*In vivo* Hyperthermia Enhances Plasma Antiviral Activity and Stimulates Peripheral Lymphocytes for Increased Synthesis of Interferon-gamma." *Lymphokine Research* 7(2):185–93, April, 1987.

Downing, J. F., et al. "Hyperthermia in Humans Enhances Interferon-gamma Synthesis and Alters the Peripheral Lymphocyte Population." *Journal of Interferon Research* 8(2):143–50, April, 1988.

Felter, H. W. and J. U. Lloyd. (1898.) *King's American Dispensatory* (18th ed., 3rd rev.). Portland, OR: Eclectic Medical Publications, 1983.

Graham, N. M., et al. "Adverse Effects of Aspirin, Acetaminophen, and Ibuprofen on Immune Function, Viral Shedding, and Clinical Status in Rhinovirus-infected Volunteers." *Journal of Infectious Disease* 162:1277–82, 1990.

Kluger, M. J. "Fever." *Pediatrics* 66:720–24, 1980.

Kluger, M. "The Evolution and Adaptive Value of Fever." *American Scientist* 66:38–43, 1978.

Knudsen, F. U., et al. "Long-term Outcome of Prophylaxis for Febrile Convulsions." *Archives of Disease in Childhood* 74:13–18, 1996.

Martinez, F. and J. W. Coleman. "The Effects of Selected Drugs, Including Chlorpromazine and Non-steroidal Anti-inflammatory Agents, on Polyclonal IgG Synthesis and Interleukin Production by Human Peripheral Blood Mononuclear Cells." *In Vitro. Clinical and Experimental Immunology* 75:252–57, 1989.

Rothrock, S. G., et al. "Do Oral Antibiotics Prevent Meningitis and Serious Bacterial Infections in Children with *Streptococcus pneumonia* Occult Bacteremia? A Meta-analysis." *Pediatrics* 99(3):438–44, 1997.

Silver, H. K., H. C. Kempe, and H. B. Bruyn. *Handbook of Pediatrics.* Los Altos, CA: Lange Medical Publications, 1980.

Soman, M. "Diagnostic Workup of Febrile Children Under 24 Months of Age: A Clinical Review." *Western Journal of Medicine* 137:1–12, 1982.

Chapter 9: Colds

Cowan, P. F. "Patient Satisfaction with an Office Visit for the Common Cold." *Journal of Family Practice* 24: 412–13, 1987.

Czarnetzki, B. M., et al. "Immunoreactive Leukotrienes in Nettle Plants (*Urtica urens*)." *International Archives of Allergy and Applied Immunology* 91(1):43–46, 1990.

English, J. A. and K. A. Bauman. "Evidence-based Management of Upper Respiratory Infection in a Family Practice Teaching Clinic." *Family Medicine* 29:38–41, 1997.

Felter, H. W. and J. U. Lloyd. (1898.) *King's American Dispensatory* (18th ed., 3rd rev.). Portland, OR: Eclectic Medical Publications, 1983.

Graham, N. M., et al. "Adverse Effects of Aspirin, Acetaminophen, and Ibuprofen on Immune Function, Viral Shedding, and Clinical Status in Rhinovirus-infected Volunteers." *Journal of Infectious Diseases* 162:1277–82, 1990.

Hemila, H. "Vitamin C and the Common Cold." *British Journal of Nutrition* 67:3–16, 1992.

Hutton, N., et. al. "Effectiveness of an Antihistamine-decongestant Combination for Young Children with the Common Cold: A Randomized, Controlled Clinical Trial." *Journal of Pediatrics* 118:125–30, 1991.

Kogan, M. D., et al. "Over-the-counter Medication Use Among U. S. Preschool-age Children." *Journal of the American Medical Association* 272:1025–30, 1994.

Mainous III, A. G. and W. J. Hueston, et al. "Antibiotics and Upper Respiratory Infection: Do Some Folks Think There Is a Cure for the Common Cold?" *Journal of Family Practice* 42: 357–61, 1996.

Mossad, S. B. and M. L. Macknin. "Zinc Lozenges for Treating the Common Cold." *Annals of Internal Medicine* 125:81–8, 1996.

Schoenberger, D. "The Influence of Immune-stimulating Effects of Pressed Juice from *Echinacea purpurea* on the Course and Severity of Colds." *Forum on Immunology* 8:2–12, 1992.

Steinweg, K. K. "Natural History and Prognostic Significance of Purulent Rhinitis." *Journal of Family Practice* 17:61–64, 1987.

Todd, J. K., et al. "Bacteriology and Treatment of Purulent Nasopharyngitis: A Double-blind, Placebo-controlled Evaluation." *Pediatric Infectious Disease Journal* 3:226–32, 1984.

Wald, E. R., et al. "Frequency and Severity of Infections in Day Care." *Journal of Pediatrics* 112:540–46, 1988.

Yang, G. and Y. Yu. "Immunopotentiating Effect of Traditional Chinese Drugs-Ginsenoside and Glycyrrhiza Polysaccharide." *Proceedings of the Chinese Academy of Medical Sciences and the Peking Union Medical College* 5(4):188–93, 1990.

Zakay-Rones, Z., et al. "Inhibition of Several Strains of Influenza Virus *In Vitro* and Reduction of Symptoms by an Elderberry Extract (*Sambucus nigra* L.) During an Outbreak of Influenza B Panama." *Journal of Alternative and Complementary Medicine* 1(4):361–69, 1995.

Chapter 10: Flu

Belshie, R. B. "The Efficacy of Live Attenuated, Cold-adapted, Trivalent, Intranasal Influenzavirus Vaccine in Children." *New England Journal of Medicine* 338:1405–12, 1998.

Braunig, B., et al. "*Echinacea purpurea* Radix for Strengthening the Immune Response in Flu-like Infections." *A Zeitchrift fur Phytotherapie* 13:7–13, 1992.

Duke, J. *Green Pharmacy.* Emmaus, PA: Rodale Press, 1997.

Kuchi, F., et al. "Inhibition of Prostaglandin and Leukotriene Biosynthesis by Bingerols and Diarylheptanoids." *Chemical Pharmaceutical Bulletin* 40:387–91, 1992.

Lopez-Bazzocchi, I., et al. "Antiviral Activity of the Photoactive Plant Pigment Hypericin." *Photochemistry and Photobiology* 54:95–98, 1991.

Lu, H. and G. T. Liu. "Antioxidant Activity of Dibenzocyclooctene Lignans Isolated from *Schisandraceae.*" *Planta Medica* 58:311–13, 1992.

Mumcuoglu, M. "*Sambucus nigra* L. Black Elderberry Extract: A Breakthrough in the Treatment of Influenza." Skokie, IL: RSS Publishing, 1995.

Nagai, T., et al. "*In Vivo* Anti-influenza Virus Activity of Plant Flavonoids Possessing Inhibitory Activity for Influenza Virus Sialidase." *Antiviral Research* 19(3):207–17, Sep. 1992.

Peng, T., et al. "The Inhibitory Effect of *Astragalus membranaceus* on Coxsackie B-3 Virus RNA Replication." *Chinese Medical Science Journal* 10:146–50, 1995.

Pompei, R., et al. "Antiviral Activity of Glycyrrhizic Acid." *Experientia* 36:304, 1980.

Shimizu, N., et al. "The Core Structure and Immunological Activities of Glycyrrhizan UA, the Main Polysaccharide from the Root of *Glycyrrhiza uralensis.*" *Chemical and Pharmaceutical Bulletin* 40(8):2125–58, Aug. 1992.

Stimpel, M., et al. "Macrophage Activation and Induction of Macrophage Cytotoxicity by Purified Polysaccharide Fractions from the Plant *Echinacea purpurea.*" *Infection and Immunity* 46(3):845–49, Dec. 1984.

Tang, J., et al. "Virucidal Activity of Hypericin Against Enveloped and Non-enveloped DNA and RNA Viruses." *Antiviral Research* 13:313–25, 1990.

Udintsev, S. N., et al. "[Correction by Natural Adaptogens of Hormonal-metabolic Status Disorders in Rats During the Development of Adaptation Syndrome Using Functional Tests with Dexamethasone and ACTH]." *Biulleten Eksperimentalnoi Biologii I Meditsiny* (*Bulletin of Experimental Biology in Medine*) (Russian) 112(12):599–601, Dec. 1991.

Wagner, H. "Immunostimulant Action of Polysaccharides (Heteroglycans) from Higher Plants." *Arzneimittelforschung* 34:659–61, 1984.

Weber, N. D., et al. "*In Vitro* Virucidal Effects of *Allium sativum* (Garlic) Extract and Compounds." *Planta Medica* 158:417–23, 1992.

Wichtl, M., ed. Tr. N. G. Bisset. *Herbal Drugs and Phytopharmaceuticals A Handbook for Practice on a Scientific Basis.* Stuttgart: Medpharm Scientific Publishers, 1989. Distr. Boca Raton, FL: CRC Press, 1994.

Yoshida, Y., et al. "Immunomodulating Activity of Chinese Medicinal Herbs and *Oldenlandia diffusa* in Particular." *International Journal of Immunopharmacology* 19:359–70, 1997.

Zakay-Rones, Z., et al. "Inhibition of Several Strains of Influenza Virus *In vitro* and Reduction of Symptoms by an Elderberry Extract (*Sambucus nigra* L.) During an Outbreak of Influenza B Panama." *Journal of Alternative and Complementary Medicine* 1(4):361–69, 1995.

Zgorniak-Nowosielska, I., et al. "Antiviral Activity of *Flos verbasci* Infusion Against Influenza and Herpes Simplex Viruses." *Archiuum Immunologiae et Theraiae Experimentalis* 39(1–2):103–08, 1991.

Zhao, K. S., et al. "Enhancement of the Immune Response in Mice by *Astragalus membranaceus.*" *Immunopharmacology* 20:225–33, 1990.

Zimmerman, R. K., et al. "Influenza, Influenza Vaccine, and Amantadine/ritadine." *Journal of Family Practice* 45:107–112, 1997.

Chapter 11: Sinusitis

Brinker, F. "Botanical Medicine Research Summaries: *Tancetum parthenium.*" *Eclectic Dispensatory of Botanical Therapeutics.* Sandy, OR: Eclectic Medical Publications, 1995.

Hayes, N. A. and J. C. Foreman. "The Activity of Compounds Extracted from Feverfew on Histamine Release from Rat Mast Cells." *Journal of Pharmacy and Pharmacology* 39(6):466–70, 1987.

Hobbs, C. *Usnea: The Herbal Antibiotic.* Capitola, CA: Botanica Press, 1986.

Hou, Y., et al. "Effect of *Radix astragali seu hedysari* on the Interferon System." *Chinese Medical Journal* 94(1):35–40, 1981.

Hutton, N., et al. "Effectiveness of an Antihistamine-Decongestant Combination for Young Children with the Common Cold: A Randomized, Controlled Clinical Trial."

Journal of Pediatrics 118:125–30, 1991.

Masterova, I., et al. "Royleanones in the Roots of *Salvia officinalis* L. of Domestic Provenance and Their Antimicrobial Activity." *Ceskoslovenska Farmacie* 45:242–45, 1996.

Mittman, P. "Randomized, Double-blind Study of Freeze-dried *Urtica dioica* in the Treatment of Allergic Rhinitis." *Planta Medica* 56(1):44–47, 1990.

Neubrauer, N. and R. W. Marz. "Placebo-controlled, Randomized Double-blind Clinical Trial with Sinupret Sugar-coated Tablets on the Basis of a Therapy with Antibiotics and Decongestant Nasal Drops in Acute Sinusitis." *Phytomedicine* 1:177–81, 1994.

Pompei, R., et al. "Antiviral Activity of Glycyrrhizic Acid." *Experientia* 38:304, 1980.

Poole, M. D. "Antimicrobial Therapy for Sinusitis." *Otolaryngology Clinics of North America* 30:331–39, 1997.

Wald, E., et al. "Comparative Effectiveness of Amoxicillin and Amoxicillin-Clavulanate Potassium in Acute Paranasal Sinus Infections in Children: A Double-blind, Placebo-Controlled Trial." *Pediatrics* 77:795–800, 1986.

Wald, E., et al. "Upper Respiratory Tract Infections in Young Children: Duration and Frequency of Complications." *Pediatrics* 87:129–33, 1991.

Weiss, R. F. .Tr. A. R. Meuss. *Herbal Medicine*. Beaconsfield, England: Beaconsfield Publishers, 1988.

Chapter 12: Ear Infections

Aligne, C. A. and J. J. Stoddard. "Tobacco and Children: An Economic Evaluation of the Medical Effects of Parental Smoking." *Archives of Pediatric and Adolescent Medicine* 151:648–53, 1997.

Bluestone, C. D. "Pathogenesis of Otitis Media: Role of the Eustachian Tube." *Pediatric Infectious Disease Journal* 15:281–91, 1996.

British Herbal Medicine Association. *British Herbal Pharmacopoeia*. West Yorks, England: British Herbal Medicine Association, 1979.

Buckley, G. and A. Hinton. "Otitis Media with Effusion in Children Shows a Progressive Resolution with Time." *Clinical Otolaryngology* 16:354–57, 1991.

Cantekin, E. I., E. M. Mandell, et al. "Lack of Efficacy of a Decongestant-antihistamine Combination for Otitis Media in Children." *New England Journal of Medicine* 308:297–301, 1983.

Diamant, M. and B. Diamant. "Abuse and Timing of Use of Antibiotics in Acute Otitis Media." *Archives of Otolaryngology* 100: 226–32, 1974.

Dowell, S. F., et al. "Otitis Media—Principles of Judicious Use of Antimicrobial Agents." *Pediatrics* (supplement) 101:165–71, 1998.

Duncan, B., J. Ey, et al. "Exclusive Breast Feeding for at Least 4 Months Protects Against Otitis Media." *Pediatrics* 91:867–72, 1993.

Froom, J., L. Culpepper, et al. "Diagnosis and Antibiotic Treatment of Acute Otitis Media: Report from International Primary Care Network." *British Medical Journal* 300:582–86, 1990.

Hardy, A. M. and M. G. Fowler. "Child-care Arrangements and Repeated Ear Infections in Young Children."

American Journal of Public Health 83:1321–25, 1993.

Kleinman, L. C., J. Kosecoff, et al. "The Medical Appropriateness of Tympanostomy Tubes Proposed for Children Younger than 16 Years in the United States." *Journal of the American Medical Association* 271:1250–55, 1994.

Moore, M. *Medicinal Plants of the Desert and Canyon West*. Santa Fe, NM: Museum of New Mexico Press, 1989.

Murray, M. T. "What Is the Best Treatment for Otitis Media?" *Natural Medicine Journal* 1(2):1–4, Mar 1998.

Mygind, N., K. I. Meistrup-Larsen, et al. "Penicillin in Acute Otitis Media: A Double-blind Placebo-Controlled Trial." *Clinical Otolaryngology* 6 5–13, 1981.

Niemela, M., et al. "Pacifiers Increase the Risk of Recurrent Acute Otitis Media in Children in Daycare Centers." *Pediatrics* 96:884–88, 1995.

Nsouli, T. M., et al. "Role of Food Allergy in Serous Otitis Media." *Annals of Allergy* 73: 215–19, 1994.

Pichichero, M. E. and R. Cohen. "Shortened Course of Antibiotic Therapy for Acute Otitis Media, Sinusitis and Tonsillopharyngitis." *Pediatric Infectious Disease Journal* 16:680–95, 1997.

Saarinen, U. M. and M. Kajosaari. "Breast Feeding as Prophylaxis Against Atopic Disease: Prospective Follow-up Study until 17 Years Old." *Lancet* 346:1065–69, 1995.

Schappert, S. M. *Office Visits for Otitis Media: United States, 1975–1990: Advance Data*. Hyattsville, MD: National Center for Health Statistics, 1992.

Uhari, M., et al. "Xylitol Chewing Gum in Prevention of Acute Otitis Media: A Double-blind, Randomized Trial." *British Medical Journal* 313:1180–84, 1996.

Uhari, M., et al. " A Novel Use of Xylitol Sugar in Preventing Acute Otitis Media." *Pediatrics* 102(4):879, 1998.

Van Buchem, F. L., et al. "Acute Otitis Media: A New Treatment Strategy." *British Medical Journal* 290:1033–37, 1985.

Van Buchem, F. L., et al. "Therapy of Acute Otitis Media: Myringotomy, Antibiotics, or Neither?" *Lancet* 81: 883–887, 1981.

Chapter 13: Sore Throats

Bisno, A. L. "Nonsuppurative Poststreptococcal Sequelae: Rheumatic Fever and Glomerulonephritis." In G. Mandell, R. Douglas, J. Bennett (eds.) *Principles and Practice of Infectious Disease* (4th ed.). New York: Churchill Livingstone, 1995.

Brinker, F. "*Melissa officinalis*." *Eclectic Dispensatory of Botanical Therapeutics* (vol. 2). Sandy, OR: Eclectic, 1995.

Darmstadt, G. L. "Scarlet Fever and its Relatives." *Contemporary Pediatrics* 15:44–46, 1998.

Dobrescu, D., et al. "Contributions to the Complex Study of Some Lichens-*Usnea* Genus. Pharmacological Studies on *Usnea barbata* and *Usnea hirta* Species." *Romanian Journal of Physiology* 30:101–07, 1993.

Gwaltney Jr., J. M. "Pharyngitis." In G. L. Mandell, et al (eds.) *Principles and Practice of Infectious Diseases* (4th ed.). New York: Churchill Livingstone, 1995.

Hobbs, C. *Usnea: The Herbal Antibiotic*. Capitola, CA: Botanica Press, 1986.

Lauro, L. and D. Rolih. "[Observations and Research on an Extract of *Inula viscosa* Ait]." *Bollettino-Societa Italiana Biologia Sperimentale* 66(9):829–34, Sep 1990.

Shulman, S. T. "Streptococcal Pharyngitis: Clinical and Epidemiologic Factors." *Pediatric Infectious Disease Journal* 8:816–19, 1989.

Zheng, M. S. "An Experimental Study of the Anti-HSV-II Action of 500 Herbal Drugs." *Journal of Traditional Chinese Medicine* 9(2):113–16, June 1989.

Chapter 14: Coughs

Black, S. "Epidemiology of Pertussis." *Pediatric Journal of Infectious Disease* 16(4):S85–S89, 1997.

Chapman, R. S., et al. "The Epidemiology of Tracheobronchitis in Pediatric Practice." *American Journal of Epidemiology* 114:786–97, 1981.

Cressman, W. R. and C. M. Myer, "Diagnosis and Management of Croup and Epiglottitis." *Pediatric Clinics of North America* 41(2):265+, 1994.

Foster, S. and J. Duke, *A Field Guide to Medicinal Plants.* Boston: Houghton Mifflin, 1990.

Johnson, D. W., et al. "A Comparison of Nebulized Budesonide, Intramuscular Dexamethasone, and Placebo for Moderately Severe Croup." *New England Journal of Medicine* 339:498–503, 1998.

Krugman, S. and S. L. Katz. "Pertussis (Whooping Cough)." *Infectious Diseases of Children.* St. Louis: Mosby, 1981.

Levy, B. T. and M. A. Graber. "Respiratory Syncytial Virus Infection in Infants and Young Children." *Journal of Family Practice* 45(6):473–81, 1997.

McCutcheon, A. R., et al. "Antiviral Screening of British Columbian Medicinal Plants." *Journal of Ethnopharmacology* 49:101–10, 1995.

McGuffin, M., et al (eds.). *American Herbal Product Association's Botanical Safety Handbook.* Boca Raton: CRC Press, 1997.

Moore, M., *Herbal Tinctures in Clinical Practice.* Santa Fe: Southwest School of Botanical Medicine, 1993.

O'Brien, K. L., et al. "Cough Illness/Bronchitis—Principles of Judicious Use of Antimicrobial Agents." *Pediatrics* 101(supplement):178–81, 1998.

Schilcher, H. *Phytotherapy in Paediatrics: Handbook for Physicians and Pharmacists.* Stuttgart, Germany: Medpharm Scientific Publishers, 1997.

Vinson, D. C. and L. J. Lutz. "The Effect of Parental Expectations on Treatment of Children with a Cough: A Report from ASPN." *Journal of Family Practice* 37:23–27, 1993.

Wichtl, M., ed. Tr. N. G. Bisset. *Herbal Drugs and Phytopharmaceuticals: A Handbook for Practice on a Scientific Basis.* Stuttgart: Medpharm Scientific Publishers, 1989. Distr. Boca Raton, FL: CRC Press, 1994.

Zakay-Rones, Z., et al. "Inhibition of Several Strains of Influenza Virus *In vitro* and Reduction of Symptoms by an Elderberry Extract (*Sambucus nigra* L.) During an Outbreak of Influenza B Panama." *Journal of Alternative and Complementary Medicine* 1(4):361–69, 1995.

Chapter 15: Hay Fever

Aberg, N., et al. "Increase of Asthma, Allergic Rhinitis and Eczema in Swedish Schoolchildren Between 1979 and 1991." *Clinical and Experimental Allergy* 25:815–19, 1995.

Fireman, P. "Otitis Media and Eustachian-Tube Dysfunction: Connection to Allergic Rhinitis." *Journal of Allergy and Clinical Immunology* 99:S787–97, 1997.

Foreman, J. C. "Mast Cells and the Actions of Flavonoids." *Journal of Allergy and Clinical Immunology* 73:769–74, 1994.

Galland, L., et al. *Superimmunity for Kids.* New York: Delacorte, 1989.

International Rhinitis Management Group (IRMWG). "International Consensus Report on the Diagnosis and Management of Rhinitis." *Allergy* 49 (supplement 19):5–34, 1994.

Johnston, C. S., et al. "Antihistamine Effect of Supplemental Ascorbic Acid and Neutrophil Chemotaxis." *Journal of the American College of Nutrition* 11:172–76, 1992.

Meltzer, E.O. "Treatment Options for the Child with Allergic Rhinitis." *Clinical Pediatrics* 37:1–10, 1998.

Mittman, P. "Randomized, Double-blind Study of Freeze-dried *Urtica dioica* in the Treatment of Allergic Rhinitis." *Planta Medica* 56:44–47, 1990.

Ojima, M., et al. "The Inhibitory Effects of Glycyrrhizin and Glycyrrhetinic Acid on the Metabolism of Cortisol and Prednisolone—*In vivo* and *in vitro* Studies." *Nippon Nibunpi Gakkai Zasshi* 66:584–96, 1990.

Ortega-Cisneros, M., et al. "Cutaneous Reactivity to Foods Among Patients with Allergic Rhiniconjunctivitis." *Revista Allergia Mexico* 44:153–57, 1997.

Weiland, S. K., et al. "Self-reported Wheezing and Allergic Rhinitis in Children and Traffic Density on Street of Residence." *Annals of Epidemiology* 4:243–47, 1994.

Wilhite, C. C. "Teratogenic Potential of Quercetin in the Rat." *Food and Chemical Toxicology* 20:75–79, 1982.

Wright, A. L., et al. "Epidemiology of Physician-Diagnosed Allergic Rhinitis in Childhood." *Pediatrics* 94:895, 1995.

Chapter 16: Asthma

Aderele, W. I., et al. "Plasma Vitamin C Levels in Athmatic Children." *African Journal of Medicine and Medical Sciences* 14 (3–4):115–20, 1985.

Balon, J., et al. "A Comparison of Active and Simulated Chiropractic Manipulation as Adjunctive Treatment for Childhood Asthma." *New England Journal of Medicine* 339:1013–20, 1998.

Bauer, K., et al."Pharmacodynamic Effects of Inhaled Dry-powder Formulations of Tenoterol and Colforsin in Asthma." *Clinical Pharmacology and Therapeutics* 53:76–83, 1993.

Bielory, L. and R. Gandhi."Asthma and Vitamin C." *Annals of Allergy* 73:89–96, 1994.

Black, P.N. and S. Sharpe. "Dietary Fat and Asthma: Is There a Connection?" *European Respiratory Journal* 10:6–12, 1997.

Brown, D. *Herbal Prescriptions for Better Health.* Rocklin, CA: Prima, 1996.

Calhoun, W. J. "Summary of Clinical Trials with Zafirlukast." *American Journal of Respiratory and Critical Care Medicine* 157: S238–45, 1998.

Christensen, P. A. and L. C. Laursen. "Acupuncture and

Bronchial Asthma." *Allergy* 39:379–85, 1984.

Collip, P. J., S. Goldzier III, et al. "Pyridoxine Treatment of Childhood Asthma." *Annals of Allergy* 35:93–7, 1975.

Courtney, R. "Asthma and Children: A New Approach." *Mothering* 87:35–41, March/April, 1998.

Crain, E. F., et al. "An Estimate of the Prevalence of Asthma and Wheezing Among Inner-city Children." *Pediatrics* 94:356–62, 1994.

Cumming, R. G., et al. "Use of Inhaled Corticosteroids and the Risk of Cataracts." *New England Journal of Medicine* 337:8–14, 1997.

Dorsch, W. and H. Wagner. "New Antiasthmatic Drugs from Traditional Medicine?" *International Archives of Allergy Applied Immunology* 94(1–4):262–65, 1991

Evans, R. "Update on Childhood Asthma." *Western Journal of Medicine* 166:340–41, 1997.

Ewer, T. C. and D.E. Stewart. "Improvement in Bronchial Hyper-responsiveness in Patients with Moderate Asthma after Treatment with Hypnotic Technique: A Randomised, Controlled Trial." *British Medical Journal* 293:1129–32, 1986.

Fung, K. P., O. K. Chow, et al. "Attenuation of Exercise-induced Asthma by Acupuncture." *Lancet* 2:1419–1422, 1986.

Ginot, P. "Effect of BN 52063, a Specific PAF-acether Antagonist, on Bronchial Provocation Test to Allergens in Asthmatic Patients." *Prostaglandins* 34:723–31, 1987.

Goodman, L. S. and A. Gilman, A. *The Pharmacological Basis of Therapeutics* (5th ed.). New York: Macmillan, 1975.

Hatch, G. E. "Asthma, Inhaled Oxidants, and Dietary Antioxidants." *American Journal of Clinical Nutrition* 61 (Suppl):625S–30S, 1995.

Homma, M., et al. "A Strategy for Discovering Biologically Active Compounds with High Probability in Traditional Chinese Herb Remedies: An Application of Saiboku-to in Bronchial Asthma." *Analytical Biochemistry* 202:179–97, 1992.

Homma, M., et al. "A Novel 11 Beta-hydroxysteroid Dehydrogenase Inhibitor Contained in Saiboku-to, a Herbal Remedy for Steroid-dependent Bronchial Asthma." *Journal of Pharmacy and Pharmacology* 46(4):305–9, April, 1994.

Internet article at www.buteykovideo.com, 4/16/98.

Jain, S.C., et al. "Effect of Yoga Training on Exercise Tolerance in Adolescents with Childhood Asthma." *Journal of Asthma* 28:437–42, 1991.

Jobst, K. A., et al. "A Critical Analysis of Acupuncture in Pulmonary Disease: Efficacy and Safety of the Acupuncture Needle." *Journal of Alternative and Complementary Medicine* 1:57–85, 1995.

Katial, R.K., et al. "A Drug Interaction Between Zafirlukast and Theophylline." *Archives of Internal Medicine* 158: 1713–5, 1998.

Kivity, S., et al. "The Effect of Caffeine on Exercise-induced Bronchoconstriction." *Chest* 97:1083–85, 1990.

Krohn, J., et al. *The Whole Way to Allergy Relief and Prevention.* Point Roberts, WA: Hartley & Marks, 1991.

Levy, B. T. and M. A. Graber. "Respiratory Syncytial Virus Infection in Infants and Young Children." *Journal of Family Practice* 45: 473–481, 1997.

Lundback, B. "Epidemiology of Rhinitis and Asthma." *Clinical and Experimental Allergy* 28, suppl 2:3–10, 1998.

Machura, E. "The Effect of Dietary Fish Oil Supplementation on the Clinical Course of Asthma in Children." *Pediatria Polska* 7: 97–102, 1997.

McGuffin, M., et al. *American Herbal Products Association's Botanical Safety Handbook.* Boca Raton: CRC Press, 1997.

Novembre, E., et al. "Incidence of Asthma Caused by Food Allergy in Childhood." *Pediatria Medica e Chirurgica* 9:399–404, 1987.

Sabbah, A. "Food Allergy in Childhood Asthma." *Allerg Immunol* (Paris), 22:325–31, 1990.

Schmidt, M. *Smart Fats.* Berkeley, CA: Frog Ltd., 1997.

Schultz, V., R. Hansel, and V. Tyler. *Rational Phytotherapy.* New York: Springer, 1998.

Schwartz, J. and S. T. Weiss. "Caffeine Intake and Asthma Symptoms." *Annals of Epidemiology* 2:627–35, 1992.

Shimizu, T., et al. "Relation Between Theophylline and Circulating Vitamin Levels in Children with Asthma." *Pharmacology* 53:384–89, 1996.

Simons, F. E. "A Comparison of Beclomethasone, Salmeterol, and Placebo in Children with Asthma." *New England Journal of Medicine* 337:1659–65, 1997.

Stevenson, D. D. and R. A. Simon. "Sensitivity to Ingested Metabisulfites in Asthmatic Subjects." *Journal of Allergy & Clinical Immunology* 68:26–32, 1981.

Unge, G., J. Grubbstrom, et al. "Effect of Dietary Tryptophan Restrictions on Clinical Symptoms in Patients with Endogenous Asthma." *Allergy* 38:211–12, 1983.

Vedantha, P. K., et al. "Clinical Study of Yoga Techniques in University Students with Asthma: A Controlled Study." *Allergy & Asthma Proceedings* 19:3–9, 1998.

Weiss, R. F. *Herbal Medicine.* Stuttgart: Hippokrates Verlag, 1988.

Wilkens, J. H., et al. "Effects of a PAF-antagonist (BN52063) on Bronchoconstriction and Platelet Activation During Exercise-Induced Asthma." *British Journal of Pharmacology* 29:85–91, 1990.

Yu, D. Y. and S. P. Lee. "Effect of Acupuncture on Bronchial Asthma." *Clinical Science and Molecular Medicine* 51:503–9, 1976

Chapter 17: Nausea and Vomiting

Bone, M. E. and D. J. Wilkinson. "Ginger Root: A New Antiemetic." *Anaesthesia* 45:669–71, 1990.

McGuffin, M., et al (eds.). *American Herbal Product Association's Botanical Safety Handbook.* Boca Raton: CRC Press, 1997.

Mowrey, D. B. "Motion Sickness, Ginger, and Psychophysics." *Lancet* 1:655–657, March 1982.

Murray, M. "Ginger (*Zingiber offinale*)." *American Journal of Natural Medicine* 3:12–16, Sep. 1996.

Sharma, S. S., et al. "Antiemetic Efficacy of Ginger (*Zingiber offinale*) Against Cisplatin-induced Emesis in Dogs." *Journal of Ethnopharmacology* 42:111–20, 1997.

Chapter 18: Diarrhea and Constipation

Addiss, D. G., et al. "Epidemiology of Giardiasis in Wisconsin: Increasing Incidence of Reported Cases and

Unexplained Seasonal Trends." *American Journal of Tropical Medicine and Hygiene* 47:13–19, 1992.

Barnard, J. "Gastrointestinal Disorders Due to Cow's Milk Consumption." *Pediatric Annals* 26: 244–250, 1997.

Bastidas, G. J. "Effect of Ingested Garlic on *Necator americanus* and *Ancylostoma canium*." *American Journal of Tropical Medicine and Hygiene* 18:920–23, 1969.

Bhatnagar, S., et al. "Efficacy of Milk-based Diets in Persistent Diarrhea: A Randomized, Controlled Trial." *Pediatrics* 98: 1122–26, 1996.

De Simone, C., et al. "Enhancement of Host Resistance Against *Salmonella typhimurium* Infection by a Diet Supplemented with Yogurt." *Immunopharmacology and Immunotoxicology* 10:399–415, 1988.

Gotz, V., et al. "Prophylaxis Against Ampicillin-associated Diarrhea with a Lactobacillus Preparation." *American Journal of Hospital Pharmacy* 36:754–757, 1979.

Guggenbichler, J. P. "Adherence of Enterobacteria in Infantile Diarrhea and its Prevention." *Infection* 11(4):239–42, July 1983.

Gupte, S. "Use of Berberine in Treatment of Giardiasis." *American Journal of Diseases of Children* 129:866, July 1975.

Heinerman, J. *Heinerman's New Encyclopedia of Fruits and Vegetables.* West Nyack, NY: Parker Publishing, 1995.

Iacono, G., et al. "Intolerance of Cow's Milk and Chronic Constipation in Children." *New England Journal of Medicine* 339:1100–1104, 1998.

Jacobs, Jennifer, et al. "Treatment of Acute Childhood Diarrhea with Homeopathic Medicine: A Randomized Clinical Trial in Nicaragua." *Pediatrics* 93:719–25.

Joensuu, J., et al. "Randomized, Placebo-controlled Trial of Human Reassortant Rotavirus Vaccine for Prevention of Severe Rotavirus Gastroenteritis." *Lancet* 350:1205–9, 1997.

Kneepkens, C. M., et al. "Apple Juice, Fructose, and Chronic Nonspecific Diarrhoea." *European Journal of Pediatrics* 148: 571–73, 1989.

Louhiala, P. J., et al. "Day-care Centers and Diarrhea: A Public Health Perspective." *Journal of Pediatrics* 131: 476–79, 1997.

McGuffin, M., et al (eds.). *American Herbal Product Association's Botanical Safety Handbook.* Boca Raton: CRC Press, 1997.

Mowrey, D. *Herbal Tonic Therapies.* New Canaan, CT: Keats, 1993.

Mowrey, D. *The Scientific Validation of Herbal Medicine.* Lehi, Utah: Cormorant Books, 1986.

Rennels, M.B., et al. "Efficacy and Safety of High-dose Rhesus-human Reassortant Rotavirus Vaccines—Report of the National Multicenter Trial." *Pediatrics* 97:7–13, 1996.

Santosham, M., et al. "Efficacy and Safety of High-dose Rhesus-human Reassortant Rotavirus Vaccine in Native American Populations." *Journal of Pediatrics* 131:632–8, 1997.

Sharma, R., et al. "Berberine Tannate in Acute Diarrhea." *Indian Pediatrics* 7:496–501, 1970.

Speer, F. "The Allergic Child." *American Family Physician* 11:88–94, 1975.

Yolken, R. H., et al. "Human Milk Mucin Inhibits Rotavirus Replication and Prevents Experimental Gastroenteritis." *Journal of Clinical Investigation* 90:1984–91, 1992.

Chapter 19: Colic

Adams, L. M. and M. Davidson. "Present Concepts of Infant Colic." *Pediatric Annals* 16:817–20, 1987.

Balon, A. J. "Management of Infantile Colic." *American Family Physician* 55:235–42, 1997.

Hill, D. J., et al. "A Low-allergen Diet Is a Significant Intervention in Infantile Colic: Results of a Community-based Study." *Journal of Allergy and Clinical Immunology* 96:886–92, 1995.

Hunziker, U. A. and R. G. Barr. "Increased Carrying Reduces Infant Crying: A Randomized, Controlled Trial." *Pediatrics* 77:641–48, 1986.

Jakobsson, I. and T. Lindberg. "Cow's Milk Proteins Cause Infantile Colic In Breast-fed Infants: A Double-blind Crossover Study." *Pediatrics* 71:268–71, 1983.

Metcalf, T. J., et al. "Simethicone in the Treatment of Infant Colic: A Randomized, Placebo-controlled, Multicenter Trial." *Pediatrics* 94:29–34, 1994.

Weizman, Z., et al. "Efficacy of Herbal Tea Preparation in Infantile Colic." *Journal of Pediatrics* 122:650–52, 1993.

Chapter 20: Bladder Infections

Avorn, J., et al. "Reduction of Bacteriuria and Pyuria after Ingestion of Cranberry Juice." *Journal of the American Medical Association* 271:754, 1994.

Brinker, F. *Eclectic Dispensatory of Botanical Therapeutics* (Vol. 2). Sandy, OR: Eclectic Medical Publications, 1995.

Loening-Baucke, V. "Urinary Incontinence and Urinary Tract Infection and Their Resolution with Treatment of Chronic Constipation of Childhood." *Pediatrics* 100:228–32, 1997.

McGuffin, M., et al (eds.). *American Herbal Product Association's Botanical Safety Handbook.* Boca Raton: CRC Press, 1997.

Reid, G., et al. "Prevention of Urinary Tract Infection in Rats with an Indigenous *Lactobacillus casei* Strain." *Infection and Immunity* 49: 320–24, 1985.

Schilcher, H. *Phytotherapy in Paediatrics.* Stuttgart: Wissenschaftliche Verlagsgesellschaft, 1992.

Silva de Ruiz, C., et al. "Effect of Lactobacilli and Antibiotics on *E. coli* Urinary Infections in Mice." *Biological and Pharmaceutical Bulletin* 19:88–93, 1996.

Sobel, J. D. and D. Kaye. "Urinary Tract Infections." In Mandell, G.L., et al. *Principles and Practice of Infectious Diseases* (4th ed.). New York: Churchill Livingstone, 1995.

Sobota, A. E. "Inhibition of Bacterial Adherence by Cranberry Juice: Potential Use for the Treatment of Urinary Tract Infections." *Journal of Urology* 131:1013–16, 1984.

Sun, D., et al. "Influence of Berberine Sulfate on Synthesis and Expression of Pap Fimbrial Adhesion in Uropathogenic *Escherichia coli*." *Antimicrobial Agents and Chemotherapy* 32:1370–74, 1988.

Walker, E. B., et al. "Cranberry Concentrate: Urinary Tract Infection Prophylaxis." *Journal of Family Practice* 45: 167, 168, 1997.

Wichtl, M. and N. G. Bisset. *Herbal Drugs and Phytopharmaceuticals: A Handbook for Practice on a Scientific Basis.* Stuttgart: Medpharm GmbH Scientific Publishers, 1989.

Yarnell, E. "Botanical Medicine for Cystitis." *Alternative & Complementary Therapies* pp. 269–273, August, 1997.

Chapter 21: Skin Problems

Arnsmeier, S. L. and A. S. Paller. "Getting to the Bottom of Diaper Dermatitis." *Contemporary Pediatrics* 14:115–29, 1997.

Bassett, I. B., et al. "A Comparative Study of Tea-tree Oil versus Benzoyl Peroxide in the Treatment of Acne." *Medical Journal of Australia* 153:455–58, 1990.

Bjorneboe, A., et al. "Effect of Dietary Supplementation with Eicosapentaenoic Acid in the Treatment of Atopic Dermatitis." *British Journal of Dermatology* 117:463–69, 1987.

Bordoni, A., et al. "Evening Primrose Oil (Efamol) in the Treatment of Children with Atopic Eczema." *Drugs Under Experimental and Clinical Research* 14:29–7, 1988.

Buesing, K. H. "Inhibition of Hyaluronidase by Echinacin." *Arzneimittel-Forschung* 2:467–69, 1952.

Burks, A. W., et al. "Atopic Dermatitis and Food Hypersensitivity Reactions." *Journal of Pediatrics* 132:132–36, 1998.

Evans, F. Q. "The Rational Use of Glycyrrhetinic Acid in Dermatology." *British Journal of Clinical Practice* 12:269–79, 1958.

Hederos, C.-A. and A. Berg. "Epogam Evening Primrose Oil Treatment in Atopic Dermatitis and Asthma." *Archives of Disease in Childhood* 75:494–97, 1996.

Leyden, J. J. "Therapy for Acne Vulgaris." *New England Journal of Medicine* 336:1156–62, 1997.

Lin, C. C., et al. "Anti-inflammatory and Radical Scavenge Effects of *Arctium lappa.*" *American Journal of Chinese Medicine* 24(2):127–37, 1996.

Marroquin, E. A., et al. "Clinical Trial of *Jatropha curcas* Sap in the Treatment of Common Warts." *Fitoterapia* 68:160–62, 1997.

McNally, N. J., et al. "The Problem of Atopic Eczema: Aetiological Clues from the Environment and Lifestyles." *Social Science Medicine* 46:729–41, 1998.

McNally, N. J., et al. "Atopic Eczema and Domestic Water Hardness." *Lancet* 352:527–31, 1998.

Mowrey, D. B. "Next Generation Herbal Medicine." Lehi, UT: Comorant Books, 1988.

Ojima, M., et al. "The Inhibitory Effects of Glycyrrhizin and Glycyrrhetinic Acid on the Metabolism of Cortisol and Prenisolone-*In vivo* and *In vitro* Studies." *Nippon Naibunpi Gakkai Zasshi* 66:584–96,1990.

Sheehan, M. P. and D. J. Atherton. "A Controlled Trial of Traditional Chinese Medicinal Plants in Widespread Non-exudative Atopic Eczema." *British Journal of Dermatology* 126:179–84, 1992.

Sheehan, M. P. and D. J. Atherton. "One-year Follow-up of Children Treated with Chinese Medicinal Herbs for Atopic Eczema." *British Journal of Dermatology* 130:488–93, 1994.

Chapter 22: Chicken Pox and Herpes

Advisory Committee on Immunization Practices. "Prevention of Varicella." *Mortality and Morbidity Weekly Report* 45:1–36, 1996.

Amir, J., et al. "Treatment of Herpes simplex Gingivostomatitis with Acyclovir in Children: A Randomized Double-blind, Placebo-controlled Study." *British Medical Journal* 314:1800–03, 1997.

Azimove, M. M., et al. "Pharmacological Study of the Anti-inflammatory Agent Glyderinine." *Farmakologiia I Toksikologiia (Pharmacology and Toxicology)* 51(4):90–93, July-Aug., 1988.

Balfour, H., et al. "Acyclovir Treatment of Varicella in Otherwise Healthy Children." *Pediatric Pharmacology and Therapeutics* 116:633–39, 1990.

Brody, I. "Topical Treatment of Recurrent Herpes Simplex and Post-herpetic Erythema Multiforme with Low Concentrations of Zinc Sulphate Solution." *British Journal of Dermatology* 104:191–213.

Brunell, P. "Varicella in the Womb and Beyond." *Pediatric Infectious Disease Journal* 9(10):770–72, October, 1990.

Doran, T. F., et al. "Acetaminophen: More Harm than Good for Chicken Pox?" *Journal of Pediatrics* 114:1045–48, 1989.

Fitzherbert, J. "Genital Herpes and Zinc." *Medical Journal of Australia* 1:399, 1979.

Fleming, D. T., et al. "Herpes Simplex Virus Type 2 in the United States, 1976 to 1994." *New England Journal of Medicine* 337:1105–11, 1997.

Griffith, R. S., et al. "Success of L-lysine Therapy in Frequently Recurrent Herpes Simplex Infection." *Dermatologica* 175:183–90, 1987.

Griffith, R., et al. "Relation of Arginine-lysine Antagonism to Herpes Simplex Growth in Tissue Culture." *Chemotherapy* 27:209–13, 1981.

Hovi, T., et al. "Topical Treatment of Recurrent Mucocutaneous Herpes with Ascorbic Acid-containing Solution." *Antiviral Research* 27:263–70, 1995.

Moore, D. and R. Hopkins. "Assessment of a School Exclusion Policy during a Chicken Pox Outbreak." *American Journal of Epidemiology* 133:1161–66, 1991.

Pompei, R., et al. "Glycyrrhizic Acid Inhibits Virus Growth and Inactivates Virus Particles." *Nature* 281:689–90, 1979.

Preblud, S. R. "Varicella: Complications and Costs." *Pediatrics* 78:728–35, 1986.

Prober, C., et al. "Consensus: Varicella-zoster Infections in Pregnancy and the Perinatal Period." *Pediatric Infectious Disease Journal* 9:865–69, 1990.

Rapprich, M. K. "The *Melissa* plant-An Old Medicinal Plant with a New Profile of Effectiveness." *Der Deutsche Dermatologe (The German Dermatologist)* 10:1318–28, 1983.

Slagowska, A., et al. "Inhibition of Herpes Simplex Virus Replication by *Flos verbasci* Infusion." *Polish Journal of Pharmacology and Pharmacy* 39(1):55–61, Jan.-Feb. 1987.

Tang, J. "Virucidal Activity of Hypericin Against Enveloped and Nonenveloped DNA and RNA Viruses." *Antiviral Research* 13:313–25, 1990.

Tyring, S. K., et al. "A Randomized, Placebo-controlled Comparison of Oral Valacyclovir and Acyclovir in

Immunocompetent Patients with Recurrent Genital Herpes Infections." *Archives of Dermatology* 134:185–91, 1998.

Wacker, A. and W. Hilbig. "Virus Inhibition of *Echinacea purpurea*: Inhibition of Influenza, Herpes, and Vescular Stomatitis." *Planta Medica* 33:89, 1978.

Woelbling, R. H. and K. Leonhardt. "Local Therapy of Herpes Simplex with Dried Extract From *Melissa officinalis*." *Phytomedicine* 1:25–31, 1994. www.ars-grin.gov/~ngrlsb, 5/14/98.

Chapter 23: Headaches

Awang, D. "Feverfew Trials: The promise of—and the Problem with—Standardized Botanical Extracts." *HerbalGram* 41:16–17, 1998.

Barsby, R. W. J., et al. "Feverfew and Vascular Smooth Muscle: Extracts from Fresh and Dried Plants Show Opposing Pharmacological Profiles, Dependent upon Sesquiterpene Lactone Content." *Planta Medica* 59:20–25, 1992.

Bettistella, P. A., et al. "Beta-endorphin in Plasma and Monocytes in Juvenile Headache." *Headache* 36:91–94, 1996.

Bogduk, N. "Headaches and Cervical Manipulation." *Patient Management* 11:163–167, 1987.

Egger, J., et al. "Is Migraine Food Allergy? A Double-blind Controlled Trial of Oligoantigenic Diet Treatment." *Lancet* 2(8355):865–9, 1983.

Fusco, B. M. and M. Giacovazzo. "Peppers and Pain. The Promise of Capsaicin." *Drugs* 53:909–14, 1997.

Fusco, B. M., et al. "Preventative Effect of Repeated Nasal Applications of Capsaicin in Cluster Headache." *Pain* 59:321–25, 1994.

Gallai, V., et al. "Magnesium Content of Mononuclear Blood Cells in Migraine Patients." *Headache* 34:160–65, 1994.

Glueck, C. J. "Amelioration of Severe Migraine with Omega-3 Fatty Acids: A Double-blind, Placebo-controlled Clinical Trial." *American Journal of Clinical Nutrition* 43:710, 1986.

Gobel, H., et al. "Essential Plant Oils and Headache Mechanisms." *Phytomedicine* 2:93–102, 1995.

Hansen, P. E. and J. H. Hansen. "Acupuncture Treatment of Chronic Tension Headache—A Controlled, Cross-over Trial." *Cephalalgia* 5:137–42, 1985.

Johnson, E. S., et al. "Efficacy of Feverfew as Prophylactic Treatment of Migraine." *British Medical Journal* 291:569–73, 1985.

Lewis, D. W. "Migraine and Migraine Variants in Childhood and Adolescence." *Seminars in Pediatric Neurology* 2:127, 1995.

Longo, G., et al. "Treatment of Essential Headache in Developmental Age with L-5-HTP (Crossover, Double-blind Study Versus Placebo)." *Ediatria Medica E Chirurgia* 6: 241–5, 1984.

Maissen, C. P. and H. P. Ludin. "Comparison of the Effect of 5-hydroxytryptophan and Propranolol in the Interval Treatment of Migraine." *Schweizerische Medizinishe Wochenschrift* 121: 1595–90, 1991.

McCarren, T. "Amelioration of Severe Migraine by Fish Oil (n-3) Fatty Acids." *American Journal of Clinical Nutrition* 41:874a, 1985.

Murphy, J. J., et al. "Randomised Double-blind Placebo-controlled Trial of Feverfew in Migraine Prevention." *Lancet* 23, 2:8604: 189–92, 1988.

National Headache Foundation, http://www.headaches.org: 4/22/98.

O'Hara, J. and T. K. Koch. "Heading Off Headaches." *Contemporary Pediatrics* 15:97–116, 1998.

Onogi, T., et al. "Capsaicin-like Effect of (6)-shogaol on Substance P-containing Primary Afferents of Rats: A Possible Mechanism of its Analgesic Action." *Neuropharmacology* 31:1165–69, 1992.

Palevitch, D. G., et al. "Feverfew (*Tanacetum parthenium*) as a Prophylactic Treatment for Migraine: A Double-blind Placebo-controlled Study." *Phytotherapy Research* 11 (7):506–11, 1998.

Peikert, A., et al. "Prophylaxis of Migraine with Oral Magnesium: Results from a Prospective, Multi-center, Placebo-controlled and Double-blind Randomized Study." *Cephalalgia* 16:257–63, 1996.

Rasmussen, B.K., et al. "Epidemiology of Headache in a General Population: A Prevalence Study." *Journal of Clinical Epidemiology* 44:1147–57, 1991.

Scheller, J. M. "The History, Epidemiology, and Classification of Headaches in Childhood." *Seminars in Pediatric Neurology* 2:102, 1995.

Schwartz, B. S., et al. "Epidemiology of tension-type Headache." *Journal of the American Medical Association* 279:381–83, 1998.

Titus, F., et al. "5-Hydroxytryptophan Versus Methsergide in the Prophylaxis of Migraine. Randomized Clinical Trial." *European Neurology* 25:327–29, 1986.

Chapter 24: Sleep

Anders, T. F. and L. A. Eiben. "Pediatric Sleep Disorders: A Review of the Past 10 Years." *Journal of the American Academy of Child and Adolescent Psychiatry* 36:9–20, 1997.

Blader, J. C., et al. "Sleep Problems of Elementary School Children." *Archives of Pediatric and Adolescent Medicine* 151:473–80, 1997.

Dahl, R. E., et al. "Sleep Disturbances in Children with Atopic Dermatitis." *Archives of Pediatric and Adolescent Medicine* 149:856–60, 1995.

Dressing, H., et al. "Insomnia: Are Valerian/Melissa Combinations of Equal Value to Benzodiazepine?" *Therapiewoche* 42:726–36, 1992.

Hobbs, C. and S. Foster. "Hawthorn: A Literature Review." *HerbalGram* 22:19–33, Spring, 1990.

Holm, E., et al. "The Action Profile of D, L-kavain. Cerebral Sites and Sleep-Wakefulness-Rhythm in Animals." *Arzneimittel-Forschung* 41:673–83, 1991.

Kinzler, E., et al. "Efficacy of Kava Special Extract in Patients with Conditions of Anxiety, Tension, and Excitation of Non-psychotic Origin." *Arneim-Forschung Drug Research* 41:584–88, 1991.

Kleber, E., et al. "Modulation of Key Reactions of the Catecholamine Metabolism by Extracts from *Eschscholtzia californica* and *Corydalis cava*." *Arzneimittel-Forschung* 45(2):127–33, Feb., 1995.

Leathwood, P. D., et al. "Aqueous Extract of Valerian Root (*Valeriana officinalis* L.) Improves Sleep Quality in Man."

Pharmacology, Biochemistry, and Behavior 17:65–71, 1982.

Lindahl, O. and L. Lindvall. "Double-blind Study of a Valerian Preparation." *Pharmacology, Biochemistry, and Behavior* 32:1065–66, 1982.

Sadeh, A., et al. "Sleep in Stable, Asymptomatic Asthmatic Children." Presented at the 10th Annual Meeting of the Association of Professional Sleep Societies. Washington, D.C.: May, 1997.

Schmidt, B. D. "When Baby Just Won't Sleep." *Contemporary Pediatrics* (no volume):38–52, May, 1985.

Viola, H., et al. "Apigenin, a Component of *Matricaria recutita* Flowers, is a Central Benzodiazepine Receptor Ligand with Anxiolytic Effects." *Planta Medica* 61:213–16, 1995.

Wolfman, C., et al. "Possible Anxiolytic Effects of Chrysin, a Central Benzodiazepine Receptor Ligand Isolated from *Passiflora coerulea*." *Pharmacology Biochemical Behavior* 47:1–4, 1994.

Chapter 25: Attention Disorders

Boris, M. and F. S. Mandel. "Foods and Additives Are Common Causes of the Attention Deficit Hyperactive Disorder in Children." *Annals of Allergy* 72:462–68, 1994.

Cantwell, D. P. "Attention Deficit Disorder: A Review of the Past 10 Years." *Journal of the American Academy of Child and Adolescent Psychiatry* 35:978–87, 1996.

Crook, W. G. "The Yeast Problem." *Nutrition Science News* 3:256–60, 1998.

Efron, D., et al. "Side Effects of Methylphenidate and Dexamphetamine in Children with Attention Deficit Hyperactivity Disorder: A Double-blind, Crossover Trial." *Pediatrics* 100:662–66, 1997.

Egger, J., et al. "Controlled Trial of Hyposensitization in Children with Food-induced Hyperkinetic Syndrome." *Lancet* 339:1150–53, 1992.

Egger, J., et al. "Controlled Trial of Oligoantigentic Treatment in the Hyperkinetic Syndrome." *Lancet* 1(8428):540–45, March 9, 1985.

Farnsworth, N. R., et al. "Siberian Ginseng (*Eleutherococcus senticosis*): Current Status as an Adaptogen." *Economics of Medicinal Plant Research* 1:156–215, 1985

Field, T. J., et al. "Adolescents with Attention Deficit Hyperactivity Disorder Benefit from Massage Therapy." *Adolescence* 33:103–08, 1998.

Fotherby, K. J. and J. P. Hunter. "Symptoms of Food Allergy." *Clinical Gastroenterology* 14(3):615–29, July, 1985.

Girardi, N. L., et al. "Blunted Catecholamine Responses After Glucose Ingestion in Children with Attention Deficit Disorder." *Pediatric Research* 38:539–42, 1995.

Hagerman, R. J. and A. R. Falkenstein. "An Association Between Recurrent Otitis Media in Infancy and Later Hyperactivity." *Clinical Pediatrics* 26:5, 1987.

Kozielec, T. and B. Starobrat-Hermelin. "Assessment of Magnesium Levels in Children with Attention Deficit Hyperactivity Disorder (ADHD)." *Magnesium Research* 10:143–48.

Peiper, H. and R. L. Hoffman. "ADD: The Natural Approach." *Natural Pharmacy* 1(9):15–17, Sept., 1997.

Schilcher, H. *Phytotherapy in Paediatrics: Handbook for Physicians and Pharmacist*. Stuttgart: Medpharm Scientific Publishers, 1992.

Starobrat-Hermelin, B. and T. Kozielec. "The Effects of Magnesium Physiological Supplementation on Hyperactivity in Children with Attention Deficit Hyperactivity Disorder (ADHD). Positive Response to Magnesium Oral Loading Test." *Magnesium Research* 10:149–56, 1997.

Stevens, L. J., et al. "Essential Fatty Acid Metabolism in Boys with Attention-deficit Hyperactivity Disorder." *American Journal of Clinical Nutrition* 62:761–68, 1995.

Wender, E. H. and M. V. Solanto. "Effects of Sugar on Aggressive and Inattentive Behavior in Children with Attention Deficit Disorder with Hyperactivity and Normal Children." *Pediatrics* 88(5):960–66, Nov., 1991.

Wender, E. H. "Attention Disorders: The Advance Is a Return to Basics." *Western Journal of Medicine* 166:343–44, 1997.

Werbach, M. R. "Does Sugar Make Kids Hyper?" *Nutrition Science News* 3(5):270, May 1988.

Wolraich, M. L. and A. Baumgaertel. "The Practical Aspects of Diagnosing and Managing Children with Attention Deficit Hyperactivity Disorder." *Clinical Pediatrics* 497–504 Sept., 1997.

Chapter 26: Psychological Disorders

Allen, A. J., et al. "Case Study: A New Infection-triggered, Auto-immune Subtype of Pediatric OCD and Tourette's Syndrome." *Journal of the American Academy of Child and Adolescent Psychiatry* 34:307–11, 1995.

Dressing, H., et al. "Insomnia: Are Valerian/Melissa Combinations of Equal Value to Benzodiazepine?" *Therapiewoche* 42:726–36, 1992.

Greenberg, P. E., et al. "Depression: A Neglected Major Illness." *Journal of Clinical Psychiatry* 54:419–24, 1993.

Kowatch, R. A., et al. "Mood Disorders." In Parmelee, D. (ed.), *Child and Adolescent Psychiatry*. St. Louis: Mosby, 1996.

Leathwood, P. D., et al. "Aqueous Extract of Valerian Root (*Valeriana officinalis*) Improves Sleep Quality in Man." *Pharmacology, Biochemistry, and Behavior* 17:65–71, 1982.

Levine, J. "Controlled Trials of Inositol in Psychiatry." *European Neuropsychopharmacology* 7:147–55, 1997.

Lindahl, O. and L. Lindvall. "Double-blind Study of a Valerian Preparation." *Pharmacology, Biochemistry, and Behavior* 32:1065–66, 1982.

March, J. S. and H. L. Leonard. "Obsessive-compulsive Disorder in Children and Adolescents: A Review of the Past 10 Years." *Journal of the American Academy of Child and Adolescent Psychiatry* 34:1265–71, 1996.

McGuffin, M., et al (eds.). *American Herbal Product Association's Botanical Safety Handbook*. Boca Raton: CRC Press, 1997.

No author. "Health Agencies Update: St.-John's-wort Study Launched." *Journal of the American Medical Association* 278:1563, 1997.

Schmidt, M. A. *Smart Fats*. Berkeley: Frog Ltd., 1997.

Valleni-Basile, L. A., et al. "Frequency of Obsessive-compulsive Disorder in a Community Sample of Young Adolescents." *Journal of the American Academy of Child and Adolescent Psychiatry* 33:782–91, 1994.

Resources

Herbal And Natural Medicine Associations

American Association of Naturopathic Physicians (AANP)
601 Valley Street, Suite 105
Seattle, WA 98109
(206) 298-0125
http://www.naturopathic.org

American Botanical Council
PO Box 201660
Austin, TX 78720
(512) 331-8868

American Herbalists Guild
PO Box 70
Roosevelt, UT 84066
http://www.earthlink.net

American Holistic Health Association
P.O. Box 17400
Anaheim, CA 92817-7400
(714) 779-6152
Email: ahha@healthy.net
http://www.healthy.net/pan/chg/ahha/

Flower Essence Society
PO Box 459
Nevada City, CA 95959
(800) 548-0075
www.flowersociety.org

Herb Research Foundation
1007 Pearl Street, Suite 200
Boulder, CO 80302
(303) 449-2265
http://www.herbs.org

La Leche League
1400 N. Meacham Road
Schaumburg, IL 60173-4048
(800) LA-LECHE
http://www.lalecheleague.org

United Plant Savers
PO Box 420
Barre, VT 05649
http://www.plantsavers.org

Herbal Products

Frontier Herb Co-op
PO Box 299
Norway, IA 53218
(800) 669-3275

Herbs for Kids
151 Evergreen Drive
Bozeman, MT 59715
(406) 587-0180
www.herbsforkids.com

Herb Pharm
PO Box 116
Williams, OR 97544
(541) 846-7178

Horizon Herbs
P.O. Box 69
Williams, OR 97544
(541) 846-6704
Fax: (541) 846-6233

Zand Herbal Formulas
1722 14th Street, Suite 230,
Boulder, CO 80302
(303) 786-9435
www.zand.com

Vitality Works
134 Quincy Street
Albuquerque, NM 87108
(505) 268-9950

Schools of Herbal Education

California School of Herbal Studies
9309 HWY 116, Box 39,
Forestville, CA 95436
(707) 887-7457
www.cshs.com

Rocky Mountain Center for Botanical Studies
PO Box 19254
Boulder, CO 80308
(303) 442-6861
http://www.herbschool.com

Sweetgrass School of Herbal Medicine
1627 W. Main, Suite 116
Bozeman, MT 59715
www.wtp.net/~rrr

Allergy products and information

Allergy Control Products
89 Danbury Rd.
Ridgefield, CT 06877
(800) 422-DUST

Priorities: Allergy and Asthma supplies
1451 Concord Street
Framingham, MA 01701
(800) 553-5398
http://www.priorities.com

Food Allergy Network
10400 Eaton Place, Suite 107
Fairfax, VA 22030-2208
(800) 929-4040
www.foodallergy.org

Harmony catalog (formerly Seventh Generation)
360 Interlocken Blvd., Suite 300,
Broomfield, CO 80021
(800) 869-3446

Parasite testing

Great Smokies Diagnostic Laboratory
Tests available: Comprehensive Parasitology
Comprehensive Digestive Stool Analysis (CDSA)
63 Zillicoa Street
Asheville, NC 28801
(800) 522-4762

Publications

Herbs for Health
Herb Companion Press, LLC
201 East Fourth Street
Loveland, CO 80537-5655
www.interweave.com

For subscriptions:
PO Box 7708
Red Oak, IA 51591
(800) 456-6018

The Herb Companion
Herb Companion Press, LLC
201 East Fourth Street
Loveland, CO 80537-5655
www.interweave.com

For subscriptions:
PO Box 7714
Red Oak, IA 51591
(800) 456-6018

HerbalGram
American Botanical Council
P.O. Box 144345
Austin, TX 78714-4345
(800) 373-7105 for orders,
www.herbalgram.org
e-mail: custserv@herbalgram.org

Mothering
PO Box 1690
Santa Fe, NM 87504
(505) 984-8116
Fax (505) 986-8335
email: mother@ni.net
www.mothering.com

Medical Herbalism Magazine
PO Box 20512
Boulder, CO 80308
http://www.medherb.com

INDEX